WORLD
Medicine

The East West Guide to
Healing Your Body

WORLD Medicine

The East West Guide to Healing Your Body

TOM MONTE
and The Editors of *EastWest Natural Health*

A Jeremy P. Tarcher/Putnam Book
published by
G. P. PUTNAM'S SONS
New York

A Jeremy P. Tarcher/Putnam Book
Published by G. P. Putnam's Sons
Publishers Since 1838
200 Madison Avenue
New York, NY 10016
http://www.putnam.com/putnam

Most Tarcher/Putnam books are available at special quantity discounts for bulk
purchases for sales promotions, premiums, fund-raising, and educational needs.
Special books, or book excerpts, can also be created to fit specific needs.

For details, write or telephone Special Markets, Putnam Publishing Group, 200
Madison Avenue, New York, NY 10016. (212) 951-8891.

Published simultaneously in Canada

Library of Congress Cataloging-in-Publication Data

Monte, Tom.
    World Medicine: The East West guide to healing your body /
by Tom Monte and the editors of Natural Health.
       p.   cm.
    Includes bibliographical references.
    ISBN 0-87477-733-X (paper); ISBN 0-87477-755-0 (case)
    1. Alternative medicine.   2. Medicine.   3. Healing.   I. Natural Health.
II. Title.
R733.M65   1993   92-43052 CIP
615.5'3—dc20

Illustration Credits:

Page 23: Illustration by Polly Jordan. Page 24: Copyright © 1990 by Terry
Oleson, Ph.D. Page 32: Illustration copyright © 1984, Dr. Vasant Lad.
Reprinted with permission of Lotus Light, Box 1008, Silver Lake, Wisconsin,
53170. Page 40: Courtesy of Health and Homeopathy Publishing, publisher
of *The Family Guide to Homeopathy* by Alan Horvilleur, M.D. Pages 134-35:
Reprinted with permission from *The Yellow Emperor's Classic of Internal
Medicine,* translated by Ilza Veith, copyright © 1947, 1975 Ilza Veith. Page
179: Copyright © 1987, Organica Press. Reprinted with permission. Page 295:
Illustration copyright © 1988, Windpfered Verlag. Reprinted from *The Chakra-
Handbook* with permission of Lotus Light, Box 1008, Silver Lake, Wisconsin,
53170. Page 325: From *The Principles of Light and Color* by Edwin Bobbitt,
copyright © 1992 Sun Publishing Company. This book is available from Sun
Publishing Company.

Anatomical drawings are by Nancy Kriebel, medical illustrator.

Design by Susan Shankin

Cover illustration of venous system © M. Kulyk, Science Source/Photo
Researchers

Printed in the United States of America
                7   8   9   10

This book is printed on acid-free paper.

To the memory of Rob Allanson,
teacher and friend

CONTENTS

ILLUSTRATIONS

ACKNOWLEDGMENTS

IT IS IMPOSSIBLE for me to acknowledge all of the friends who supported me in the writing of this book. Nevertheless, I wish to express my heartfelt thanks to the following people, whose assistance was essential to making this book a reality.

To Leonard Jacobs, who has helped me in countless ways throughout my professional life.

To the teachers, healers, and visionaries—many of whom are represented in the pages of this book—who have empowered lay people with the knowledge and the tools to heal themselves. Especially to Michio and Aveline Kushi, Nathan and Ilene Pritikin, who taught me new ways of seeing health and how it could be enhanced.

To Robert Allanson and William Tims, who in the early 1980s wrote a series of articles for *East/West Journal* that revealed the first synthesis of an East-West view of the body.

To editors Mark Mayell and Connie Zweig, at *Natural Health* magazine and Jeremy P. Tarcher, Inc., respectively, who kept me on track during the writing of this book.

To my wife, Toby, and my three children, who each day give me the inspiration and support to do this work.

THE MAGIC AND MYSTERY OF THE HUMAN BODY

$\mathcal{T}$HE HUMAN BODY is a realm of wonder and dread. Inside each of us is a greater magic than anything contrived by human imagination. The workings of the body can barely be comprehended, much less matched, by human invention. The heart beats 100,000 times a day, 2.5 billion times in the average lifetime. The eyes perceive ten million gradations of light. The nose can differentiate among thousands of odors and fragrances. The brain takes in billions of bits of information, organizes them, and offers a staggering array of responses. Who can consider the turbulence of human emotions, the insight and comprehension of a single mind, or the purity of a child's love without standing back in awe that so much magic can be contained in so finite a package?

No artist yet has managed to fully capture the mystery reflected in the eyes, the grace and strength in the hands, or the allure in the legs. The body is the realm in which art and utility become one.

Yet, it isn't only with wonder that one approaches the human form, but with trepidation, too. You need only to listen to your heart beat, or consider all those electrical impulses flashing across your rippled brain, to awaken to the terrible fragility of life. In-

In modern Western society biomedicine not only has provided a basis for the scientific study of disease, it also has become our own culturally specific perspective about disease, that is, our folk model.

GEORGE ENGEL

deed a child can listen to a conch and say he hears the ocean roar, but when an adult places his ear to another human chest, he listens to the sounds of life and death, and the whisper of immortality. It is the presence of this ultimate reality that takes the body beyond the limits of science and into the worlds of ethics, culture, religion, and spirit.

The body is many worlds in one. Consequently, if you ask an anatomist, a psychologist, an artist, and a priest for their views on the body, you will likely receive four distinct answers, all of them correct. Travel to other cultures and ask the same question of Middle Eastern, Chinese, and Native American healers, and each will give you a vastly differing description of the human form. Each of these accounts also will be correct. In fact, no single view of the body offers a definitive understanding.

The people of each culture are tempted to believe that they possess the only "true" way of seeing the body and life itself. At best, this is a quaint human trait. At worst, it is a form of blind arrogance. There is no ultimate view of the body, any more than there is an ultimate language. There are, in fact, many ways of understanding the great mystery that resides in the human form. Each approach has its strengths and weaknesses, its insights and limitations.

We live at a time when people crave information about the human body. We yearn for greater self-sufficiency when it comes to our health and health care. Many of us would like to heal ourselves of illness or prevent disease, using methods that have fewer toxic side effects than many of today's modern pharmaceuticals. So we are turning increasingly to the tools of the ancient past, and combining them with the techniques and understanding of modern science.

Today, people are transcending their cultural borders to understand the views of other traditions, other peoples. In medicine we are building bridges between East and West, ancient and modern, spirit and matter. One of the challenges that confronts us in our bridge-building is crossing the chasm that exists between worldviews. The ancients—both of East and West—saw the world as a unified whole in which all phenomena are intimately connected. We moderns see life as a series of disconnected parts, most of which have nothing to do with each other.

Today, we are struggling to reconcile these two fundamental

philosophies, especially in the field of healing. We want to understand our individual organs and functions, but also to see how each relates to the whole body, mind, and spirit. We search for knowledge to better understand ourselves, our bodies, and thereby live more fully satisfying lives.

YOUR BODY: FRIEND OR FOE?

One of the shortcomings of the modern approach to health care is the belief that we are victims of either our body's planned obsolescence or of germs—tiny agents that are invisible, pernicious, and arbitrarily infectious. We "catch" a cold, or we "come down" with the flu, as if the illness descends mysteriously from above. Other clichés reveal our thinking: "He was never sick a day in his life and then suddenly he got this!" In other words, our friend was going along fine, minding his own business, when bingo—his body broke down. He was an innocent victim of some mysterious illness.

Our methods of treatment reveal even more deeply this ingrained set of attitudes. Most treatments are designed to suppress symptoms or kill the invader. How often do we stop to think that perhaps those symptoms are really the body's way of telling us that something in our behavior is causing an underlying disease, or that the common cold may have a beneficial effect on our health? How many of us believe that the body has the power to heal itself?

To understand your body's language and to learn from your illnesses, you must learn to see the body as a friend with its own operating system, its own healing powers, and its own laws for maintaining health. Too often people think of the body as an enemy, failing us when we least expected it, or when we needed it most.

This book explores the vastly different ways of looking at your body and your health. We're going to show you that there are many ways to understand your body—ways you hadn't thought of before, but that make a difference in how you see yourself, how you treat your body, and how well it works. We hope to place you on better terms with your body, to help you recognize your body as a friend.

That is not as difficult as you might think. It requires nothing

The mechanistic view of the human organism has encouraged an engineering approach to health in which illness is reduced to mechanical trouble and medical therapy to technical manipulation.

FRITJOF CAPRA

3

Western scientific medicine is largely concerned with objective, nonpersonal, physiochemical explanations of disease as well as its technical control. In contrast, many traditional systems of healing are centered on the phenomenon of illness, namely, the personal and social experience of disease . . . Where Western scientific medicine focuses on curing the disease, traditional medicine aims primarily at healing the illness—that is, managing the individual and social response to disease.

DAVID S. SOBEL

more than what you would give to any friend: attention, understanding, intelligence, and love. And why not? Your body is the best gift that's ever been given to you. It is also one of the greatest paradoxes you will face in life. On one hand, it is an infinite mystery. On the other, it is so simple and self-revealing that even a child can understand how it works, and what can be done to support its health and well-being. Throughout the pages of this book, we'll be confronting that paradox—the mystery and the simplicity of the human form. We'll introduce you to many of the wonders of your body. We'll also show you many of the simple steps you can take to keep yourself well, or to overcome illness when it appears.

We're going on a journey through a remarkable kingdom, a place in which miracles and magic are everyday occurrences. In no other place in this world are more wondrous things happening than inside each of us.

Let's begin our journey with an ordinary tour: a walk in the park. Our park is both beautiful and commonplace. Expanses of green grass; groves of trees here and there; a lake. Sunlight tints the leaves on the trees and the grass below your feet with a hint of golden color. The park is filled with people: a Little League baseball game is going full tilt over there; periodically, a runner lopes by at your elbow; an elderly couple strolls arm-in-arm over there, while a pair of young lovers sit at a park bench to your right. Ahead, a father and son attempt to get their kite up into the air, while under a stately oak to your left is a young mother entertaining her infant daughter with a rattle. At another bench is a young man nursing a cold, passing a tissue frequently to his nose. Finally, on the other side of the park, in the pools of sunlight and shadow, an elderly Chinese man performs a solitary, slow-moving dance called tai chi.

At the baseball game, a boy of about thirteen, fully decked out in baseball regalia, approaches the plate. Baseball chatter chirps from the onlookers in the bleacher seats, from the players in the field, and from those sitting on the bench. The batter takes his stance in the batter's box, raises the bat above his right shoulder, and fixes his gaze upon the pitcher. The pitcher takes in the measure of the batter and settles into his stance. He turns his gaze to the catcher who signals the pitch to throw. The wind kicks up some dust from the mound as the umpire—dressed like a benign

Darth Vadar—crouches behind the catcher and awaits the pitch. The duel is engaged. The pitch is on the way. The batter has less than a second to assess the pitch and accurately direct his bat to strike the ball.

The act of hitting a speeding baseball with a bat is one of the most difficult challenges in sport, but the accomplishment seems even greater when you realize what the body must do almost instantaneously to accomplish that feat.

The baseball is visible to the batter because it reflects waves of energy, known as electromagnetic radiation or light. Those light waves, traveling at 186,000 miles per second, reach the batter's eye before the ball reaches the plate. The eyes instantly focus on the waves of light by precisely adjusting various parts of the eye: the cornea, which is the clear, convex window at the front of the eye; the pupil, the opening right before the lens; and the lens itself. All of these adjustments are performed in concert by muscles within the eye that respond to orders from the brain. The brain will tell the various parts of the eye to contract or expand, depending upon whether or not it is receiving a clear image.

Once the light enters the eye, it strikes the retina, a membrane of nerves the size of postage stamp that sits at the back of each eye. The retina binds the light to certain chemicals within the nerves, sparking an electrical impulse that travels from the retina to the brain, via the optic nerve. The visual cortices are located in the back of the brain, in both the left and right hemispheres. The brain receives multiple images because the left and right eyes perceive the light from slightly different vantage points. Also, the image is upside down, thanks to the fact that the light is refracted, or bent, within the eye. The brain puts these images together instantly and, voilà!, here comes the baseball.

It's a fastball, about belt-high and, yes, it's in the strike zone. The batter assesses the pitch and decides to swing. He's got a fraction of a second left to bring the bat around and hit the ball. No problem. He can do it.

Electrical nerve impulses start to flash from the visual cortices to other parts of the brain. First, the signals speed to the most primitive parts, the cerebellum and the pons, both located at the top of the spinal cord, at the base of the brain. Here are located computer-like programs that coordinate muscles and bones to move in graceful harmony. These programs have been established during the many hours the boy has spent practicing his swing. Next, electrical impulses fly to the motor section of the cerebral cortex, located within a thin layer of gray cells that covers the entire surface of the brain. The motor cortex is located at the very top of the brain, in a band that stretches across the left and right hemispheres. The cerebral cortex is the most advanced part of the brain. It refines the programmed movements of the cerebellum and pons to make them more finely tuned to the behavior of this particular pitch. From the motor cortex, nerve impulses—the actual orders—are sent to the spinal cord and then to the respective parts of the body, such as the shoulders, arms, hands, hips, legs, and feet. Each signal provides specific orders to each part of the body, which must perform its act in concert with the whole. No one knows exactly how this is accomplished, but it is.

Our young friend's eyes follow the ball as it rockets toward him. Suddenly, the bat is in motion. His body is centered at the waist, head down, shoulders and arms flowing through the pitch. Crack! The young player is all elbows and knees as he hurries to first base. Heads in the bleachers and on the field turn in unison to follow the ball as it arcs gracefully to the gap in left-center field. The batter rounds first base and slides into second, disappearing in a cloud of dust. Safe. He can't suppress a big smile. He's elated that he hit the ball, as is half the crowd, but even he doesn't realize what magic he just performed.

MAKING SENSE OF THE MAGIC

Magic was humanity's earliest explanation for how the body worked. Long before systematized approaches to health and the body were organized some 6,000 years ago, humanity's ancestors used potions, amulets, rings, and charms to rid the body of harmful demons and spirits that brought illness and suffering. The eyes, especially, were seen as sites of power and magic. Warrior tribesmen of New Zealand ate the eyes of tribal chiefs because they believed the deity lived within them. The eyes of animals were routinely used medicinally to treat eye problems. One ancient Egyptian potion for blindness was made up of the water from hogs' eyes, honey, and lead, all of which was injected into the eyes of the blind. (The success rate of this treatment has understandably gone unrecorded.) Shamans used the fierce "powers" in the eyes to frighten demons, which were believed to be the source of illness. To this day, many traditional peoples still believe that shamans have the ability to cure and harm people with the powers in their eyes.

Humankind's understanding of the body began to emerge from the mists of superstition some 5,000 years ago, when the body began to be studied extensively in China, India, Greece, and Egypt. Despite their differences in language and metaphors, all of these early cultures approached the body from the same basic worldview. These traditional peoples saw life as an integrated whole, a unity. The body was approached as a unified system in which the physical, mental, and spiritual aspects of life were one. Moreover, each life was united with the life of the universe itself. It is one life, which all things share.

In China, this ultimate unity was seen as the creator of two archetypal forces, called yin and yang. These two forces manifest in everything in the material universe and make the relative world possible. Like poles of a magnet, yin and yang attract each other and thus produce movement and energy. In China, that universal life energy is called chi, or qi.

The idea of a universal life force was common among virtually all traditional peoples. In India it is called prana, in Japan ki, and in ancient Greece, pneuma.

In a number of ancient societies the healers performed crude surgeries, did autopsies, and investigated the structure and function of organs and tissues. But their investigations were often guided by a simple question: What causes this mass of flesh to function? What gives an organ life? Their answer was that in addition to the corporeal body, there is a more fundamental entity, which is this underlying energy that is life itself. This life energy infuses the entire human being, causing the body to have vitality, movement, and function. The life force also gives the body the power to heal wounds, to overcome disease, and succeed in the face of difficulty and challenge.

Death is seen as the moment the life force leaves the flesh. Without the life force, none of the bodily functions continue. The flesh is revealed as merely a matrix of earthly substances that immediately decay and return to the earth.

The idea of a life force points to a major difference between

Modern medicine is already in its twilight years. It is about forty or fifty years old, and by now there's been a chance for the ill effects to catch up with the originally heralded benefits. The breakthroughs have turned out to be breakdowns, and most of the shiny metal has turned out to be tarnished.

ROBERT MENDELSOHN

7

these early traditional societies and modern ones dominated by the tools and techniques of scientific medicine, and especially between East and West. In traditional systems, such as the Chinese and Greek, the body is seen as having the ability to cure itself of illness. The physician serves only to assist the body's own healing powers. Conversely, modern medicine uses drugs and surgery to overcome disease. Antibiotics, for example, kill a pathogen, while surgery removes organs and their related problems altogether. Rather than encourage the body's healing powers, the modern medical doctor uses medicine to deal directly with the illness.

In the Chinese system, the life force flows through the body in specific channels, or meridians. These channels of energy unite the entire body into an organized whole, much like integrated circuitry unites an electrical unit. But the channels of energy also make certain organs and senses particularly intimate and mutually dependent upon each other.

Opposing Worldviews in Everyday Life

Let's return to the park and see how the ancient and modern systems approach the same problem from differing angles. Just ahead of us a boy and his father are flying a kite. The kite is up in the air and waving gently in the wind. Occasionally, a gust blows the kite toward some trees to the left. As father and son follow the kite with their eyes, the father admonishes the boy to keep the kite away from the trees. We notice that the boy is wearing thick glasses; he's nearsighted, which means he has trouble focusing on objects at a distance. He's probably having a hard time seeing the kite clearly and judging its proximity to the trees.

The Chinese say that the health of the eyes is directly dependent on the condition of the liver. The liver, say the Chinese, rules the eyes by nourishing them with qi. The liver is regarded as the root of vision, in that it continually sends qi to the eyes. An unhealthy liver will be unable to provide the eyes with adequate life force, causing degeneration in the muscles and parts of the eye, thus affecting clarity of vision. Almost all eye problems, including lack of visual acuity, glaucoma, and cataracts, are related to liver imbalances, say the Chinese. This relationship is evidenced when jaundice and other liver disorders cause the eyes to yellow.

It's more important to know what kind of patient has a disease than what kind of disease a patient has.

Hippocrates

8

The system works in both directions. Eye strain can cause liver disturbances.

In a traditional medicine such as the Chinese system, the body is seen in ever-widening relationships. The workings of any single organ is seen within the context of the whole. Thus, an eye problem will be approached as a symptom of an underlying imbalance in the body, particularly in the liver. A Chinese healer will address an eye problem by treating the eyes and the liver, and whatever might affect these organs. This would include an examination of the person's environment, food choices, relationships, emotional life, and working patterns. All of these areas would be looked at for their effects on the flow of qi within the body. The concentric circles ripple outward, until the healer and the patient have arrived at a specific set of causes. The healer will then prescribe an array of herbs, dietary recommendations, perhaps massage or acupuncture, and exercises to reestablish harmony within the body. The Chinese healer is working to strengthen the underlying life force, though he or she may also provide some symptomatic relief as well. Once the life force is reestablished, the body's own healing mechanisms have the ability to overcome any illness or disorder, including many forms of eye impairments.

In the West, the body is seen as a biochemical machine in which the parts are separate and distinct. It is understood in ever-smaller units—that is, as tissues, organs, cells, molecules, and atoms. For this reason, Western science is often referred to as reductionist, meaning it is searching for the single underlying unit that makes up the body or, in the case of disease, a single pathogen or physical impairment that gives rise to symptoms.

A Western physician, therefore, sees an eye problem as confined largely to the eye and its related parts. Treatment consists of eyeglasses to compensate for weak vision, or drugs or surgery to correct the malfunctioning eye.

The understanding of a life force has larger applications—it even applies to a baseball player's swing. An athlete's performance, or any action, for that matter, is not merely an act of biochemistry, but an attunement with this all-pervasive life force, which is the underlying power of the universe. The player who is attuned to the universe in this way cannot help but be perfect in the moment. But in order to achieve that perfect unity between the body and the life force, the mind must be "empty."

The human organism is much larger than we imagine, for as a living entity it is inseparable from a "personal ecology," its working balances with the world. The body is also a much more porous entity than we see, through which millions of microorganisms and foreign molecules circulate. These cohabitors and invaders are held in check by the body's homeostatic, immunological, and detoxification systems and by the benign flora of the gut and other ecological forces.

JOSEPH D. BEASLEY

Biological explanations for what happens when you hit a baseball are not only useless, say modern practitioners of traditional Chinese medicine, but serve to get in the way of your ability to attune yourself to the power of the universe. Explanations are the work of the "mind," the concept-forming aspect of your identity. The mind fragments and interprets experience. It tells you which parts of experience are important and which parts are unimportant. But the perfect swing lies in a state in which you are empty of "mind," empty of labels or concepts, and free to apply your skill unfettered to the task at hand. You don't think about the act. You simply do it, and thereby come into harmony with the underlying life force that is creating the moment itself. By being attuned to the underlying power or truth, the batter and ball become one.

In his introduction to Eugene Herrigal's book, *Zen in the Art of Archery*, Daisetz T. Suzuki explains this principle as it applies to archery: "In the case of archery, the hitter and the hit are no longer two opposing objects, but are one reality. The archer ceases to be conscious of himself as the one who is engaged in hitting the bull's-eye which confronts him. The state of unconsciousness is realized only when, completely empty and rid of the self, he becomes one with the perfecting of his technical skill, though there is in it something of a quite different order which cannot be attained by any progressive study of the art." Suzuki goes on to explain that when the archer eliminates self-consciousness or mind, he or she comes into "contact with the ultimate reality."

From this perspective, hitting a speeding baseball has little to do with the ball itself, but with coming into right relationship with the underlying truth—the ultimate reality—that guides the movements of the ball, the pitcher, the batter, and the bat.

Coming into relationship with that reality depends in part on one's own sensitivity and spiritual development. As Herrigel says about archery: "The Japanese does not understand [archery as] a sport but, strange as this may sound at first, a religious ritual. And consequently, by the 'art' of archery he does not mean the ability of the sportsman, which can be controlled, more or less, by bodily exercises, but an ability whose origin is to be sought in spiritual exercises and whose aim consists in hitting a spiritual goal, so that fundamentally the marksman aims at himself and may even succeed in hitting himself." Thus, the game becomes a means of self-development.

Just as archery is regarded as a spiritual exercise in the Orient, so too is self-defense. The man performing that slow dance under the trees in the park is actually meditating. Tai chi, an ancient martial art, is a way of experiencing the central current of life, often called Tao, that flows all around and through us. He moves as if he is gracefully pushing masses of air to slow-moving music. Every action is a study in balance: a forward push is rounded off and turned into retreat; retreat stimulates advancement. He is attempting to align himself with the yin and yang of qi, trying to experience the power that drives the universe. By moving in harmony with that subtle yet all-powerful force, he not only experiences the source of health, but also learns to draw it toward him and influence it. He is thus protected from negative influences, and he himself becomes a force for regeneration and health wherever he goes.

Even from the standpoint of Western science, the notion of an underlying energy that animates the body is not so far-fetched. In fact, the body itself is an electrical unit. Every organ and, indeed, the entire nervous system works on the basis of electrical currents. The heart is an electrical pump. It beats by virtue of electrical impulses generated within the heart muscle by two nodes, one at the top of the heart and the other in the wall that separates the two sides of the heart. The electrical charges fired by these nodes flow through fibrous bands that permeate the heart muscle and stimulate the familiar expansion and contraction of the heart. Indeed, that expansion and contraction is created by two oppositely charged ions which together cause electrons to flow along these bands of muscle fibers. As we will see in the last chapter, the concept of an underlying life force composed of electromagnetic energy is now being seriously explored by Western scientists, and receiving surprising support.

We appear to be individual bodies, but this individuality is also a constant state of equilibrium between a true personal authenticity and a continuous participation with the collective energy of all humanity and all existence.

RICHARD MOSS

PART ONE

Six Systems of Healing

VARIOUS TRADITIONAL PEOPLES around the world have long included among their medicinal practices such therapies as diet and herbs, compresses and poultices, massage techniques and acupuncture, purgatives and sweats. They have been particularly well developed in four major medical systems: Chinese, Ayur-Veda of India, Greek medicine, and homeopathy.

But beyond the efficacy of specific herbs or techniques lies a more fundamental understanding of health. Health is typically defined in traditional medical systems as a state of balance and wholeness. These systems are based on the belief that humans are unified with—even the product of—the vast forces that maintain the cosmos. Illness is caused when one or more of these forces within a person is imbalanced. Medicine is the means of restoring balance.

For the Chinese, health is achieved by creating harmony between the opposing powers of yin and yang. When the organs maintain a balanced condition, when they do not become too contracted or too expanded, the life force or qi flows smoothly throughout the body. Each organ receives optimal life force; it is capable of warding off illness and efficiently eliminating waste. When one or more organs, however, becomes excessively contracted or expanded, qi flow becomes blocked. Once the life force is diminished, the organ becomes sluggish, inefficient, and stagnant—a perfect host for disease.

Organs, blood vessels, or tissues can become excessively contracted by any number of influences, including stress, emotional turmoil, excessive amounts of animal foods and salt, excessive work and not enough play, injury, or lack of exercise. Organs can become overly expanded through emotional imbalance, dietary influences such as excessive sugar or alcohol, drugs, the absence of work and an excess of inactivity, and lack of exercise. Health is established by restoring balance to one's lifestyle, and thus to the organs or system of the body. This, in turn, causes the life force to flow freely and optimally once again. Once the life force flows optimally throughout the body, the organs themselves can throw off the underlying causes of disease. They are capable of healing themselves. In such a system, the illness is itself a symptom of a diminished life force.

Balance is the means to health and long life, say the Chinese, Greeks, and Indians. By eliminating extremes in behavior, life can be enjoyed fully, without excessive burdens.

The oldest medical book in the world is *The Yellow Emperor's Classic of Internal Medicine,* the basis of Chinese medicine. It describes the balance of yin and yang this way: The sages of old used "temperance in eating and drinking. Their hours of rising and retiring were regular and not disorderly and wild. By these means the ancients kept their bodies united with their souls, so as to fulfill their allotted span completely, measuring unto a hundred years before they passed away.

"Nowadays people are not like this; they use wine as a beverage and they adopt recklessness as usual behavior. They enter the chamber [of love] in an intoxicated condition; their passions exhaust their vital forces; their cravings dissipate their true [essence]; they do not know how to find contentment within themselves; they are not skilled in the control of their spirits. They devote their attention to the amusement of their minds, thus cutting themselves off from the joys of long [life]."

Protection of the life force through moderation was the key to health and long life. Hippocrates, the Greek physician known today as the father of medicine, had a similar view. He taught that health is achieved by balancing four humors, or fluids, within the body. As long as these fluids remained in harmony among each other, an individual experienced good health. When they became imbalanced, one suffered illness.

In both the Greek and the Chinese systems, imbalances are often corrected by the body by merely "discharging" the stagnation or excesses stored within. Hippocrates referred to this discharge as catharsis (derived from the Greek *katharsis* or *katharmos*), which means the purging or cleansing of the system, especially the bowels. The common cold could, for example, serve to eliminate toxins and excesses that are the basis for disease.

NATURE CURES, PHYSICIANS ASSIST

To a conventional medical doctor, the runny nose, sneezing, cough, and watery eyes of a typical cold are seen as merely irritating symptoms that should preferably be eliminated as quickly as possible. Medication is designed to do just that. But from the point of view of most traditional medicines, the common cold, with its sneezing, runny nose, and frequent urination, is a highly efficient way of eliminating accumulated toxins and waste.

Hippocrates said that although health is the natural state of humans, disease is also a natural process that follows an organic pattern. During that illness there are key points at which the physician can intercede and assist the patient in restoring health. Hippocrates called these points of "crisis" or "opportune moments" at which balance and the forces of health can be restored. Hippocrates also implied that disease seems to serve some kind of evolutionary or maturing process. According to Philip Wheelwright,

University of California scholar and author of *The Presocratics,* illness can serve to create what Hippocrates called a new "blended maturity" among the elements within.

Like the Chinese, Hippocrates developed an extensive array of foods, herbs, and physical therapies (such as poultices and compresses) to restore balance to the body. "Proper food and drink, calmness of mind and body, suitable exercise, and the like, are among the chief ways in which the bodily conditions can be made as favorable as possible to the speedy and firm completion of the cycle through illness and back again to health," writes Wheelwright.

Today, scientists are demonstrating the effectiveness of such methods, especially herbs. Said John Hopkins University researcher Erwin Ackerknecht: "It is amazing what an enormous number of effective drugs is known to the primitives. From twenty-five to fifty percent of their pharmacopoeia is often found to be objectively active." This should not be as amazing as it sounds. The World Health Organization has identified 121 modern drugs made totally from plant compounds. Ackerknecht points out that our modern knowledge of a vast array of drugs comes chiefly from traditional peoples. University researchers are now studying the powerful healing properties found in herbal remedies from the natives of the Brazilian rain forest and other traditional cultures.

How did traditional people discover their methods? The easy answer is trial and error, but you will not get that response when you ask a Chinese sage or a Native American medicine man how they arrived at their information.

"From ancient times the communication with Heaven has been the very foundation of life," said the Yellow Emperor. "This foundation exists between yin and yang and between heaven and earth. Therefore the sages preserved the natural spirit and were in harmony with the breath of Heaven and were thus in direct communication with Heaven."

In *Planet Medicine,* Richard Grossinger quotes a Native American who explains how members of his tribe came to understand nature and its healing arts: "We know what the animals do, what are the needs of the beaver, the bear, the salmon, and other creatures, because long ago men married them and acquired this knowledge from their animal wives. Today the priests say we lie, but we know better."

The Cherokee Indians say that animals invented disease to reduce the human population. But the plant kingdom discovered the animals' plot and called a council meeting at which the plants decided to provide healing remedies to humanity when stricken by illness. All plants were to have some healing properties, no matter how common or seemingly useless they might appear to be.

To traditional peoples, the world was alive with powers, life forces, and spirits. Mountains, rivers, trees, and boulders all possessed personality and even soul. Their oneness of nature was not an abstract concept, but a deep and personal relationship in which people talked to the four winds, the sun, the stars, and the moon. These were minor deities, the emissaries of the Great Spirit.

The healer mediated between the human world and the world of the transcendent powers. Healers, therefore, served as both physician and priest. Shamans the world over called upon the powers of healing implicit in the universe to rid the sick of evil or noxious spirits. There were no conceptual boundaries between mind and body and soul. Whatever was in the spirit became manifest in the body, and vice versa. The perception of life was not linear, but circular. Thus, treatment included the physical and the spiritual—food, herbs, and physical therapy, along with ritual, jewels and crystals, and prayer.

Today, scientists know that such methods work. The powers of the mind have just begun to be explored, but studies are showing that the invisible realm of thoughts, emotions, and belief systems dramatically influences health in positive and negative ways. Studies have shown that belief in recovery can be as powerful as any medication.

At Mount Sinai School of Medicine in New York, Dr. Steven J. Schliefer and his coworkers have found that highly emotional states, such as bereavement, have a deadening effect on the immune system. One type of immune cells, the lymphocytes, often fail to respond in the presence of a pathogen in people who have recently suffered the loss of a loved one. Men who suffer the loss of a spouse have a 40 percent higher mortality rate within their own age groups than those who do not experience such loss. Dying of a broken heart might just as well be expressed as a broken immune system. If these people pass through the bereavement period, their immune systems rebound.

But even subtle changes in mood and behavior affect internal chemistry. The power of laughter to heal is now well documented, but science is showing that even a smile can change both mood and internal chemistry. Dr. Robert Zajonc, a psychologist at the University of Michigan, has found that certain facial muscles have the ability to raise and lower the temperature of the blood flowing to the brain. Such changes can affect brain chemistry, particularly the function of the hypothalamus gland, located in the brain. Other research has shown that changes in the hypothalamus, in turn, alter the function of the immune, endocrine, cardiovascular, and respiratory systems.

Thus, a new form of shamanism is emerging called psychoneuroimmunology, or the study of how the mind affects the body. Clearly, the boundaries between body, mind, and spirit— once thought to be inviolate—are giving way.

Today, a new set of views is taking hold, a belief system that looks much like our ancient traditions, but is supported and transformed by our modern sciences. The sciences of medicine and physics are building bridges, too. When the physicist looks deeply into the world of the atom and its even tinier realms, he or she is discovering a unity that the ancients would have agreed with, and understood. The words of eminent physicist David Bohm are strangely reminiscent of the Yellow Emperor or Lao Tsu: "Ultimately, the entire universe (with all its 'particles,' including those constituting human beings, their laboratories, observing instruments, etc.) has to be understood as a single undivided whole, in which analysis into separately and independently existent parts has no fundamental status."

Though they differ in language and metaphor, most traditional medical systems are based on these principles of health as a state of balance or wholeness, governed by a universal life force, with illness resulting from imbalances within the body that block the life force from flowing optimally and freely within the body. Also, the symptoms of disease are seen as the body's effort at self-healing. Let's now have a closer look at each healing system, including the conventional modern medical one, to understand their respective metaphors and see beyond them.

CHAPTER 1

CHINESE MEDICINE

O OTHER MEDICAL SYSTEM deserves the title "traditional" more than Chinese medicine. Modern Western medicine, which we often refer to as "traditional," is only two centuries old. Chinese medicine, on the other hand, is at least 3,000 years old, and is still being used to treat tens of millions of people in China and other places around the world. From the view of a traditional Chinese healer, modern medicine is the "experimental" system because people have relatively little experience with it, and certainly the "alternative" because it is far from the precepts upon which the Chinese system is built.

Chinese medicine is based on the view that humanity is part of a larger creation, a greater body, that is the universe itself. Each of us is subject to the same laws that govern the stars, the planets, the trees, and the soil. In this way, Chinese medicine is essentially "macroscopic," in that its understanding of health begins with an understanding of nature, and the laws that govern it. To follow the laws of nature is to be blessed with good health, long life, and good fortune, say the Chinese. Ultimately, this path leads to a revelation about one's own life and the life of the universe itself.

To investigate the workings of the body is, for the Chinese, to

Nature, time, and patience are the three great physicians.

CHINESE PROVERB

explore the nature and origin of the universe. All the forces that created and shaped the universe are present in the human being, and consequently rule our health and destiny. Health care is, therefore, a spiritual pursuit in which the healer serves as both physician and priest.

Chinese medicine is based on *The Yellow Emperor's Classic of Internal Medicine,* written at least 2,500 years ago. The *Yellow Emperor's Classic* formed the basis of Chinese medicine and the foundation for most of Asian medicine, including the systems adopted by Japan, Korea, the Philippines, and other Asian countries. (The exception is India, which may have been influenced by the Chinese, but developed its own system, called Ayur-Veda.) Indeed, virtually all of the Oriental health systems flourishing in the West today—including acupuncture, shiatsu, acupressure massage, macrobiotics, Do–In, and sotai—are based upon Chinese medicine.

The first law that Chinese medicine is based upon is the law of yin and yang. According to the Chinese, all life and the entire material universe originated from a single unified source, called Tao, which is an integrated and undifferentiated whole that is present in everything. Tao created two opposing forces—yin and yang, which are archetypal opposites that combine to create everything in the relative world. The chart below lists their respective characteristics.

	YIN	YANG
Cosmic Bodies	earth	heavenly realms
	moon	sun
Temperament	passive	aggressive
	mentally active	physically active
	following	leading
	asleep	awake
Time of day	night	day
Season	fall and winter	spring and summer
Magnetic pole	negative	positive
Temperature	cold	hot
Density	contracted to solid	expanded and hollow

Speed	slow	fast
Relative moisture	moist to saturated	dry
Body location	feet lower extremities	head upper extremities
Organs	dense, internal organs: kidneys, lungs, heart, liver, bones	hollow, surface organs: intestines, spleen, gall bladder, skin
Height	low	high
Distance	near	far
Sides	left	right
Light	darkness	light
Sexual characteristics	female	male
Constitution	female	male

Yin and Yang, the two principles in nature, and the four seasons are the beginning and the end of everything and they are also the cause of life and death. Those who disobey the laws of the universe will give rise to calamities and visitations, while those who follow the laws of the universe will remain free from dangerous illness, for they are the ones who have obtained Tao, the Right Way.

THE YELLOW EMPEROR

Yin and yang are relative terms. Individual women and men can be more or less yin or yang. Some women are far more yang than some men. Each gender has an inherent or archetypal nature, according to the Chinese. Men are constitutionally more yang, women constitutionally more yin.

Yin and yang are each incomplete without the other. By combining, they create all phenomena. Thus, everything is composed of a unique mix of both. Take the moon, for example. The moon is yin in comparison with the sun. However, the moon possesses both yin and yang characteristics, because it has both a dark side (yin) and a light side (yang).

Individuals, too, have both yin and yang aspects. Certain characteristics within the same person can reflect both yin and yang. A passive person (yin) can be stubborn (yang), for example, or a chaotic person (yin) can be domineering (yang).

As the chart shows, Chinese divided the body into yin and yang parts. Certain organs are considered yin, some others more yang. The attraction of yin and yang creates movement and energy, an energy known in China as qi, or the life force. Qi energy is all around us and infusing us. The life force permeates the entire universe; it is an infinite resource available to all.

THE BODY'S ENERGY CHANNELS

As the twentieth century draws to a close, China faces a historic choice. How will it preserve the riches of its traditional medicine while embracing the specific technologies and interventions of Western medicine? For our part, we in the West are now looking more carefully, and less condescendingly, at alternative practices of medicine and mind-body interactions. We are using scientific technologies to investigate nonspecific therapies and placebo effects.

HERBERT BENSON

Qi flows through the body in precise and orderly patterns called meridians. They can be understood as deep rivers of energy running through the body. There are fourteen meridians, twelve of which are associated with organs in the body, while two have the responsibility of unifying various systems.

Each meridian runs vertically, bringing qi to specific parts of the body. No part is left unnourished of qi, unless a meridian becomes blocked or stagnant. This causes an imbalance in the flow of life force. Such imbalances can be compared to placing a big rock in a river: behind the rock, the water becomes excessive and powerful; in the lee of the rock, the water is diminished.

This imbalance—one side yang, the other yin—causes an imbalance among organs. Certain organs can become excessive or hyperactive (yang), while others can become deficient and hypoactive (yin). There can be excessive swelling or expansion (yang), or too much contraction (yin).

Without adequate life force, tissues and organs become stagnant. They can no longer eliminate waste from cells. As waste products accumulate, the blood-cleansing organs become stressed. Eventually, their capacity to clean the blood is exceeded. Accumulation of toxins (such as fat, cholesterol, ammonia, uric acid, triglycerides, and carbon dioxide) creates an environment for disease to manifest.

The Chinese, Greeks, and Indians believed that the symptoms of disease are actually the body's efforts to cure itself. Fever, runny nose, diarrhea, frequent urination, sweating, and other "symptoms" are actually the body's way of throwing off the underlying conditions that cause disease.

The underlying accumulation of toxins weakens the immune system sufficiently to allow a virus to take hold within the system. But more specifically, the accumulation of toxins diminishes the life force, which is the foundation of health. The continued diminution of the life force results in death.

In Chinese medicine, all health care is designed to balance qi. Treatment is meant to bring harmony between deficiency and excess, between yin and yang.

Virtually all behavior can affect the flow of qi in the body. Too much rest or complacency can make one loose and weak (yin), which can be balanced and healed by greater amounts of work and activity (yang). People who work excessively and experience too much stress, on the other hand, need relaxation to restore equilibrium and health to life.

The Chinese categorized virtually every activity, food, and herb according to the yin and yang spectrum. Because these are relative values, a single object or activity can be more yang than some things, more yin than others. For example, exercise is considered more yang than writing, but both would be considered yang activities compared to watching television, eating, or sleeping, each of which is progressively more yin.

The Chinese used the effects of foods, herbs, and other therapeutic techniques to restore balance and harmony to the body. If a person's condition is too contracted, for example, expansive foods and activities restore balance; if the condition is too expanded, contracting foods and activities create balance.

The preeminent form of therapy in Chinese medicine, of course, is acupuncture. Acupuncture is the one part of Chinese medicine that nearly all Westerners have heard of or seen, though few Westerners understand its purpose.

Since qi energy is an infinite resource permeating the entire environment, it can be directed into the body to restore health. An acupuncturist uses needles as antennae to direct qi to organs or functions of the body. However, the needles also can be used to drain qi where it is excessive; to warm parts of the body that are cool or stagnant; to decrease or increase moisture; and to reduce excessive heat. The acupuncturist does this by selecting specific points along specific meridian lines and then applying various needling techniques to bring about the desired results. There are as many as 2,000 points, but traditional acupuncturists use somewhere between 150 and 200 points.

Diagnosis of health and illness is done by using several techniques, including physiognomy, or relating facial and body features to internal organs; examining the tongue, iris, and sclera of the eye; and palpating the pulse.

Pulse diagnosis was raised to a high art in China. The pulse is sensed by placing three fingers with varying amounts of pressure on the radial artery at the wrist. With pulse diagnosis, the Chinese physician is said to read six organs on each wrist, or a total of twelve organs and meridians. According to a number of acupunc-

Pulse Points on the Wrist

Three points on each wrist correspond with certain organs. The left wrist reveals the condition of (1) heart and small intestine; (2) liver and gall bladder; and (3) kidney and bladder. The pulses of the right hand reveal the condition of (1) lungs and large intestine; (2) spleen and stomach; and (3) heart governor and triple heater.

How the Ear Reveals the Body

The Chinese first recognized some four millennia ago that manipulating acupuncture points on the ears could relieve certain illnesses. Ear acupuncture treatments have been further developed by both the Chinese and the French.

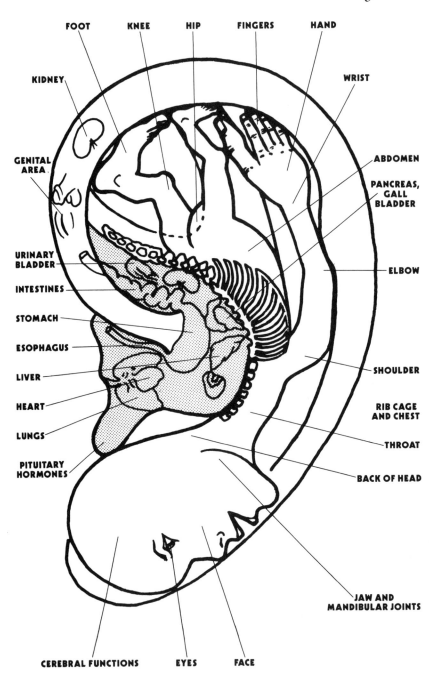

FOOT KNEE HIP FINGERS HAND

KIDNEY

WRIST

GENITAL AREA

ABDOMEN

PANCREAS, GALL BLADDER

URINARY BLADDER

ELBOW

INTESTINES

STOMACH

ESOPHAGUS

LIVER

HEART

SHOULDER

LUNGS

RIB CAGE AND CHEST

PITUITARY HORMONES

THROAT

BACK OF HEAD

JAW AND MANDIBULAR JOINTS

CEREBRAL FUNCTIONS EYES FACE

ture practitioners, it takes years to master the art of reading the pulse.

Beyond the law of yin and yang is the most all-encompassing tool in traditional medicine: The Five Element Theory, the basis of Chinese medicine and the central tool for diagnosis and treatment.

THE FIVE ELEMENT THEORY

Nowhere in the Chinese philosophy is the relationship between the macrocosm and the microcosm more precisely detailed than in the Five Element Theory. This links the seasons of the year, aspects of nature, and the body's organs, as well as specific foods, herbs, and treatments that will cure disease. It is also used for agricultural planning, healing, psychology, maintaining harmony in relationships, and even divination. This incredible tool single-handedly demonstrates the Chinese talent for seeing the unity within apparent diversity.

For our purposes, we'll examine the Five Elements from the perspective of understanding the body and healing. According to the theory, all change occurs in five distinct stages. Each of these stages can be associated with a particular time of the year; a particular element in nature; and a pair of organs within the body. Energy moves within the body in the same pattern that it does in nature, say the Chinese—the seasonal cycles. In the Chinese system, however, there are five seasons: fall, winter, spring, summer, and late summer, the latter proceeding from mid-July to mid-September. The five stages of change, their related seasons, aspects of nature, and related organs are as follows:

Summer is associated with fire and the heart and small intestine. These organs and season are, therefore, referred to as the Fire Element.

Late summer, proceeding from July to mid-September, is a time between the intensity of summer and the decline of fall. It is regarded as a stable time of the year and, hence, associated with the earth. The Earth Element is also associated with the stomach and spleen. (Many modern interpretations of the Five Elements also link the pancreas with the Earth Element.)

Fall is associated with metal and the lungs and large intestine. This is the Metal Element.

The differences between traditional Chinese and Western medicine have to do with the ways in which diseases are perceived, diagnosed, and treated. It remains to be seen how the two systems compare in terms of efficacy. But the systems need not be mutually exclusive. There is no reason why physicians cannot combine the finest elements of both schools. A Chinese proverb says, "The methods used by one man may be faulty; the methods used by two men will be better."

DAVID EISENBERG

Winter is associated with the kidneys and bladder and the winter months, from December 21 to March 21. It is known as the Water Element.

Spring is associated with the liver and gall bladder and the tree or wood. It is known as the Wood Element.

If you plot these five stages on a circle, as we have below, you will see that each stage leads to the next. Each stage of element nourishes those related organs within the element, and then passes qi on to the next stage. For example, the Fire Element provides qi to the heart and small intestine and then passes qi onto the Earth Element, the stomach, spleen, and pancreas. For this reason, Fire is called the mother of the Earth Element, because it provides life force to the Earth organs. This is called the nourishing or creative cycle.

At the heart of traditional Chinese medicine is the Five Elements Theory, which healers use both to diagnose and treat illness. The Five Elements—Fire, Wood, Water, Metal, and Earth— link the seasons of the year, aspects of nature, the body's organs, and specific foods, herbs, and treatments. It is also used for agricultural planning, healing, psychology, maintaining harmony in relationships, and even divination. This incredible tool typifies the Chinese talent for seeing the unity within apparent diversity.

The Five Elements

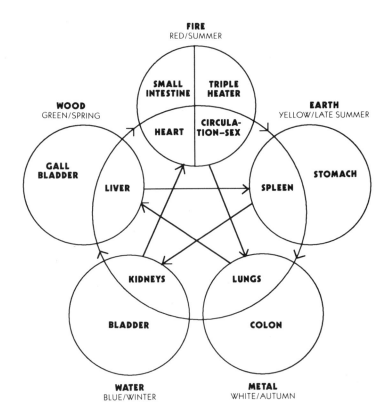

Wood nourishes Fire. Thus, the liver and gall bladder nourish the heart and small intestine with qi.

Fire nourishes Earth. The heart and small intestine nourish the spleen and stomach (and pancreas) with qi.

Earth nourishes Metal. The spleen and stomach provide qi to the lungs and large intestine.

Metal nourishes Water. The large intestine and lungs provide qi to the bladder and kidneys.

Water nourishes Wood. Kidneys and bladder pass qi on to the liver and gall bladder.

There is more than just nourishment in life, however. There are also limitations. Organs must be governed, too. Thus, there is also a controlling cycle. To illustrate this need, consider that a river is powerful because of the quantity of its water and the presence of its banks, which direct the flow of water by providing limits. Without such limits, the water overflows its banks and floods, thus destroying the river and the surrounding geography. As long as there are limits imposed on the water, the river has power to move obstacles out of the way, eliminate waste, or even drive a turbine to generate hydroelectric power. The water itself would be considered the nourishing power of the river, while the banks would be considered the controlling influence.

It is the same in the body. Organs must be nourished and governed. In this way, they have sufficient power and energy to eliminate waste and maintain harmony. The controlling cycle is as follows:

Fire controls Metal. Thus, the heart and small intestine control or limit energy within the lungs and large intestine.

Earth controls Water. The stomach, spleen, and pancreas limit or control the energy flowing within the kidneys and bladder.

Metal controls Wood. The lungs and large intestine control or limit the energy flowing in the liver and gall bladder.

Water controls Fire. The kidneys and bladder control the energy within the heart and small intestine.

Wood controls Earth. The liver and gall bladder control the energy flowing in the stomach, spleen, and pancreas.

The analysis goes even further. Each element and organ group is nourished by specific foods and herbs, while other foods and herbs control this specific organ group. Just as each organ grouping is associated with a season, so it is also associated with a particular time of day or night. The liver, for example, is most active between the hours of 1 A.M. and 3 A.M.; the heart is most active between 11 A.M. and 1 A.M.; the kidneys are most active between 3 P.M. and 5 P.M.

Traditional Oriental healers use this information to diagnose and treat. If every element is working optimally, there are no symptoms and there is optimal health. If, on the other hand, one or more of the organs is blocking energy, the organ system which is nourished by it will suffer. Consequently, those who damage their liver often suffer from heart or small intestine troubles, while those who damage their spleen, stomach, and pancreas also suffer from diseases of the large intestine and lungs.

Chinese medicine embodies a remarkable union of technical competence and spiritual force. Because it is also a successful method of alleviating suffering, Chinese medicine may succeed in bringing popular attention to the unifying concepts of the East more quickly and completely than any other manifestation of Oriental thought.

LEON HAMMER

Looking at the body according to the Five Elements, one can easily see the harmony within our systems, and come to know the importance of each organ to the body as a whole. For example, typically we would say that digestion is performed by the stomach and intestines, but according to the Five Elements, digestion is absolutely dependent on the healthy functioning of the spleen.

Biologically, we know that the spleen filters the blood of broken and dead cells and infuses the blood with immune cells, such as lymphocytes and other white cells. In Western medicine, the spleen is not considered essential to life and is often surgically removed in the case of certain cancers and other disorders.

However, Oriental medicine regards the spleen as one of the supremely important organs and essential to the orderly functioning of life. Spleen energy—that is, qi emanating from the spleen—governs the movement of food through digestion. Spleen energy helps to transport the food through the intestinal tract. As it does this, it also assists the small intestine in turning the essence of food—that is, the essential nutrients—into blood and qi energy. The spleen sends qi to the lungs and large intestine. In this way, it nourishes these two organs with life force, making possible both breathing and elimination of waste.

To understand how the controlling cycle influences the body, let's look at the relationship between the Water and Fire Elements.

Very often, people eat too much salt, which causes kidney disorders. Kidney and bladder (the Water Element) control the heart and small intestine function (Fire Element). Consequently, kidney disorders, especially those arising from excess salt intake, cause illnesses of the Fire Element, such as heart disease and high blood pressure. If we wish to treat this condition, we must treat the controlling element, which in this case is the Water Element. By sharply reducing salt, oils, and fats and by increasing mild aerobic exercise (Fire Element), we strengthen both the Water and Fire Elements and their corresponding organ systems.

Chinese medicine is such an extremely complex and sophisticated healing system that any summary must ultimately do it an injustice. In addition to its two fundamental principles—the law of yin and yang and the Five Elements—is an array of other diagnostic and medicinal tools that are themselves refinements upon this foundation. Illnesses arise out of imbalances within the body that are characterized as "too dry," or "too moist." An organ can contain excessive "heat," or "fire." It can be "cool," or "damp." The body can also contain too much "wind," meaning that there is excessive movement or instability in organs or systems that should be still. These refinements upon yin and yang and the Five Elements are applied to every condition, so that constipation, for example, does not arise merely from stagnation, but from too much "cold," perhaps, or excess "dryness."

Every imbalance, however, ultimately arises from a person's way of life, which is to say, a person's relationship with the universe itself. Thus, the Chinese healer restores balance by combining appropriate herbs, diet, and medicinal practices, along with changes in the patient's personal way of living.

CHAPTER 2

AYURVEDIC MEDICINE

All diseases of the body can be destroyed at the root by regulating the Prana; this is the secret knowledge of healing.

SWAMI VISHNU-
DEVANANDA

LEGEND SAYS THAT the system known as Ayur-Veda, or the knowledge of long life, was given to one of the Hindu rishis, or "seers," by the god Indra. When that may have happened, no one knows, but scholars do know that the Ayurvedic system goes back at least to the fifth century B.C. and is based on the Vedas, the oldest known philosophical and spiritual writings.

Like the Chinese and Greek systems, Ayur-Veda sees health within a universal context. Human life, say the Hindus, is an extension of the life of the creator, or what the Vedas refer to as "cosmic consciousness." Health is based upon one's relationship with cosmic consciousness. The healer serves to reestablish harmony between the individual and the life of the universe by balancing universal forces within each person. These forces are both complementary and unique: they complete each other and yet maintain their own identities and natures.

As with most traditional health systems, Ayurvedic medicine is also based upon a creation myth. From a single, unified and cosmic consciousness two forces emerged, one male, the other female, called Shiva and Shakti, respectively. These two forces combined to create multiple levels of being that include cosmic intelligence, ego and physical forms, including humankind.

Cosmic consciousness is also manifest as a life force, which the Hindus call "prana." This life force is the animating power of life. It not only provides vitality and endurance to each living being, but is also the basis of healing. The life force manifests in physical form as the Five Elements, which are bound together by three forces, called the Three Doshas. Let's consider the Five Elements first.

Ayur-Veda teaches that the body is composed of the Five Great Elements: Earth, Water, Fire, Air, and Ether. These elements are not seen in the purely material sense, but are metaphorical categories that describe functions and aspects of the human body. For example, the breakdown and absorption of food during digestion can be seen as a Fire function. The human digestive tract is the body's crucible, its oven, in which food is "prepared" for assimilation and utilization by the body. The Earth Element stands for all the mineral substances that make up the body, including those that combine to create bone, cartilage, and contribute to muscle formation (such as calcium). Earth is also associated with the body's solid waste. Water, of course, would represent all the liquid substances of the body, including blood, mucus, lymph, hormones, semen, fat, urine, and other fluids. It is also associated with the kidneys and genitals. Air is the substance that animates the body and gives it the ability to move, and thus is linked to the nervous system. Ether, the most subtle and abstract of the Five Elements, is the principle of form and idea from which the body draws its archetypal design; it thereby holds the body together.

Since the elements are seen as interdependent functions, they are often present in the same activity. For example, while Earth is responsible for bones, the activity of walking, which involves both bone and muscle, includes Earth and Fire—Fire, because this element is responsible for the expenditure of energy.

Each of these Five Elements is responsible for the creation of individual senses and their ongoing functions. Fire is associated with the eyes and seeing; Air with touch and the skin; Water with taste and the tongue; Earth with smell and the nose; and Ether with hearing and the ear.

If you take a scalpel and start to dissect the human body, you will get past the level of organs, tissues, cells, molecules, atoms, and elementary particles, only to end up with a handful of nothing. All physical matter is basically a bundle of energy waves vibrating in the void. Yet is this void really a nothingness, or is it the very womb of reality?

DEEPAK CHOPRA

The Seats of Vata, Pitta, and Kapha

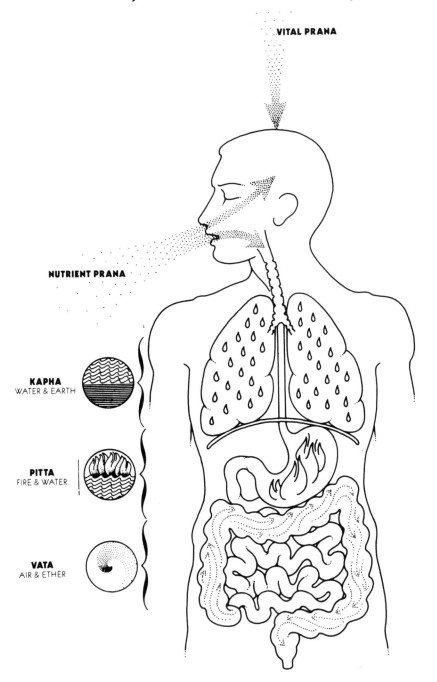

VITAL PRANA

Like the Chinese and Greeks, the traditional healers of India developed a healing system based on an underlying life energy. The system is called Ayur-Veda, and the life energy prana. Prana activates the body and mind, and is manifested in the human body according to the five basic elements (Ether, Air, Fire, Water, and Earth) and the three basic principles or doshas (vata, pitta, and kapha).

NUTRIENT PRANA

KAPHA
WATER & EARTH

PITTA
FIRE & WATER

VATA
AIR & ETHER

THE THREE DOSHAS

Having achieved form and substance, the body maintains harmony and health by balancing the three forces within it—the three doshas or vata, pitta, and kapha. Vata and kapha are seen as opposites, while pitta is the mediating force between the two extremes. The three doshas act on the Five Elements. They are the moving forces behind the substances and functions represented by the Five Elements. When the three doshas are balanced, the body functions harmoniously. When there is an imbalance among the doshas, illness results.

Vata represents the force of kinetic energy within the body. It ceaselessly stimulates motion, including the function of the nervous system, muscles, heart, blood flow, and thoughts. It is the vata activity in the brain that stimulates thought; the vata activity in the heart that stimulates beating; in the muscles that creates movement; in the nervous system that sparks electrical impulses and communication. Vata is associated with the Air Element.

Kapha is the source of potential energy. It is responsible for stability, groundedness, holding, and physical strength. Kapha causes tissues to be moist and lubricated. It is, therefore, associated with the lymph and with mucus. It is closely linked with the elements Earth and Water.

Pitta is most closely associated with Fire. It causes the burning of energy and the creation of heat within the body. It governs digestion, assimilation, and the metabolic processes of cells. It is linked with all the fiery aspects of life—hunger, curiosity, and thirst. Pitta mediates between kinetic energy (vata) and potential energy (kapha). Just as a fire burns and endures by transforming potential energy into kinetic, so pitta utilizes the two opposite forces to bring movement and endurance to bodily function.

If left to itself, vata would burn itself up; it would consume life in an intense blaze of ceaseless activity. Kapha, on the other hand, would decline into indolence and inactivity. Pitta must mediate between the two; but if either kapha or vata is excessive, pitta also will suffer, because both movement and rest must be equally available in order for pitta to function properly.

As we have seen, each of the three doshas may be present in the same organ, depending on whether it is currently active or at rest. However, individual organs are more closely aligned with

The Buddhists admonish us not to confuse the finger with that to which it points. Not only have we forgotten that the finger is pointing, or toward what it is pointing, but we believe that our reality can be resolved and understood by dissecting the finger, by breaking it down to its atoms and molecules as though somehow that is the ultimate reality and that's going to answer those questions for us. It's not that it's wrong, it's just incomplete.

KENNETH PELLETIER

specific doshas. Below are the three doshas and their corresponding organs:

Vata

Bones, including bone marrow
Brain, especially motor activity
Colon, when active
Heart
Lungs, specifically in the act of breathing
Nervous system

Pitta

Blood
Brain, in the synthesis of stored information, memory, and learning
Eyes, when awake
Hormones, in their active phase, as when stimulating an activity
Liver
Small intestine, especially during digestion and assimilation
Spleen

Kapha

Brain, especially in its capacity to store information
Joints
Lymph
Mouth
Stomach
Chest cavities

The three doshas give rise to and stimulate physical functions, and also create individual states of consciousness. In general, a balance between the doshas will create a high state of aliveness in which intellect and emotions are balanced; activity is governed by awareness of one's limitations; desire is balanced with understanding and forgiveness. Imbalance among the doshas, especially when one of them is excessive, will create distortions within the personality.

At its best, kapha represents emotional stability, "centeredness," and forgiveness. A kapha-type person recognizes his or her

The Theory of Tridoshas is one of the grandest and noblest contributions of ancient India to world culture. Although it has been known and practiced in India for over 3,000 years, its tenets are unknown or little known in the different parts of the civilized world. In the various medical systems of the world, for understanding diseases—and the diseased— the Tridosha doctrine is unique and supreme. Its practical value in diagnosis and treatment is without a parallel. It should be studied, grasped and applied in all medical systems without exception.

B. BHATTACHARYA

place in the larger configuration and can draw nourishment from work, relationships, and environment. He or she has a natural understanding of limits and boundaries.

When kapha is imbalanced, there is a tendency toward acquisitiveness, accumulation, and greed. The person has an inability to forgive, a possessiveness toward relationships and resources, and a desire to receive more than one has worked for.

Vata provides natural grace in movement and healthy motor function. The person with a balanced vata understands the needs of the body and its natural urges. He or she has a healthy ability to move on to the new and the untried, to let go of outdated relationships and behaviors.

When vata is imbalanced, a person has a hunger for sensory experiences, especially sex. He or she also has a heightened fear, anxiety, and skepticism toward others and may be controlled by nervous energy. He or she may be unable to feel "grounded" or emotionally stable and often gets exhausted.

Pitta provides a yearning for knowledge, for new experience, and understanding. Pitta causes one to see the broad picture, to understand divergent needs and to harmonize people's seemingly conflicting desires. Pitta types have a willingness to delve into details, to break down resistances, to work hard, and play hard. However, when pitta is imbalanced, a person feels great physical hunger, digestive problems, and thirst. There is a lack of gratitude for what is given, because it never seems enough, and much anger as a result of unfilled expectations. Pitta people may feel considerable hatred and jealousy.

The human body is the universe in miniature. That which cannot be found in the body is not to be found in the universe. Hence the philosopher's formula, that the universe within reflects the universe without. It follows, therefore, that if our knowledge of our own body could be perfect, we would know the universe.

MAHATMA GANDHI

CONSTITUTIONAL BODY TYPES

The doshas manifest in unique combinations in each person, thus giving rise to individual body types that lean toward one dosha or another. Some people have a body type that was more influenced by vata prenatally, while another will have more pitta characteristics. Each dosha creates tendencies within each of us, but because no one is perfectly balanced, one or two of the doshas will have dominated during the shaping of the constitution and the personality.

These imbalances will provide unique strengths and weaknesses, and thus create tendencies toward specific kinds of disorders and illnesses. Below is an overview of the three dosha types. No one is entirely a vata, pitta, or kapha person. People tend to be combinations of these three archetypal constitutions. But each of us has leanings toward one or the other. Ayurvedic physicians maintain that the three doshas combine to create eight basic constitutional types, which represent most people.

Those who have the kapha body type are stocky and often heavy-set, but frequently are surprisingly agile and athletic. If they overeat or avoid exercise, they can easily become overweight. They tend to be slow-moving, slow to excite or rile, and emotionally stable. They sleep like babies, are generally jolly, and can accumulate much wealth. Their approach to life is steady and slow. They like the status quo. They do not have a strong physical hunger for food or drink; rather, they derive emotional satisfaction from what they consume.

Kapha people have a tendency toward illnesses afflicting the kapha-related organs, especially the lungs, lymph, and stomach. Because of their weight and the kapha tendency to reduce movement and circulation, they also can suffer from heart disease. Peter Ustinov, former Secretary of State George Schultz, and George Simenon's famous detective, Maigret, are good examples of the kapha body type.

The pitta body type is often athletic, muscular, extremely active, and ruddy-skinned. Those who have this kind of body are intense people, hard-working and smart. They have excellent digestion, lots of energy, and usually do most things quickly. They tend to have fiery natures, be inspirational to others, and are leadership-oriented. Pitta people have excellent appetites; they hunger for food, experience, and learning. They can be easily irritated and impatient. They are often highly focused and directed in life. Once they desire something or lock onto a goal, they can be very committed and determined. However, this tendency gives pitta people the capacity for obsession and fanaticism. They must learn to lighten up. They can lose perspective, becoming jealous and violent. Vladimir I. Lenin and Margaret Thatcher are examples of pitta people.

Pitta body types are prone to illnesses affecting the pitta organs, especially the liver and gall bladder, blood, small intes-

How does Ayurveda achieve [its] noble aim and difficult task? Not by discovering and then destroying the various germs or bacilli, worms and viruses, but by the simple device of raising the individual resistance of the body and providing active immunity by vigorous discipline—not only on the physical and mental levels, but also at the spiritual and supra-mental levels.

R. K. GARDE

tine, and spleen. They can easily suffer from ulcers, as well. They should beware of cancer and stroke.

Since vata is continually moving, those with a vata body type are prone to dryness—dry skin, dry hair, and a humorless outlook on life. Vata people are small-boned, thin, and narrow-chested. They do not have a lot of flesh and are often so thin that their ribs and hips protrude. They are often nervous people and unable to sit still. Others sense that they are being consumed by something. They have little interest in food or drink, and often eat on the run. This leads to constipation, a chronic problem with vata types. They can be very cerebral, intellectual, and smart, though their thinking tends toward abstraction rather than concrete or practical ideas. The vata type is susceptible to illness of the vata organs, as well as arthritis, lower back problems, and lung disorders. Don Knotts (Barney Fife) and Woody Allen are examples of vata people.

The three doshas affect how the life force, prana, flows through the body, whether it is balanced, excessive, or deficient in certain organs. Ayur-Veda also maintains that this life force flows through the body in a definite pattern of meridians, or rivers of energy. These meridians correspond roughly to the Chinese system of acupuncture. And like the Chinese, the Ayurvedic physician uses the pulse and physiognomy to diagnose the patient. For foods, herbs, and treatments related to each dosha and element, see the specific chapter for each organ.

GREEK MEDICINE

HIPPOCRATES WAS A TOWERING and even revolutionary figure of his day. Born on the Greek island of Cos in 460 B.C., he founded the first school of medicine dedicated to the scientific understanding of health and the body. He refused to consider health and illness as a gift or punishment visited upon humanity by the gods. Instead, he regarded each as the consequence of "natural" and "orderly" processes that could be understood and, in the case of illness, treated.

There is debate over whether Hippocrates wrote any of the materials attributed to him. What most scholars believe is that Hippocrates wrote some of the texts penned under his name, and that many of the rest were transcribed from his lectures. In any case, much of his general understanding and many of his methods have been preserved. Ironically, the man who today is called "the father of medicine" has little influence over modern medical thinking. He is more apt to be cited as an inspiration by practitioners of alternative medicine, many of whom regard his fundamental precepts as still valid.

For Hippocrates, all living things move toward specific and knowable goals. Each living thing plays a part in a more grand cycle, which is essentially healthy and constructive. When illness manifests, the body's natural tendencies are to heal itself and restore the individual to its larger social purpose.

Health is the natural state of humanity, Hippocrates believed. Illness is also natural, however, and is governed by natural laws that are understandable. As such, illness follows a specific pattern. The physician's job is to intervene in that process at precise moments to assist the body in healing. The healing process thus consists of a triad: physician, patient, and the conditions surrounding the patient. All three must participate in the recovery process. "It is not enough for the physician to do his duty," Hippocrates said. "He must also receive cooperation from the patient, from the attendants, and from the external circumstances."

Like the early pioneers of Eastern medical systems, Hippocrates understood health and illness as relative states of balance. Elements exist within the body that must be balanced for health to exist. Illness, therefore, is a state of imbalance.

In one of the fragments of his writings, entitled *The Nature of Man,* Hippocrates described the basic constitution of human beings, and the fundamental elements that must be balanced to reestablish health.

"The human body contains blood, phlegm, yellow bile, and black bile," Hippocrates wrote. "These constitute the nature of the body, and through them a man suffers pain or enjoys health. A man enjoys the most perfect health when these elements are duly proportioned to one another in power, bulk, and manner of compounding, so that they are mingled as excellently as possible. Pain is felt when one of these elements is either deficient or excessive, or when it is isolated in the body without being compounded with the others."

According to Philip Wheelwright, Greek scholar and author of *The Presocratics,* the "excessive element is an intruder and a usurper: it must be either expelled or sent back to its proper place in the bodily complex." The body accomplishes this feat through the disease process itself, which is seen as the corrective action taken by the body to heal itself. The physician assists this process, says Wheelwright, through the use of "proper food and drink, calmness of mind and body, suitable exercise, and the like," which assists the "completion of the cycle through illness and back again to health."

Wherever the art of medicine is loved, there also is love of humanity.

HIPPOCRATES

Hippocrates

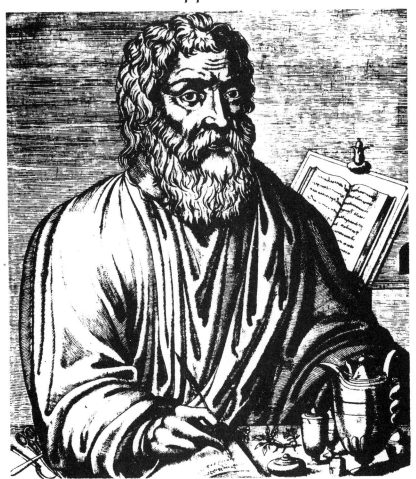

The great Greek physician Hippocrates (c. 460–377 B.C.) is a pioneering figure in medicine who termed healing "the noblest of all the arts." His ideas on the balance of health and illness, and the role of the healer in the healing process, are still studied by alternative practitioners.

Though scientific in his approach, Hippocrates had no hesitation in calling medicine an art. "The healing art is the noblest of all the arts," he said. As such, the physician must study each patient individually and adapt to the conditions of the illness.

"Nature was at work before any teaching began, and it is the part of wisdom to make adjustments to the situation that nature has provided," he told his students. Specifically, Hippocrates maintained that the physician must intercede at only the right moment in the process of healing. Once the moment has been reached, the physician must act quickly. "Time is that in which there are opportune moments, and an 'opportune moment' is that in which there is not much time." Hippocrates called these moments *kairos,* the root for "crisis." It was during such "healing crises" that the body reached a moment of truth in which restoration of health or death hung in the balance. At this moment, *pepsis* or the forces of healing could be assisted and illness overcome.

"The wise physician will know when to try to aid and accelerate the peptic process and when to let it alone," says Wheelwright. The doctor "must watch for the 'opportune moment' when the situation is exactly right for the exercise of his art."

Hippocrates maintained that the whole process could have beneficial effects. Illness could serve to create a new order among the four humors, as well as eliminate poisons and wash away impurities within the system. The Greek word that was used was *katharsis,* meaning to purify, especially the digestion. Once this purification was complete, one could achieve a new state of being, "a blended maturity" as Hippocrates called it.

Like his Asian counterparts, Hippocrates encouraged his students and fellow physicians to be humble and to recognize the true source of healing. "The healing art involves a weaving of a knowledge of the gods into the texture of the physician's mind . . . For it is not by individual cleverness that a physician is effective. Although he has his hands on many aspects of an ailment, it may still happen that the cure comes about quite spontaneously. Of course, whatever contributions the healing art is able to make should be accepted from it. But the path of wisdom in the art lies in making final acknowledgment to Those Very Ones."

Ancient Hippocratic medicine is no longer practiced as such, but its influence formed the basis of a medical tradition that flowed from Galen to Parascelsus to Avicenna, and thus to many traditional healers practicing today. Among modern healers, Hippocratic principles are most clearly in evidence in the system known as naturopathy.

We are bound to our bodies like an oyster is to its shell.

PLATO

HOMEOPATHY

All we know is still infinitely less than all that still remains unknown.

WILLIAM HARVEY

LATE IN THE EIGHTEENTH CENTURY, the German physician Samuel Hahnemann became discouraged by the prevailing practice of medicine, which in his day used such techniques as bloodletting and blistering to treat illness. Doctors of the time also employed a number of substances, such as mercury, now recognized to be extremely toxic. Hahnemann found that these methods were not only ineffective, but made the patient sicker and often caused death.

A deeply spiritual man, Hahnemann believed that physicians were meant to assist the body's natural healing mechanisms, rather than administer chemicals that would override those mechanisms. His lifelong dream was to discover "if God had not indeed given some law, whereby the diseases of mankind would be cured."

Disenchanted, Hahnemann decided to drop the practice of medicine and earn his living by translating. He was translating medical texts when he came upon one by William Cullen, a Scottish physician. Cullen maintained that cinchona bark cured fever by virtue of its astringent and bitter qualities. Hahnemann was incredulous and decided to test the hypothesis on himself. He took a dose of the cinchona, which contains quinine, a well-known medicine for fever and malaria. Instead of producing astringency, the cinchona caused fever and the symptoms of malaria in the healthy Hahnemann. He repeated the same experiment using other medicines, with similar results.

Based on these experiments, Hahnemann stated, "A substance that produces a certain set of symptoms in a healthy person has the power to cure a sick person manifesting those same symptoms." He thus articulated the first of several principles of what would be the new medicine of homeopathy. He called the principle the Law of Similars, which in essence states that like cures like. The name homeopathy joined the Greek words *homoios,* which means like, and *pathos,* for pathology or sickness.

The Law of Similars revealed to Hahnemann how the body reacts to disease. He maintained that the presence of an illness stimulates the body's defense system to eliminate the illness. That defensive reaction produces symptoms, which are part of the body's effort at eliminating the underlying disease. The symptoms are not the illness, said Hahnemann, but part of the curative process.

Hahnemann maintained that the effective medicines actually produce a condition similar to the illness itself, which arouses the body's defense system against the underlying disease. In effect, the medicine makes it easy for the body to recognize the underlying disease and mobilize its defenses against the illness. The outward manifestations of this effort are symptoms. A cough, for example, is the body's attempt at expectorating the pathogen; fever is hostile to the underlying pathogen; mucus attempts to isolate it and allow it to be driven from the body as a runny nose, sneezing, and watery eyes. This was, of course, an ancient understanding of symptoms, as was his belief that the body was animated by an underlying life force, which Hahnemann called the "vital force."

Strictly speaking, the Law of Similars was not by itself a new principle either. It was known among Ayurvedic physicians two thousand years earlier, and was central to the medical approaches of Hippocrates and Paracelsus, the sixteenth-century philosopher, alchemist, and physician. Still, it was in direct opposition to the prevailing medical approach of the West, which Hahnemann termed "allopathy." Allopathic healers basically prescribe drugs

The first holocaust may well have been the execution of several million women who were accused of being witches because they practiced herbal medicine.

HENRY EDWARD
ALTENBERG

43

The material organism, without the vital force, is capable of no sensation, no function, no self-preservation; it derives all sensation and performs all functions of life solely by means of the immaterial being (the vital force) which animates the material organism in health and disease.

SAMUEL HAHNEMANN

to create the opposite effect of a symptom in the body. Allopaths treat swelling, for example, by administering drugs that will directly reduce swelling. Symptoms are suppressed, which Hahnemann contended causes the disease to go deeper into the body. This leads to a more serious condition, which is harder to cure.

Hahnemann wanted to reduce the severity of the symptoms caused by medicine, and thus decided to reduce the size of the dosage. Remarkably, he found that the smaller dose was even more effective against the underlying illness. Further experimentation led Hahnemann to his next principle, which he called the Law of Potentization or the Law of Infinitesimals. This states that the smaller the dose of medicine, the greater its potency or its effect on the body's vital force. Thus, a microdose of the medication actually strengthens the vital force against the illness. Hahnemann developed a method to dilute medicines down to infinitesimal doses by diluting the quantities and then shaking them (which homeopaths call succussion). This process is done successively until, for some dosages, only molecular amounts of the original medicine remain.

CONTROVERSY AND CRITICISM

Homeopathy has drawn its most hostile criticism on the basis of its Law of Infinitesimals, because orthodox physicians have maintained that there isn't enough of the medicine left after dilution to have any effect on an illness. Homeopaths point out, first, that the body manufactures only 50–100 millionths of a gram of thyroid hormone each day—an infinitesimal amount, which, if absent, will prevent healthy metabolism. Essential trace minerals and certain vitamins also are absorbed and utilized by the body in infinitesimal quantities, yet their presence or absence determines health or illness. Yet, homeopaths also agree that the complete reason why infinitesimal amounts work is not yet fully understood.

Hahnemann's mystical bent led him to believe that dilution and succussion actually reduced the material substance to its spiritual essence, which, in his mind, accounted for the medicine's enhanced power. Like the Native American, Greek, Oriental, and Ayurvedic physicians before him, Hahnemann maintained that the underlying reality of the physical world is essentially spiritual. But unlike many modern spiritual teachers, who view such matters as abstract, Hahnemann insisted that this underlying spiritual power was physically present in the form of energy. Later, other homeopathic physicians offered similar, if more scientific, suggestions.

In 1954, Dr. William E. Boyd of Glasgow stated, "The power of the solution does not depend solely on the degree of dilution but on the special progressive method of its preparation; the energy latent in the drug is apparently liberated and increased by a forceful shaking of the liquid at each stage of the process." Other homeopathic physicians have maintained that the shaking and dilution of medicines have the same effect as rubbing a material substance until it becomes magnetized. According to homeopath Dr. F. K. Bellokossy of Denver, Colorado, "We thus produce electrical fields around every particle of the powered drug; and the more we triturate [grind], the stronger electrical fields we produce, and the more potentized becomes the triturated material."

Thus, homeopathy embraces yet another fundamental principle of ancient or traditional medicine: the presence of an underlying spiritual energy that is the governing foundation of the material world. Like its predecessors, homeopathy is at least in part spiritual medicine.

Homeopathy has been used safely since 1810, when Hahnemann first published his findings. Since then, millions of people have relied exclusively on homeopathy for the treatment of virtually all types of illnesses. In addition to these clinical experiences, numerous scientific studies have been done to test the homeopathic hypothesis, with a number of them favorably supporting the practice.

Probably the most controversial episode in the scientific testing of homeopathy took place in 1989, when a group of researchers led by French physician Jacques Benveniste reported findings that confirmed the efficacy of homeopathic medicines. After the study was published in *Nature,* the prestigious British science journal, it was attacked worldwide. *Nature* even took the unusual step of sending a team of debunkers, consisting of a magician, a journalist, and an expert on fraud (none was an immunologist familiar with the underlying medical science), to Benveniste's lab to replicate—and presumably repudiate—the original study.

Homeopathy is essentially not only many-sided but all-sided. She investigates the action of all substances, whether articles of diet, beverages, condiments, drugs or poison. She investigates their action on the healthy, the sick, animals and plants. She gives a new interpretation to that ancient, oft-quoted saying of Paul, Prove all things—*a new meaning, a new application that acts universally.*

CONSTANTINE HERING

After spending two days in his laboratory, not surprisingly they claimed that they could not reproduce his results and termed the original study's findings a "delusion." Undaunted, in the winter of 1991, Benveniste reported another series of experiments that once again validated the homeopathic thesis. His work was published in the journal of the French Academy of Sciences.

Commenting on the case, Dana Ullman, president of the Foundation for Homeopathic Education and Research in Berkeley, California, said, "The serious threat that the microdose phenomena and homeopathy poses to science and medicine is clear and evident [from] the strong antagonism that the initial research created. The fact that the critics ignored and continue to ignore the numerous other studies [that] support the action of the microdose is further evidence of this denial and ultimately of an unscientific attitude."

CHAPTER 5

NATUROPATHY

ATUROPATHY TRACES ITS ORIGINS in the U.S. to a German-born healer named Benedict Lust, who, in 1902, launched a newspaper called *The Naturopath and Herald of Health.* Lust had procured the name "naturopathy" from its originator, John H. Scheel, who ran a hospital in New York State. In his newspaper's opening editorial, Lust wrote that "'Naturopathy' is a hybrid word. It is purposely so. No single tongue could distinguish a system whose origin, scope and purpose is universal—broad as the world, deep as love, high as heaven. . . . We believe in strong, pure, beautiful bodies . . . thrilling perpetually with the glorious power of radiating health. . . . We plead for the renouncing of poisons from coffee, white flour, glucose, lard, tobacco, liquor and the other inevitable resources of perverted appetite."

Lust drew his evangelical zeal from having cured himself of tuberculosis by using the water cure of Father Sebastian Kneipp, an Austrian priest who prescribed hot and cold baths to treat disease. In 1892, Kneipp sent Lust to the U.S. as a missionary for the water cure. Once he arrived, Lust obtained doctorates in both osteopathy and medicine, and eventually opened his own school of massage, chiropractic, and naturopathy in New York.

Naturopathy, as Lust defined it, is the use of nontoxic healing

The art of medicine consists of amusing the patient while nature cures the disease.

VOLTAIRE

In Tibetan medicine, physicians and pharmacologists are not separate persons. A doctor must know all aspects of medicine. Therefore, especially during the summer, students accompany physicians to the mountains to study herbs and plants, taking particular notice of their potencies, faults, and advantageous qualities. Then during the winter, they learn how to manufacture medicines. Thereby, they learn all aspects of medical practice.

YESHI DONDEN

methods derived from the best traditional healing systems from around the world. In that sense, naturopathy did not originate with Lust, or with any single person, but has its roots in Greek, Oriental, and European medical traditions. With these systems, it shares a belief in an underlying life force, but not an explicit allegiance to a specific unifying principle such as yin and yang or the Five Elements. In his 1919 book *Philosophy of Natural Therapeutics,* Henry Lindlahr, among the pioneers of naturopathy, wrote that "every living cell in an organized body is endowed with an instinct of self-preservation which is sustained by an inherent force named *the vital force of life.*" Sounding very much like a Hippocratic or Chinese physician, Lindlahr went on to say that "every acute disease is the result of a healing effort of nature."

Today, naturopaths employ a diversity of natural therapies, including acupuncture, homeopathy, botanical remedies, chiropractic, therapeutic massage, diet and nutrition, fasting, colonics, hydrotherapy, and compresses. Naturopathic physicians who have attended an accredited four-year program (there are currently two in the U.S.) are trained in most of the same scientific disciplines taught in conventional medical schools. Consequently, a naturopath also will occasionally employ medical tests, such as blood and urine analysis, for diagnosis. Moreover, most naturopaths acknowledge that modern medicine, including drugs and surgery, has a place in crisis intervention, though they remain committed to using nontoxic and noninvasive methods.

Dr. Ross Trattler, naturopath and author of *Better Health Through Natural Healing,* summarizes the basic disease process and its causes as follows:

- Accumulation of toxic material within the body due to poor circulation, poor elimination, and lack of exercise.
- Unhealthful diet that is rich in harmful ingredients (fat, cholesterol, sugar, artificial ingredients, and excess protein) and low in essential vitamins, minerals, and fiber.
- Improper posture and body structure, including spinal misalignment, poor muscle tone, and blood and lymph stagnation.
- Destructive emotions, including fear, stress, resentment, hatred, self-pity, all of which have a debilitating effect on internal organs and the immune system.

- Suppressive drugs, such as antibiotics and vaccinations, which some studies have found depress the immune system.
- Excessive alcohol, coffee, and tobacco.
- Environmental agents in the soil, air, water, and workplace.
- Parasites, virus, and infection.
- Genetic factors that create specific weaknesses, which allow accumulated toxins and these other factors to manifest as disease.

Like the Chinese and Greek systems, naturopaths regard illness as the body's effort at self-cleansing. Sneezing, coughing, fever, sweating, diarrhea, frequent urination, and rest are all methods used by the body to eliminate the underlying conditions that promote illness. Pain is seen as a message from the body that something is wrong. Such conditions as inflammation are the body's method of localizing problems to allow the rest of the system to function unimpeded. Naturopaths say that the body will place toxins at specific places in an effort either to eliminate the poisons, or to keep them from getting to organs that are vital to life. If not appropriately dealt with early, these accumulated toxins can eventually become tumors and cancer.

The naturopathic physicians of modern times do not discard a method simply because it is old; neither do they immediately embrace a technique because it is new, popular, and heavily advertised. The methods of naturopathic medicine have been rigidly tested upon the anvil of time and experience.

JOSEPH BOUCHER

HEALING WITH HERBS

Naturopaths regard the underlying life force as the source of the body's ability to heal itself. Medicine is intended to assist this life force. Among the most frequently used remedies in natural medicine, and the oldest, are herbs. The medicinal effects of herbs are categorized by their effect on the body. For instance, some of the most common properties of herbs are:

- *Alterative:* heals and purifies the blood, without creating side effects.
- *Anodyne:* relieves pain.
- *Astringent:* causes contraction and stops discharge.
- *Antiemetic:* stops vomiting.
- *Antiseptic:* stops decay and putrefaction.
- *Antispasmodic:* relieves and prevents spasms.
- *Demulcent:* relieves inflammation.
- *Diuretic:* increases the secretion and flow of urine.
- *Emetic:* induces vomiting.

- *Emmenagogue:* promotes menstruation.
- *Emolient:* softens and soothes inflamed tissue.
- *Febrifuge:* reduces or eliminates fever.
- *Laxative:* stimulates bowel elimination.
- *Nervine:* soothes nervous system and treats nervous disorders.
- *Sedative:* promotes relaxation and sleep.
- *Tonic:* invigorates and strengthens whole body.

Herbal and dietary healing are the basis of most traditional medicines, from Asia to the Americas. The practice of using herbs and food as medicine may go back as far as 60,000 years. Yet naturopathy, like chiropractic, homeopathy, and Chinese medicine, has come under repeated attack by medical doctors who maintain that such practices are quackery. Still, scientists have been turning herbal properties into drugs for most of this century, and dietary therapy is now reaching the mainstream.

The overall diet recommended by most naturopaths is similar to what's recommended today by the U.S. Surgeon General and what China's Yellow Emperor recommended thousands of years ago: whole grains, fresh vegetables, beans, fish, and fruit, and little animal fat. Naturopaths also frequently prescribe vitamin and mineral supplements, especially to boost the immune system.

Naturopathy is a method of curing disease by releasing inner vitality and allowing the body to heal itself. The methods that the naturopath uses should be looked on only as useful tools that help release this vital healing power. In and of themselves, they are not intrinsically healing.

ROSS TRATTLER

CHAPTER 6

CONVENTIONAL MODERN MEDICINE

ODERN MEDICINE, the dominant form of health care in the world today, is poised between two trends: an increasing reliance upon technology and highly sophisticated scientific procedures for both diagnosis and treatment of illness, and a growing awareness of the importance of disease prevention and the central role of self-care and more holistic practices. Will these two seemingly opposite trends merge in the next twenty years to create a new form of medicine, which will ultimately combine the modern and the ancient, the technological and the philosophical? A closer look at the historical antecedents of modern medicine may help to answer this important question.

First, a note about terminology. Conventional, orthodox, or modern medicine is also known as allopathy. *Allo,* from the Greek for "other," and *pathos,* for "suffering, disease," combine to refer to the use of treatments that cause the opposite effect as that created by the disease. So, if an illness causes inflammation, allopathic healers prescribe remedies that directly reduce swelling. The term was coined by Dr. Samuel Hahnemann, the creator of homeopathy, the system of using minute doses of substances that induce the same effect in the body as the symptom of the disease.

The whole imposing edifice of modern medicine, for all its breathtaking successes is, like the celebrated Tower of Pisa, slightly off balance.

PRINCE CHARLES

The mainstream of medicine cannot be identified with any one medical system; rather the mainstream is formed by all the tributaries. Is it even right to assume that there should be a mainstream at all? Perhaps we need to keep the natural rivers running freely, rather than dammed and confined.

TED KAPTCHUK

Modern medicine as such is a relatively recent development. While it claims Hippocrates as "the father of medicine," that claim is rooted in only one aspect of Hippocrates' method. He was the first physician to bring scientific and analytical reasoning to health care. In the process, he set medicine apart from religion or myth. Hippocrates' method of questioning and observing the patient closely to recognize the underlying illness and its cause remains among the most important methods of diagnosis. On the other hand, few of his ideas on the stages of disease, or his healing methods—diet, herbs, and a wide variety of natural remedies—are respected or used by orthodox medical doctors today.

Despite its claim on the Greek physician, modern medicine didn't really emerge until the early sixteenth century when Andreas Vesalius, a Flemish physician, did some of the earliest experiments in anatomy. About 100 years later, in 1628, William Harvey, the great English physician, first described the circulation of blood and the functioning of the heart. In 1660, Dutch naturalist Antonj van Leeuwenhoek created the first high-powered microscope, capable of magnifying objects 300 times, which provided an essential tool for inquiry into the inner workings of the body.

Around the same time, the French philosopher René Descartes' work crystallized the concept of mechanism and dualism, effectively creating the model of the body as machine, separate and distinct from mind. Less than a century later, Isaac Newton provided the mathematical and scientific underpinnings to these concepts, which became the dominant worldview of the West for the next 300 years.

These advances formed the foundation for the pivotal medical discoveries of the nineteenth century. The most significant was by French scientist Louis Pasteur who, during the 1860s, proved that microscopic organisms, such as viruses and bacteria, could cause disease. German bacteriologist Robert Koch advanced the theory still further, positing four conditions that must be satisfied to establish the causative organism of a specific disease; these conditions became known as "Koch's Rule."

In 1895, German scientist Wilhelm Roentgen discovered X rays and led the way to the development of a practical X-ray machine. By passing X rays, highly charged waves of energy, through the body and then onto a sensitive photographic plate, scientists found that they could create an accurate image of parts of the body's interior.

THE MEDICINE OF SCIENCE AND TECHNOLOGY

X-ray diagnosis and advances in microscopes awakened scientists to the power of new technologies to provide information. Scientific medicine was increasingly looking at the body at the cellular level for the answers to health questions. This coincided with the dominant need of its day, namely, to find solutions for the leading causes of death. During the eighteenth and nineteenth centuries in the Western industrialized nations, these causes were primarily pneumonia and influenza. By contrast, heart disease and cancer were less of a concern. The discovery of bacterial and viral agents as the cause of some infectious illnesses appeared to be one step short of finding the fountain of youth.

Pasteur's work still stands as among the greatest achievements in medicine. His germ theory as the origin of disease gained overriding acceptance in the West in the early twentieth century. Since almost all illness was thought to originate from microscopic organisms, scientists began to search for the means to kill these tiny creatures. The tools that seemed to offer the most promise were synthetic drugs.

It is sometimes argued that modern pharmacology is merely a more sophisticated version of the ancient practice of herbology, but in fact the two disciplines bear only superficial resemblance to each other. Traditional herbology holds that everything about a medicinal plant is "active": its shape, which is created by specific natural or energetic forces; its taste, which will often indicate the part of the body the plant will influence; its stage of maturity; the place it was grown; the time of year and method by which it was harvested; and, finally, the plant's "spiritual origin" and mythological significance. In this sense, medicinal plants are seen to have "powers" that extend beyond the action of any single chemical constituent. They have not only material substance, but what might be termed energetic or spiritual properties.

In contrast, the practice of modern pharmacology is based on the development of concentrated, purified chemical substances that target one aspect of the disease process. In 1805, scientists

The problem here is that the practice of the art of medicine has now developed into what is called "the delivery of health-care." Health-care is a commodity and falls under, as it were, the laws of "Caesar." Caring for the sick is not and cannot be entirely a commodity for it requires of man faculties that are aspects of the movement toward inner consciousness, a movement that obeys other laws than the laws of rationalistic, societal order. It requires a nonegoistic attention and a nonegoistic intellect. The practice of medicine, therefore, places the physician between the two worlds, and it does so far more obviously and inescapably than any other profession in our culture.

JACOB NEEDLEMAN

isolated and extracted morphine from opium and thus gave medicine its first "pure" painkiller. This began the practice of extracting what chemists thought were the active ingredients in plants. In 1935, the antibacterial agents called sulfonamides were formed. These were followed by penicillin, streptomycin, and tetracycline in the 1940s (penicillin was originally discovered in 1928, but not produced as medication until a decade and a half later). Today, the pharmaceutical industry uses genetic engineering to develop some new drugs. In such cases, there is no real link with plants, except to derive some genetic material to combine with new compounds.

The realities of medical economics encourage doctors to do less and less listening to, thinking about, sympathizing with and counseling of patients—what doctors call "cognitive services." Instead, the doctor is encouraged to act, to employ procedures.

DAVID HILFIKER

Since the 1940s, new drugs followed by the thousands. The original antibiotics proved miraculous against infectious disease, and medical scientists bathed in the glory of their success. Scientists believed that a chemical cause and pharmaceutical cure for every illness would soon be found.

Looking back, however, it's clear that the eradication of many infectious diseases cannot be attributed entirely to the development of antibiotics. Improvements in sanitation and personal hygiene, which in the West took place more or less concurrently with the arrival of antibiotics, played an important role in the eradication of infectious diseases. Still, the effectiveness of these drugs convinced doctors and scientists of the power of chemistry, and set medicine on an irrevocable course that dominates Western society today.

Along with the development of the modern pharmaceutical industry came a slew of new discoveries and new machines. They quickly formed the cornerstone of medical diagnosis. Among these were the recognition in 1901 of three distinct blood groups, and the increasing understanding of blood constituents and analysis; the creation in 1906 of the electrocardiograph (EKG), used to record the electrical impulses of the heart; and the invention in 1932 of the electron microscope, capable of magnifying images to a power of five million. At the same time, lower-dose X-ray machines were developed, making X rays safer; more sensitive photographic technology provided clearer pictures; and radioactive dye was combined with X-ray technology to provide more accurate images of human organs.

Still later, scientists developed such high-tech procedures as computerized axial tomography (CAT) scanning and magnetic resonance imaging (MRI) to produce three-dimensional pictures of the interior parts of the body. Blood and urine analysis became highly sophisticated, with doctors relying heavily upon such tests for diagnosis. It is not uncommon for one doctor to send another the patient's records, and for the second doctor to confirm or offer a diagnosis without even seeing the patient. This has led critics of modern medicine to contend that tests and machines so dominate the healing profession that the *art* of healing is in danger of being lost entirely.

Concurrent with this remarkable growth in pharmacology and technology, surgery passed through a similar evolution. Surgery goes back more than 6,000 years, at least to the ancient Egyptians and Peruvians. But the principles of modern surgery originated with such innovators as Frenchman Ambroise Paré, who in 1542 bound a wound by securing strips of cloth to the skin and then joining the strips with stitches. Ether was first used as an effective anesthesia in 1842, "laughing gas" (nitrous oxide) in 1845, and chloroform in 1847.

History played a role in shaping the course of medicine during World War II, when wound treatment provided surgeons with an understanding of how the body's immune system could be suppressed to accept skin grafts, foreign implants, and transplanted organs. With this new knowledge, the first coronary bypass was performed in 1951 by Canadian Arthur Vineberg in Montreal, and the first heart transplant in 1967 by South African surgeon Dr. Christiaan Barnard.

Consistent with other branches of medicine, surgery now focuses on ever-smaller parts of the body, using microscopes and tiny instruments. It is also becoming even more technologically advanced, using such new high-tech tools as lasers and minute cameras to perform operations from within the body itself.

THE BIRTH OF A NEW MEDICINE

Today, modern Western medicine stands as a monolith on the world stage. Few other spheres of human endeavor have developed so rapidly and in so singular a fashion. In the U.S., it employs millions of people and accounts for a huge share of the country's gross national product. In terms of its sheer influence

One of the things the average doctor doesn't have time to do is catch up with the things he didn't learn in school, and one of the things he didn't learn in school is the nature of human society, its purpose, its history, and its needs . . . If medicine is necessarily a mystery to the average man, nearly everything else is necessarily a mystery to the average doctor.

MILTON MAYER

55

I see surgery as a passing fancy . . . It's a rather stupid way to treat disease. A surgical operation is nothing more than an artificial disease that is superimposed on the previously existing disease in the hope that the amalgamation of the two will redound to the benefit of the patient. It is usually a vain hope.

RICHARD SELZER

over the daily life of most people, the health care industry is perhaps unrivaled.

Ironically, modern medicine is now in the throes of a revolution, in part because the disease patterns of the Western world have changed. Today, the leading causes of death in the U.S. are no longer infectious diseases but degenerative ones, such as illnesses of the heart and arteries, cancer, and diabetes. Studies have determined that these illnesses are caused primarily by lifestyle factors, such as dietary habits, stress, and patterns of thinking, feeling, and behaving.

In other words, the leading killer diseases no longer fit into the germ theory paradigm. Modern medicine's failure to cure these illnesses, which don't really fit its worldview, and its enormous drain on many Western societies' economies, have revealed the system to be highly inflexible to the prevailing needs of modern life. The medical industry remains strongly wedded to crisis intervention, and its overreliance on extremely expensive tests, procedures, and technologies today threatens to bankrupt entire nations. At the same time, many common drugs and surgical procedures have undergone insufficient testing, or cause terrible side effects, raising doubts over the efficacy of some of medicine's methods and the veracity of its claims. Finally, because the industry in the U.S. has long served as its own watchdog, it has failed to deal adequately with such problems as overpricing and overuse.

Though most of orthodox medicine adheres stubbornly to its technological and pharmaceutical methods, a new and powerful trend is underfoot, which emphasizes the prevention of illness and the use of simpler, noninvasive methods of healing. Better diet, more active lifestyle, and healthier interpersonal relationships are the core constituents of this route to health.

Pasteur saw the future. He recognized that, although we all breathe in many pathogens, only a few of us become ill. He apparently recognized this fact as significant. On his deathbed, the great scientist is said to have told friends that his archrival, Claude Bernard, was correct in maintaining that the body withstands disease or embraces it by virtue of its overall health. "Bernard is right," Pasteur confided. "Microbes are nothing, the soil is everything."

PART TWO

The Organs

IT IS ONE THING to talk abstractly about universal forces and humanity's relationship with the cosmos, and quite another to confront the realities of specific organs, their functions, and the illnesses that afflict them. Yet, it is in this very realm that the differences between East and West are both stark and marvelous. Here, the West focuses on specific material objects. It looks at the stomach and sees muscle, mucous lining, and fibrous tissues. On the other hand, the East sees function, behavioral patterns, and metaphor. One objectifies; the other characterizes.

To best describe the body's organs, we'll combine these complementary approaches, exploring physical anatomy and personal

The Major Organs of the Body

The internal organs are layered in the body. This frontal illustration simplifies the overall anatomy by showing one kidney and the gall bladder, normally behind the liver, and the pancreas, normally behind the stomach.

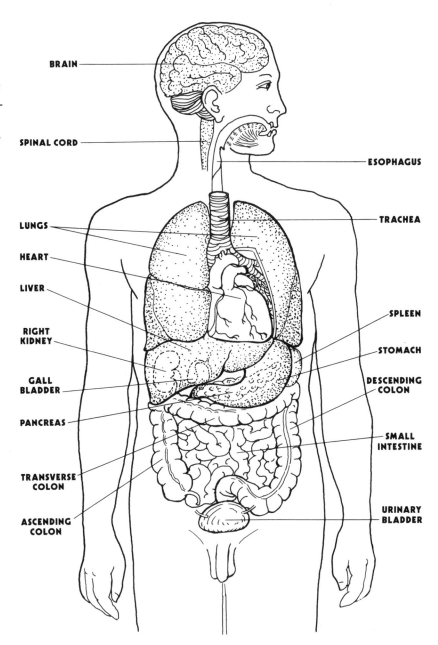

BRAIN

SPINAL CORD

ESOPHAGUS

LUNGS

TRACHEA

HEART

LIVER

RIGHT KIDNEY

SPLEEN

STOMACH

DESCENDING COLON

GALL BLADDER

PANCREAS

SMALL INTESTINE

TRANSVERSE COLON

ASCENDING COLON

URINARY BLADDER

and cultural experience. We'll consider historical reports and modern research. Throughout, we'll be referring to Eastern and ancient approaches as "traditional," meaning that they have been handed down through many centuries within specific cultures. This is, of course, somewhat of a simplification (Chinese medicine, for instance, is composed of a number of distinct healing traditions), but a useful one. Though "traditional medicine" is sometimes used to refer to modern Western medicine, we prefer the terms allopathic, conventional, or orthodox medicine.

Let's begin our cross-cultural exploration into the complex and wondrous realm of the organs with a look at how food and drink become mind and body.

CHAPTER 7

THE STOMACH

ITH A NAME that comes from the Latin *alere,* to nourish, the alimentary canal is the route that food takes in its journey through the body. It is composed of the mouth, teeth, tongue, pharynx, esophagus, stomach, small intestine, and large intestine.

The mouth, which contains thirty-two teeth and the tongue, also contains salivary glands that secrete saliva. Saliva is an alkaline liquid composed of about 99 percent water, plus some minerals, cells, and inorganic salts. It also contains the enzyme amylase, which assists in the digestion of carbohydrates. The average person produces about three pints of saliva per day.

Saliva serves many important functions, including moistening and lubricating the mouth and food, dissolving food particles to facilitate taste and swallowing, beginning digestion of carbohydrates, cleansing the mouth, and neutralizing many poisons, bacteria, and foreign agents.

The pharynx is a passageway that connects the back of the mouth and nasal passages to the esophagus. Like the esophagus, it is a muscular tube that is lined with a mucous membrane and allows both air and food to pass. At the lower portion of the phar-

To eat is human; to digest, divine.

CHARLES TOWNSEND
COPELAND

The Digestive System

The digestive system includes the entire path that food and nutrients take on their journey through the body, from the mouth and esophagus to the large and small intestines.

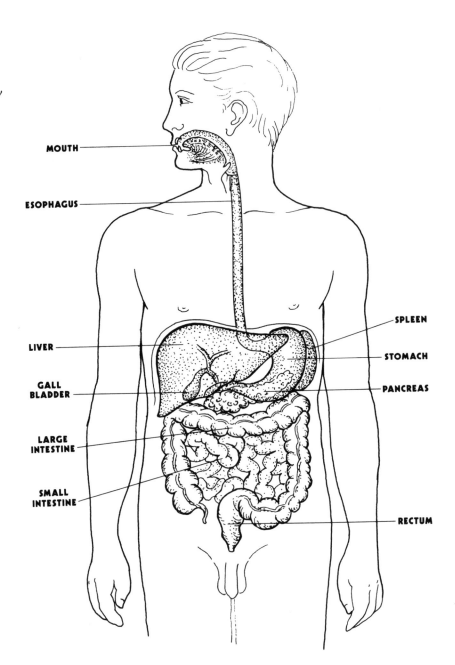

MOUTH

ESOPHAGUS

LIVER

GALL
BLADDER

LARGE
INTESTINE

SMALL
INTESTINE

SPLEEN

STOMACH

PANCREAS

RECTUM

ynx lies the larynx, the organ responsible for voice production. The larynx serves as a passageway for air from the pharynx to the trachea, or windpipe. Below the larynx is the laryngopharynx, which connects to the esophagus and permits food to pass to the stomach.

The muscles within the esophagus expand and contract, creating a peristaltic action that forces food downward to the stomach. Interestingly, gravity plays only a small part in getting food from the mouth to the stomach, as evidenced by the fact that you can drink while standing on your head.

A WINDOW ON THE STOMACH

One of the great contributions to medical knowledge of the digestive tract was made involuntarily, courtesy of an obscure French-Canadian man named Alexis St. Martin. On June 6, 1822, he was accidentally shot when a nearby musket fell and discharged both shot and wadding into his left side. The shot blew a large hole into St. Martin's stomach and lung, both of which protruded through his rib cage. Fortunately, U.S. Army surgeon Dr. William Beaumont was on the scene. Beaumont stuffed St. Martin's stomach and lung back inside the hole and proceeded to do what he could to stop the bleeding. It was touch and go for several weeks; Beaumont had to feed St. Martin through a tube inserted into his anus.

Miraculously, St. Martin made a full recovery, except that the hole in his stomach and side remained open. This presented a rather unusual problem. As long as the hole was bandaged inside the chest wall, well against the stomach, St. Martin could eat without incident. But when the bandage was removed, his food and drink escaped—and an observer could actually look right into St. Martin's stomach and see its internal workings.

Eventually, Beaumont realized the significance of St. Martin's hole and proceeded to conduct experiments to study how the stomach worked. To do this, Beaumont would put small amounts of food inside silk sacks and insert them into St. Martin's stomach for an hour or so to find out what exactly the stomach was up to when it contained food. Among his discoveries was the first positive identification of hydrochloric acid as a main constituent of stomach fluids. He also found that when a person gets angry (as

St. Martin often did when Beaumont's experiments grew tiresome), the stomach moves around a bit and becomes flushed with blood. Beaumont experimented extensively on St. Martin's gastric juices, sometimes even tasting them. He recorded his findings in *Experiments and Observations on Gastric Juice and the Physiology of Digestion* (1833).

A wanderer by nature, St. Martin moved around the country quite a bit, perhaps in the vain hope of shaking the indominable Dr. Beaumont. Alas, the good doctor followed Alexis everywhere, testing the miraculous stomach whenever possible, but often lamenting that St. Martin was a "difficult and uncooperative" subject. Their collaboration was an odd but historically important relationship. Medical historian Douglas Guthrie noted that Beaumont managed to carry off "a fine piece of research in the face of unusual difficulties." History has even given St. Martin's orifice Beaumont's name: researchers refer to it as "Beaumont's window." Today, we don't need Beaumont's window to know what the stomach looks like and what it does.

The stomach is located below the diaphragm, slightly to the left of the sternum. It is a hollow organ, shaped like a balloon or a boxing glove, with the fat end connected to the esophagus at the top, and the constricted end connected to the duodenum (the first part of the small intestine) at the bottom. The purpose of the stomach is to store food, to secrete digestive juices and churn the food into a creamy mass, to begin the digestion of proteins, and, finally, to gradually secrete the liquid mixture in slow increments into the duodenum.

The stomach's capacity is about three pints. Its ability to store food makes it possible for you to do something other than eat every twenty minutes, which is what you'd have to do to support your nutrient and energy requirements if you had no stomach. (It is actually possible to survive without a stomach.) The stomach wall is composed of longitudinal and circular muscles that enable the stomach to churn food and turn it into a thick liquid. The stomach is also lined with special glandular cells that secrete gastric juices. The muscles and glands are supplied by blood vessels and nerves. At the bottom of the stomach, where it opens into the duodenum, a powerful muscle, called a pyloric sphincter, forms a ring that opens and closes, acting as a gateway between the stomach and the small intestine.

As you've no doubt experienced, gastric juices may be released into the stomach as soon as you see or smell food. Once you eat, the stomach releases pepsin, an enzyme that breaks down proteins to make them accessible to the small intestine, and hydrochloric acid, which kills bacteria on the food and assists the pepsin. An enzyme called intrinsic factor is also released to assist in the preparation of vitamin B12, which usually accompanies protein foods, so that the vitamin can be absorbed later by the small intestine. Finally, special glands secrete mucus to form a protective lining that prevents the stomach from digesting itself or being consumed by the acid.

Within the animal kingdom, stomach sizes vary according to the kinds of diets that animals consume. Carnivores tend to have larger stomachs than herbivores, relative to the rest of their digestive tracts. The stomachs of dogs and cats, for example, make up between 60 and 70 percent of their digestive tracts, while the stomach of a horse, an herbivore, consists of only 8 percent of its digestive system. This is why you see herbivores continually grazing, while carnivores are able to avoid eating for longer periods of time.

In humans, the stomach's role in digestion depends on the kinds of foods we consume and their relative composition of carbohydrates (used by the body for immediate and enduring energy needs), fat (a secondary energy supply, stored in tissues, and used when carbohydrate reserves have been exhausted), proteins (groups of amino acids used for cell replacement and repair), and vitamins and minerals (both essential to the proper function of cells). Of these, only protein is digested by the stomach.

The mouth and small intestine digest carbohydrates. The enzymes in saliva begin to break down the carbohydrates and prepare them for further digestion and, finally, absorption into the small intestine. Thus, in order to be digested properly, carbohydrate foods must be chewed thoroughly. Chewing ensures that the carbohydrates are mixed with sufficient quantities of saliva and its enzymes. Carbohydrate-laden foods that contain little protein do not require much action by the stomach and tend to move quickly on to the small intestine. (This is why many people find that they're hungry an hour after eating Chinese food, for instance.)

Fats and oils (which are liquid fats) are digested and absorbed exclusively in the small intestine. It is a slow process that begins immediately after the fats are released into the small intestine, which forces other foods still in the stomach to wait in line to be released into the small intestine. There they are broken down by the action of bile salts from the liver. They are then turned into fatty acids and glycerol (fatty acids in an alcohol base) by a pancreatic enzyme called lipase.

Of course, fat-rich foods are often rich in protein, too, which also must be acted upon by the stomach in order to be digested. Consequently, a fat- and protein-rich meal can take as much as six hours to evacuate the stomach. The energy requirements for such an undertaking are considerable, which explains why you often want to sleep after a heavy meal.

Fat slows digestion, but a variety of foods stimulate the stomach's activity, particularly its secretion of acid. Refined grains, coffee, tea, tobacco, sugar, alcohol, spices, and fried foods increase acid production by the stomach. Many drugs, such as aspirin and steroids, also increase stomach acids. So does stress. The foods may also stimulate the organ itself, causing greater churning action and speeding the digestive process. People who have coffee, brandy, cigarettes, or cigars after a heavy meal are taking advantage of these substances' ability to stimulate stomach activity.

Vitamins and minerals are so small that they do not need to be acted upon extensively to be prepared for absorption, which takes place in the small intestine.

WHEN DIGESTION GOES WRONG

The most frequent and minor stomach disorders are, of course, indigestion, heartburn, and gas. These disorders are caused by overeating, eating too quickly, eating foods that are rich in fat or spices, or stress. Generally, all of these conditions arise from excess stomach acid. Doctors recommend an over-the-counter antacid medication, but these drugs have side effects and can disguise symptoms that may become an ulcer.

The most common form of stomach disorder is a peptic ulcer, which is a wound in the stomach wall, usually about a half inch to an inch in diameter. About 60 percent of stomach ulcers are formed in the duodenum, with the remaining occurring some-

Gastroneurologists often say, "If I could cut off his head, I could cure his ulcer." That's how powerful the mind is.

MILTON TRAGER

where in the lower part of the stomach. Ulcers can also occur in the esophagus, with rare occurrences in lower parts of the small intestine.

The typical symptom is a gnawing pain in the abdomen, especially when the stomach is empty, leading many people to complain about ulcer symptoms at night. A related problem is gastritis, which is the inflammation of the mucous membrane of the stomach, usually caused by aspirin or alcohol, infection, excessive bile acids, or stress. Gastritis may cause the same symptoms as an ulcer, though it is usually less severe.

From the perspective of conventional medical doctors, the cause of stomach ulcers is excessive stomach acid coupled with a decrease in the production of protective mucus. Most doctors acknowledge that diet plays a role in the onset of both of these factors, particularly the excessive consumption of alcohol, cigarettes, spicy foods, and aspirin, all of which increase stomach acids. Conventional treatment includes the reduction or elimination of such substances, along with the use of drugs, such as antacids, which neutralize stomach acid, and/or pharmaceuticals designed to reduce acid production, such as cimetidine, ranitidine, or famotidine.

If drugs are ineffective, surgery is often required. Surgeons may perform a vagotomy, which involves cutting the fibers of the vegas nerve that control acid production, or they may do a partial gastrectomy, which is the surgical removal of part of the stomach.

Another common stomach disease is cancer. Malignancies of the stomach kill about 15,000 Americans annually. Studies consistently show that diet is the leading cause of stomach cancer, especially diets rich in salted, smoked, and pickled foods. The Japanese, who consume large amounts of such foods, suffer the highest rate of stomach cancer in the world. Orthodox medical treatment may include the complete removal of the stomach.

THE STOMACH AS ENERGY SYSTEM

From the traditional Chinese perspective, organs have both physiological and psychological functions. Those functions are associated with particular aspects of nature, where those characteristics are demonstrated. For example, the stomach and spleen are asso-

You can only cure retail but you can prevent wholesale.

BROCK CHISHOLM

ciated with the Earth Element. According to this understanding, the stomach receives food and separates the gross matter, or nutrients, from the qi, or life force. It sends nutrients downward to the small intestine to be further digested and absorbed. Qi is sent to the spleen, which disperses it to a number of other organs, including the large intestine and the lungs.

The stomach is seen as the source of emotional stability or centeredness, having the characteristics of solidity associated with the earth. This is further reflected by the fact that the stomach is located in the center of the body, and is therefore seen as a kind of psychological center, a balancing point, around which our lives revolve. A strong stomach gives a person the sense of being emotionally balanced ("grounded") in the midst of changing conditions. A weak stomach makes a person nervous and anxiety-prone.

The stomach, which is the receiver or accepter of food, is further seen as a metaphor for humanity's ability to embrace and accept life. In this sense, food is a metaphor for human experience. Those who can eat and digest a wide variety of foods have a great capacity to enjoy life and adapt to many different kinds of experiences. Those whose tastes are highly restricted or picky tend to live more narrowly and censor much of what life offers. In the same way, those who have chronic stomach problems tend to be cautious about what they can and cannot eat or do; they are understandably afraid of what might upset their stomachs. On the other hand, those who can eat everything tend to be sense-oriented and to want new experiences.

The Chinese maintain, however, that the law of paradox is always at work. Those who have strong stomachs are prone to overindulge in food and drink. They are, therefore, vulnerable to illness and death due to food-related causes. Those with weak stomachs, if they are wise, have an incentive to take good care of themselves, limit their eating, and thus enjoy long life. In the former case, a person's strength becomes his or her weakness; in the latter case, a person's weakness becomes his or her strength. Traditional systems emphasize moderation as the key to wisdom, health and longevity, no matter how strong an individual's stomach is.

The Earth Element organs are associated with the emotions of "sympathy." A strong stomach will be revealed in a person as compassion and understanding for other people. Such a person will not be weak, however. He or she sees the larger issues involved in situations, and therefore has balance and perspective.

A weak stomach, on the other hand, can give rise to one of two extremes: excessive sympathy, or a lack of compassion and understanding, which shows itself in extreme selfishness or boorishness. In either case, people with weak stomachs tend to see themselves as victims to a far greater extent than those with stronger stomachs. So, a person with a weak stomach may demonstrate excessive self-pity, self-preoccupation, or hypochondriasis, for example. Such people have little care or understanding for others, simply because they are preoccupied with what may affect their health adversely. So, they lack compassion.

The spleen is sometimes referred to as the mother of the large intestine because it provides life energy to the organ. Consequently, foods, behavior, and emotions that upset the stomach and spleen will have a direct effect on large intestine function. When the spleen is upset or imbalanced, its ability to send qi to the large intestine will be impaired. If the stomach and spleen become excited, it will send excess qi to the large intestine, causing diarrhea. If the spleen and stomach become deficient, it will send an inadequate amount of qi to the large intestine, causing constipation.

The movement of life energy by the stomach and spleen are seen as taking opposite directions. The stomach rules the descending movement—that is, to the small intestine—while the spleen controls the ascending movement. Because the stomach and spleen function interdependently, any stomach disorder is seen as a spleen imbalance as well. Vomiting is a classic example. Vomiting occurs when the stomach becomes too contracted at the duodenum, while the spleen becomes expanded and excited. This represents a set of extremes. The stomach does not allow energy and food to pass downward into the small intestine. Meanwhile, the spleen's excited condition forces energy and food upward. This condition is brought about by excesses in eating or stress or poor habits. For example, foods that are overly contractive, such as meat, hard cheeses, salt, or eggs, cause the stomach to become contracted and the duodenum to close. Extremely expansive foods, such as spices, sweets, or alcohol, excite and expand the spleen. So, a night of pepperoni pizza and wine is usually followed by heartburn and/or a quick trip to the bathroom.

69

The digestion of fats after a meal can be seen as a purely biochemical process involving only the breakdown of the fat particles (chylomicra) by the appropriate enzymes. But observations made on a teacher of anatomy in his forties revealed that the mere prospect of having to lecture to medical students slowed down the rate at which chylomicra disappeared from his bloodstream. The digestion of fat particles is retarded by almost any disturbance in the life routines. Thus, mental processes can affect the course of physiological processes as seemingly simple as the digestion of food.

RENÉ DUBOS

In general, traditional Chinese healers see heartburn, belching, and stomachaches as stomach and spleen disorders. For the Chinese, the life force moves in orderly and specific cycles, as with the seasons or the course of a day. Each organ-group is associated with a particular time of the year. The stomach is associated with late summer, roughly mid-July to mid-September. At this time of the year, the stomach and spleen receive the most qi. This can be a time of healing for these organs, or a time in which symptoms arise if underlying problems exist in the Earth Element organs.

Each day, with its alternating periods of light and dark, is a microcosm of larger cycles taking place during the course of the year. The Chinese maintain that the stomach is most active between 7 A.M. and 9 A.M., generally the breakfast hours. Then the stomach receives the most abundant amount of qi that it will receive during the day.

The Chinese also associate each organ with a particular sense, such as taste, smell, or hearing. When the organ functions optimally, the corresponding sense will be acute. Also, each organ is stimulated more by one particular taste than by another. Not surprisingly, the sensation associated with the stomach is taste, and the flavor that stimulates it most is the sweet flavor. Thus, moderate use of sweet-tasting foods can heal the Earth Element, while overconsumption can weaken the Earth Element organs.

The stomach and spleen rule the imagination or the world of ideas. People with sparkling or creative ideas are said to have strong stomachs.

Singing is thought to have a strengthening and medicinal effect on the Earth Element organs. The combination of harmonious vibration (song) and deep, rhythmic breathing soothes and calms the Earth Element. People who sing well are said to have strong stomachs, and a traditional Chinese healer may encourage those with weak stomachs to sing more.

RESTORING HARMONY TO YOUR EARTH STOMACH

The above information is used by Chinese healers to diagnose and treat the stomach. If, for example, a patient suffers symptoms during the early morning hours, the stomach is suspected of being involved in the illness. Also, excessive sympathy, a lack of compassion, a generalized inability to taste food, excessive nervousness, or anxiety (the Woody Allen type) all suggest a stomach imbalance.

That imbalance is the result of a diminution or an excess of qi. The organ is either hypoactive or hyperactive. Either type of imbalance can be caused by an excess of certain foods or certain conditions in life. For example, there can be too much sugar in your diet, or too much stress in your life. The restoration of qi and balance to the organs begins by harmonizing or moderating the various conditions in one's life. Moderate eating, sleeping, working, and playing, along with the use of foods that heal the stomach, will restore balance and health.

Excess consumption of the following foods is frequently at the root of a stomach imbalance, according to Chinese healers, who'll usually encourage the person to reduce or abstain from the foods so that the stomach can heal itself.

- Spices, including foods such as hot green or red peppers.
- Salt, including foods such as pickles.
- Refined grains, such as white bread and other white flour products.
- Alcohol, especially sweet wines, which are said to injure the stomach and spleen.
- Sweets, especially refined sweets, such as white sugar.
- Artificial ingredients, such as food colors, preservatives, and flavors.

The Chinese also warn against eating too much animal food, such as red meat, dairy products, and eggs, because of the high protein content, which requires greater effort on the part of the stomach to digest, and the fact that they are typically rich in fat, which further stresses digestion. They also point out that frequent use of most drugs, ranging from caffeine in coffee, nicotine in tobacco, and alcohol in beer and wine, to prescription pharmaceuticals and recreational drugs, have an adverse effect on stomach function.

Lifestyle issues related to stomach disorders include:

- Excess stress.
- Chronic anxiety or nervous tension.

- Exclusivity, haughtiness, or arrogance.
- The refusal to engage in life's ups and downs (which may be a cover for a general fear of life, nervousness, and tension).
- Irregular hours, such as retiring late to bed, or rising late in the morning.
- Poor or chaotic eating habits, such as eating on the run, failing to chew food properly, eating right before bed (which requires the stomach to be active while the rest of the body gets to rest), and mixing foods together on the same plate and then eating foods at once.

HEALING THE STOMACH

In general, foods that grow in late summer and early fall are said to be healing to the Earth Element, including the stomach, because these foods are the product of the same forces that produce and nourish the stomach. In other words, the qi in the following foods enhances stomach qi:

- Grains: millet, sweet corn, and kudzu.
- Vegetables: collard greens, all types of squash, and rutabaga.
- Chickpeas.
- Fruits: apple, raisins, orange, sweet cherry, figs, and honey-dew melon.
- Fish: salmon, tuna, and swordfish.
- Sweeteners: barley malt and rice syrup.
- Shiitake mushrooms.

For stomach problems, including indigestion, here are three Japanese folk remedies: a quarter-teaspoon or so of umeboshi plum, to alkalize the stomach; a cup of hot bancha tea with two drops of shoyu; and boiled and puréed squash, carrot, and onion, drunk at room temperature.

Some stomach-healing recommendations from the naturopathic realm include:

- Carrot, celery, and cabbage juice, especially when symptoms arise; drink two to four times per day.

- Cabbage juice, especially when symptoms arise; drink two to four times per day, unless already taking carrot, celery, and cabbage juice.
- Herbal teas with comfrey, licorice, goldenseal, or aloe vera juice; one cup two times per day.
- Whole grains, boiled and well chewed.
- Squash, broccoli, collard greens, carrots, or other foods rich in vitamin A.
- Vitamins: A and B complex.
- Minerals: zinc and iron.

Now good digestion wait on appetite.
And health on both!

WILLIAM SHAKESPEARE

No other organ is so intimate with food as the stomach. It's commonly recognized that various kinds of foods cause the stomach to suffer, but you may not realize that food also can heal the stomach. The approaches described above have been used for centuries to do just that.

Homeopathic remedies for indigestion:

CHAMOMILLA: When an attack of indigestion follows a fit of anger and irritability. Stomach distended with gas, abdomen cramping, bitter mouth, flushed cheeks, aversion to warm drinks.

NUX VOMICA: For the hard-driving type who indulges in too much food, coffee, liquor, tobacco. Heartburn, belching, bloating after eating. May be constipated.

PULSATILLA: Wake up feeling like you have stones in your stomach. Peevish. Dry mouth, bad taste, not thirsty. Pain one-half hour after eating, aversion to fatty foods and snug clothing.

Homeopathic remedies for nausea and vomiting:

ARSENICUM: Nausea, vomiting, diarrhea due to spoiled food. Burning pain after eating relieved by warm drinks.

IPECAC: Nausea, gripping pains in the intestines. Nausea from moving objects or reading in a car.

NUX VOMICA: "Wants to and can't." Could refer to vomiting, moving bowels, or urinating. Patient is awake after 3 A.M. and falls asleep toward morning. Wakes feeling wretched.

Herbs for the stomach:

GINGER: Relieves indigestion, nausea, vomiting.

BASIL: Treats stomach cramps.

CATNIP: Treats upset stomach.

CHAPTER 8

THE SPLEEN

THE SPLEEN HAS baffled people for centuries. In his 1876 book *Doctors and Patients,* Dr. John Timbs recalled the lament of a Scottish physician who one day confessed, "I wish more people would die of diseases in the spleen, that men might know what purpose the spleen is intended to answer."

In the absence of knowledge came myth. In the literature of both East and West, the spleen ranks second only to the heart as the organ cited as a major source of human feelings. Unfortunately, early anatomists and etymologists must have seen the spleen as the shadow of the heart, for they have ascribed to it a host of unpleasant characteristics. The *American Heritage Dictionary* notes the obsolete and archaic definitions of the word *spleen* as the seat of mirth, caprice, melancholy, and ill-temper. To be spleenful, says the dictionary, is to be "ill-humored, peevish, and irritable." To "vent one's spleen" connotes the unlovely act of spouting venom at one's neighbor.

Shakespeare attempted to lift the spleen out of its murky depths by acknowledging its finer side. In the first act of *A Midsummer Night's Dream,* he intoned that in the spleen are felt the paradoxes of love, its quickly passing joys and its lingering sorrows:

The body is not only more mysterious than we know, it is more mysterious than we can know.

ANONYMOUS

75

Making it momentary as a sound,
Swift as a shadow, short as any dream,
Brief as the lightning in the collied night,
That, in a spleen, unfolds both heaven and the earth . . .

In the Talmud, Jewish scholars note that the spleen produces laughter. When the spleen is ill, states one scholar, a person is given to foolish laughter, but when one "extirpates the splenic tumor, laughter ceases and such people always have a serious demeanor."

The Oriental and Occidental always have seen things from opposing points of view, and no organ demonstrates this better than the spleen. If the Biblical axiom that "the last shall be first" applies to any organ of the body, then, according to the Chinese, it applies best to the spleen. To the Chinese mind, which has always elevated the lowly and celebrated the hidden, the spleen is responsible for an array of important functions, not the least of which is to act as a receiver of ideas. The spleen, say the Chinese, picks up the refined vibrations, the very thoughts, of the universe.

Western medical science knows a lot more about the spleen than it once did, but the organ is still shrouded in mystery. To an orthodox medical doctor, the spleen has a limited array of functions. Like the appendix and the tonsils, the spleen is largely considered expendable and not essential to life. When the spleen is removed, other organs, principally the liver and the lymphatic system, are said to take up its responsibilities. According to the American Medical Association, the removal of the spleen "has no known ill effects."

In a number of traditional medical systems, however, the spleen is invested with great worth. The spleen is seen as the ruler of everything from joy and laughter (by the Hebrew and Greek systems), to balancing potential and kinetic energy (Ayurvedic), to "transformation and transportation" within the body and spirit (Chinese).

FORM AND FUNCTION

The spleen is located on the left side of the abdomen. It is fist-sized and weighs approximately seven ounces. It is a spongy, dark red organ, composed of fibrous tissue that gives it the capacity to expand and contract, and it thus can contain a variable amount of blood. Between its fibrous bands are tissues called splenic pulp.

This pulpy material produces lymphocytes and phagocytes, two types of immune cells that are essential to immune function.

The organ is surrounded by smooth muscle. During exercise, or when stimulated by nerves or hormones, the organ can contract, sending more blood into the system. In the center of the spleen is an indentation, called a hilius, where the organ receives oxygen-rich blood via the splenic artery. The splenic vein runs out of the hilius, transporting blood filled with carbon dioxide out of the organ and back to the heart.

The spleen filters the blood of broken and worn-out red blood cells and bacteria. These cells are destroyed by phagocytes and lymphocytes. Hemoglobin and iron are recovered from the worn-out cells and stored in the spleen, to be used in the formation of other cells and bilirubin, the pigmentation in bile. The spleen also stores blood and can control the amount of blood available to the body by its capacity to expand and contract.

During fetal life, the spleen creates red blood cells. Shortly after birth, however, this role is passed on to the bone marrow.

Medical doctors are beginning to recognize an important immune function for the spleen. The immune cells that it produces create specialized antibodies designed for specific antigens or illnesses. The spleen introduces these immune cells into the bloodstream as blood passes through the organ, and thus increases the number of immune cells in the body. People who have their spleens removed have weaker immune systems, and are more vulnerable to infections and disease.

The spleen can become enlarged due to a variety of illnesses, including malaria, infectious mononucleosis, tuberculosis, typhoid fever, hemolytic anemia, and some forms of cancer, including leukemia, Hodgkin's disease, and lymphomas. The spleen also can be ruptured when it receives a severe blow, as from a fall or an auto accident, which can cause severe bleeding and death. In such cases, doctors will often surgically remove the spleen and tie off the splenic artery.

TRANSFORMING THE QI FROM FOOD

Traditional Chinese healers maintain that the spleen is a primary organ of digestion. They say that it transforms the foods' nutrients into qi, governs the orderly flow of blood throughout the body, nourishes the four limbs with qi, and helps the body discern the five tastes (bitter, sweet, pungent, salty, and sour). Also, the spleen is responsible for the capacity to perceive creative ideas and enjoy understanding of others.

According to the Five Elements Theory, the spleen is joined by the stomach to form the Earth Element. The spleen nourishes the lungs and large intestine (the Metal Element). The stomach and spleen are nourished themselves by the small intestine and heart (the Fire Element). From this schematic, it becomes clear that the spleen is linked to the entire digestive system. While the stomach deals with foods' mass, the spleen absorbs and distributes the energy or vibration that comes from the digestive process (the actual movements of the stomach and small intestine) and the quality of energy that emerges from the food itself. Chinese healers say that spices, for example, have a particular energy all their own that affects digestion. That energy is considerable, especially when you consider that their mass is small and therefore should not present the problems to digestion that they do. Those problems emerge from the chemical nature of the spices, and the energy they release during metabolism. That energetic influence greatly affects the workings of the spleen.

The spleen distributes this qi to the small and large intestine. The quality of that energy, whether it is smooth and fluid or unstable and chaotic, will determine how well or how poorly you digest your food. Thus, Chinese healers see digestive problems, such as belching, flatulence, and a rumbling stomach, as related to the health of the spleen. So, too, are heartburn, acid indigestion, and nausea. These symptoms often indicate an excess of energy that the spleen cannot distribute in an orderly fashion. When the spleen passes excessive or chaotic energy on to the large intestine, diarrhea or spastic colon may result.

If the spleen is chronically weak or deficient, it may not be able to absorb and distribute the qi that emanates from many foods, especially spices, sugar, and wine, which the Chinese maintain are especially injurious to the spleen. Usually this kind of spleen deficiency causes intermittent or chronic constipation. In this case, the spleen is simply unable to pass sufficient qi onto the large intestine. When the intestine receives inadequate life force, it is unable to do its job.

Traditional Chinese medical theory recognizes that a healthy spleen maintains appropriate blood levels throughout the body, and also ensures that the blood remains in its normal patterns. Violations of these patterns, such as internal bleeding or excessive or deficient menstrual bleeding, are said to be related to a spleen imbalance. While obviously other organs are also involved in such cases, traditional healers contend that the spleen also must be treated if healing is to result.

In the case of the menstrual cycle, the spleen assists in maintaining its rhythm and duration. The spleen supports the process of accumulation and release of blood within the uterus. Spleen imbalances may play a role in excessively long, short, or irregular periods. Symptoms of premenstrual syndrome (PMS) are often related to spleen disharmonies.

The taste that has the strongest influence on the spleen is sweet. Mildly sweet taste tonifies and strengthens the spleen, while intense sweetness stimulates but injures it. With other Earth Element organs, the spleen helps maintain blood sugar levels. Excess consumption of sugar results in hypoglycemia or low blood sugar. Low blood sugar occurs when highly refined sugar is eaten regularly, causing blood sugar levels to increase rapidly. The pancreas secretes insulin to make the sugar available to the body as fuel in the form of glucose. The fuel is quickly burned, causing a rapid drop in available blood sugar. The resulting low blood sugar levels cause a variety of symptoms, including hunger, lethargy, fatigue, irritability, and depression.

When blood sugar levels drop, the body requires refueling. It craves carbohydrates, the principal source of energy in the food supply. If a person answers that craving, however, by eating refined or simple carbohydrates instead of complex carbohydrates (such as from whole grains, beans, and vegetables), the rollercoaster ride of elevating and rapidly declining blood sugar levels continues. Meanwhile, the spleen and pancreas become weaker. To effectively treat low blood sugar, you should try to strengthen the Earth Element by avoiding refined sugar. (See below for ways to cope with sugar cravings).

Because the spleen has difficulty dealing with acidic foods, saliva acts as a balancing agent for the spleen. In general, saliva, which is slightly alkaline, and alkaline foods are tonifying and strengthening to the spleen. Thus, the Chinese maintain that saliva is intimately connected with the spleen. The condition of the

Although analytical approaches to the body and its intake and surroundings have provided much useful information, such fragmented investigations have also obscured dynamic interrelationships which have an important bearing in medicine.

THERON RANDOLPH

79

spleen may affect how much an individual salivates. Often, when a person suffers from indigestion, the salivary glands secrete more saliva, which in turns has a medicinal effect on the spleen. Those with chronically dry mouths, on the other hand, may suffer from deficient spleens. Chewing and salivating make food more accessible to the digestion, but also to the taste buds and ability to smell. The Chinese maintain that the spleen governs the capacity to taste and smell, in part through its intimate connection with saliva.

Ayurvedic healers also see the spleen as a centering force and a place in which balance and harmony are made between opposites. The spleen is most influenced by the pitta dosha, which balances the kinetic energy of vata and the potential energy of kapha. Interestingly, the foods that Ayurvedic healers recommend as healing to the spleen coincide a great deal with the Chinese system. For example, Ayur-Veda recommends both sweet and bitter-tasting vegetables. In the Chinese system, sweet-tasting vegetables directly support the Earth Element, while bitter-tasting vegetables support the Fire Element (heart and small intestine), which in turn nourishes the Earth Element (spleen).

DELICACY AND STABILITY

As an Earth Element organ, the spleen is seen as a source of inner stability and centeredness. Paradoxically, the spleen is perhaps the most delicate of the internal organs. In a sense, it is the weak link in the body's inner chain. Therefore, when the spleen is healthy and firm, when the weakest link is strong, the whole body is healthier, more balanced, and secure.

The emotion associated with the spleen is understanding and sympathy. Spleen imbalances often result in one of two emotional extremes. Those with excited or excessive spleen conditions are prone to excessive sympathy. These people often have a saccharine sweetness about them, and may cry so easily as to constantly embarrass themselves. Such people show such abundant empathy that it seems to know no limits. They lack a certain balance or centeredness associated with a strong spleen.

Those with deficient spleens, on the other hand, may have an utter lack of compassion. They are so direct and rude as to have all the diplomacy of a loaded gun. Their brusqueness is so brutal that it indicates an almost total inability to understand or empathize with another human being.

Using the Five Elements again, we can see that understanding (Earth) controls the emotion associated with the Water Element, fear. Therefore, a strong and healthy spleen will give a person understanding and perspective when frightening events occur. However, if the spleen is weak, fear may dominate, because the controlling influence of the spleen is weak.

Often, a person experiences a combination of weak spleen energy with excessive kidney energy, causing chronic anxiety and fear. People who are perpetually anxious can be drawn to sugar to help stimulate spleen energy, but the effect of the sugar is to further weaken the spleen, once its stimulating effects have worn off.

Chinese healers say that the spleen likes dry weather rather than damp, humid, or rainy days. Those with weak spleens are particularly influenced by the weather. They detest damp, foggy, or rainy weather, which often causes them to be depressed, especially if the bad weather is extended. Conversely, sunny days have a greater than average effect on restoring hope and security to those with weak spleens. In the same vein, the Chinese say that the spleen rules skin pigmentation.

Interestingly, recent scientific research into Seasonal Affective Disorder, or SAD, has revealed that brain levels of the hormone serotonin are diminished in the absence of strong sunlight. Controlled studies have demonstrated that sunlight has an antidepressant effect on people with SAD. Researchers have noticed that such people, when deprived of sunlight, crave sweets and feel better after they have eaten sweet foods. All of this tends to confirm the Chinese perspective on the spleen's relationship to mood, weather, and the sweet taste.

The season that influences the spleen most is late summer, August and September. The time of day that the spleen is most active is 9 A.M. to 11 A.M. It is during these months and hours that the spleen can do its greatest healing, provided that the conditions are right. The spleen wants and needs a sweet taste, but excessive sweetness can injure the spleen. Paradoxically, very small amounts of salt in cooking, such as in soups and stews, helps to alkalize the food and calm and strengthen the spleen. Like too much sugar, however, too much salt harms the spleen.

Health is not so much the absence of dis-ease as it is the presence of an optimal healing process.

M. Scott Peck

Chewing food well and thoroughly mixing it with saliva is a direct way of strengthening the spleen. The following foods strengthen the spleen, when eaten in moderate amounts:

- The grains millet, sweet corn, barley, oats, rice, and wheat.
- Squash, especially acorn, butternut, buttercup, hubbard, hokkaido pumpkin, spaghetti, or pumpkin.
- Vegetables, including asparagus, squash, broccoli, brussels sprouts, cabbage, cucumber, cauliflower, celery, green beans, and leafy greens such as collards.
- The roots parsnips, sweet potato, yams, and rutabaga.
- Chickpeas.
- Shiitake and button mushrooms.
- Sweet fruits, such as apples, oranges, raisins, grapes, melons, figs, pears, plums, prunes, and cherries, and cooked fruit and compotes.
- White fish and shrimp.

Here is a sweet drink that is especially balancing to the spleen. Chop into small pieces one squash, two carrots, two parsnips, and one onion. Boil until the entire mash becomes liquid. Keep adding water to ensure that the vegetables are fully dissolved or leave only a residue of fiber at the bottom of the pot. Drink two or three times daily for hypoglycemia, sugar cravings, and spleen imbalances.

A small bowl of miso soup every day, made with wakame seaweed, also works well to establish a healthy spleen. Use about one-quarter teaspoon of miso per cup of soup, and one tablespoon-sized shard of wakame per cup.

For indigestion, gas, and upset stomach, try sucking on an umeboshi plum, a Japanese pickled plum, available in most health food or natural food stores.

For constipation, boil brown rice with carrots, onions, and grated ginger root. Cook with a pinch of sea salt until rice is soft, usually about forty-five minutes to an hour, and chew well.

There are also some lifestyle considerations for problems concerning spleen and digestion:

- Chew every mouthful thirty-five to fifty times each.
- Avoid extremely hot or cold beverages. Excessively cold beverages especially can shock the system. Also avoid drink-

ing during meals. Liquids dilute stomach juices, preventing complete digestion.

- Avoid eating while emotionally upset or under stress. Stress impairs digestion and can lead to stomach upset, constipation, or diarrhea.
- Always sit while eating, rather than standing.
- Avoid overeating and eating too frequently. Excess food burdens organs and makes all forms of indigestion, constipation, and diarrhea more likely.
- Avoid eating large amounts of highly acidic foods, including tomatoes, eggplant, citrus fruit, and spices.

While the spleen is seen as unessential in the West, it is seen as a master organ in the East. The body's ability to ward off illness depends greatly upon the health of the spleen. Because the spleen plays an important role in the immune system, the health of the spleen is central to the body's ability to deal with infection and allergic reactions.

Herbs for the spleen:

MANDARIN ORANGE PEEL: Used to treat indigestion. Especially tonic for the spleen.

SAFFLOWER: Good for delayed menses, stagnated blood, poor circulation, blood clots, lower abdominal pain caused by blood congestion.

SAFFRON: One of the finest blood vitalizers known. Stimulates circulation and regulates spleen.

CEANOTHUS (red root): Used for enlarged spleen, lymphatic congestion, despondency, melancholy.

CHAPTER 9

THE INTESTINES

If we don't take care of the body, where will we live?

ANONYMOUS

$\mathcal{A}$CCORDING TO AN EGYPTIAN LEGEND, Thoth, the god of medicine and science, descended upon the Nile in the form of an ibis, a sacred bird with a long beak. Before him was a group of priest-physicians. Thoth proceeded to fill his beak with water and then inject it into his anus. The doctors got the message, and began administering enemas to patients, including the Pharaoh himself. In fact, the physician who gave the Pharaoh enemas came to be known as "Guardian of the Royal Bowel Movement." Humanity has been administering enemas ever since, as well as trying a host of other treatments to achieve that long-sought state of intestinal health.

Concern for intestinal disorders was among the reasons that surgery was created in the West. The Western world's first secular school was a medical college established in Salerno, Italy, in 900 A.D. Both men and women taught and practiced medicine at this rarefied and prestigious institution. Scholars presented the methods of Hippocrates, Galen, and Avicenna, the revered Arabian physician, combining them with a limited range of surgical procedures, including operations to remove obstructions from the intestines. Early accounts of a renowned Salerno surgeon, Roger Frugardi, note that "Roger could cut well . . . [and] could clot

bleeding with mummy powder, or finely cut hair of the hare . . .
Torn intestines were sewn together over an elderwood tube, or an
animal's trachea."

Louis XIV of France was among the first patients to undergo
bowel surgery. Louis was a glutton and had frequent enemas,
sometimes in the presence of visitors to the throne. Eventually
Louis developed a growth in his rectum. He contacted Dr. Charles
Francois Felix to have it surgically removed. The doctor set the
date of Louis's operation six months in advance so that he could
practice his technique on folks of lower status. This was highly
advisable, as Louis was known to be harsh with bad doctors. Fortunately, for both king and doctor, the surgery was successful.

During the Victorian era, intestinal health became the rage in
England, France, and the U.S., prompting the creation of spas
that emphasized colonics and enemas. This spurred nineteenth-
century humorist Henry Wheeler Shaw to note, "A reliable set of
bowels is worth more to a man than any quantity of brains."

Today, intestinal distress continues to plague humanity. Constipation is the most common digestive problem in America, and
laxatives are a major industry. Forty million Americans purchase
them annually, 8 million of them chronically, spending more
than $250 million in the process. Ronald Reagan and Tip O'Neill
are two well-known Americans with advanced intestinal disease.
Reagan had polyps, fingerlike tumors that grow in the large intestine. O'Neill had colon cancer, a disease that strikes
110,000 Americans each year and kills over 50,000 annually.

In the Third World, 4.5 million children under the age of five
die each year of diarrhea. About 200,000 American children are
hospitalized annually for the illness, which is easily treatable. Yet,
more than 5,500 American children died from diarrhea between
the years 1973–1983.

Asian and African cultures that subsist on traditional, high-
fiber diets show little trace of intestinal disease, including cancer.
Numerous recent studies confirm that intestinal health is almost
assured by eating the right foods.

THE NUTRIENT ABSORBER

The small intestine runs from the stomach to the large intestine,
coiling throughout the lower abdomen. It is approximately 1.5

*A complete bacteriological
analysis of one tiny sample of
human feces could take a year
or more to accomplish, which
is an indication of the com-
plexity of this vast ecosystem
that lies within us all.*

LEON CHAITOW

inches in diameter and twenty-two feet long. But because it's contracted upon itself, much like an accordion, its length within the body is a little more than six feet.

The small intestine is divided into three sections. The duodenum is a short, curved tube, about ten inches long, that is attached to the stomach and receives both the bile and pancreatic ducts. It extends to the jejunum, which is about nine feet long and coils upward to the left. The jejunum attaches to the ileum, which is about twelve feet long, and coils downward to the right.

The ileum joins the large intestine at a bulblike structure called the cecum. Within the cecum is the ileocecal valve, which is a barrier created by a pair of lips within the intestinal canal that prevents food from flowing back into the small intestine once it reaches the colon.

The tube itself is composed of four layers. The innermost lining is a mucous membrane permeated with many villi, fingerlike projections that absorb nutrients. These villi are covered with millions of fronds, even tinier mounds that absorb nutrients and increase the surface area of the organ. In total, the surface area of the small intestine is roughly 100 square feet. The cells that make up the mucous membrane are shortlived. Every two to four days the entire lining is replaced. This kind of volatility makes the cells highly vulnerable to radiation, whether from X rays or radioactive particles.

The second layer is called the submucosa, and is extensively crisscrossed with blood vessels. These vessels take up the nutrients absorbed by the villi and bring the nutrient-rich blood to the liver, its first stop on its journey throughout the body.

The third layer is the muscular coat composed of longitudinal and circular muscles that create peristalsis, which moves the food particles along the intestinal canal. Finally, the entire organ is surrounded by connective tissue, which protects and supports it.

The small intestine contains trillions of bacteria, though the initial stages of the organ, the duodenum and parts of the jejunum, are essentially sterile due to the acid secretions from the stomach. Still, some bacteria do get past the stomach and, once inside the intestines and beyond the acid environment, they begin to multiply.

The types of bacteria within the intestines vary among individuals according to such factors as diet and use of antibiotics and other medications, many of which destroy intestinal bacteria. Bacteria in the intestines play a positive role by assisting in the breakdown of food and digestion, making nutrients more accessible to the bloodstream.

Among the more common species of bacteria that reside in both the small and large intestine are *E. coli,* candida albicans or yeast, and lactobacteria, of which lactobacillus is a widely known strain. Harmful bacteria, such as *E. coli* and candida albicans, secrete toxins that, if produced in sufficient quantities, can cause disease. Lactobacteria, on the other hand, are helpful to the body. They produce some vitamins, such as vitamin K, and digestive enzymes, which assist in the breakdown of foods.

Studies have shown that diets rich in animal foods, especially red meat, increase the population of harmful bacteria, and the amount of their disease-producing secretions, in the large and small intestine.

The purpose of the small intestine is to digest and absorb nutrients. Though carbohydrate digestion is begun in the mouth and the stomach digests some proteins, the vast majority of digestion and virtually all absorption are carried out in the small intestine. Here, enzymes are released to help break down foods and make them more available to the tiny villi. The small intestine also secretes mucus, which binds the food matter, called chyme, and makes it less abrasive to the organ surface.

Intestinal transit time (the time elapsed between consumption of food and elimination) depends to a great extent on the overall health of the intestines and the kinds of foods consumed. Fiber-rich foods move quickly through the organ, but heavier, fat-rich foods take far more time. On the average, food spends about four to six hours in the stomach, another five to six hours in the small intestine, and another fifteen to twenty-four hours in the large intestine before it is finally eliminated from the body.

The most common intestinal diseases are those of the large intestine. The small intestine is rarely affected by tumors, for example, and cancer of the small intestine is uncommon, at least as a point of origin. (Malignancies that originate elsewhere in the body can spread to the organ, however.)

The most common form of bacterial or viral infection is Crohn's disease, which most often affects the small intestine. The ileum is its most common site, but the disease can manifest as a series of patches throughout the small and large intestine. Crohn's disease is accompanied by a range of symptoms, including inflammation of the intestinal lining, diarrhea, fever, weight loss, anemia, loss of appetite, weakness, and fatigue. Most of these symptoms are created because the inflammation of the intestinal wall prevents efficient absorption of nutrients. In addition, ulcers can form in the intestinal wall, sometimes causing bleeding. A fistula, or a tear in the lining of the intestines, can occur, causing bleeding and infection. This is often treated by surgery. Swelling of the intestinal lining can create an obstruction and thus prevent food from passing. This, too, is treated with surgery.

According to the American Medical Association, the cause of Crohn's disease is unknown. In the U.S., Crohn's disease affects only three to six people per 100,000 population, though it has been increasing during the past thirty years.

Treatment includes anti-inflammatory drugs and other drugs, such as corticosteroids, used to control the body's use of nutrients. Those who suffer from tears in the intestinal lining may need to be hospitalized and given blood transfusions. There is no medical cure for Crohn's disease; for many, the illness becomes chronic, with periods of dormancy and flare-ups.

FIRE AND JOY

Traditional Chinese healers view the small intestine as a yang, expanded organ. In the Five Element system, its partner is the heart, a contracted organ. Both form the Fire Element. Its season is summer, during which time the small intestine receives its optimal amount of qi. Thus it is during the summer months that healers have the best opportunity to heal the small intestine of many maladies, if the patient stays in harmony with the season by not eating foods that are too fatty, heavy, or well cooked, and by not suffering excessive heat.

"The injuries caused by the heat of summer cause intermittent fever in the fall," says the Yellow Emperor, meaning that harm done to the small intestine and heart in the summer will manifest as an illness in the fall.

In the same way, the small intestine receives its optimal amounts of life force during the hours of 1 P.M. to 3 P.M. This, of

I have finally come to the conclusion that a good reliable set of bowels is worth more to a man than any quantity of brains.

HENRY WHEELER SHAW

course, is the typical siesta time in warm climates, the period after the large meal when energy is diverted to the stomach and small intestine.

The emotion associated with a balanced Fire Element is joy. Laughter is healing to the heart and small intestine. Imbalances tend to show up as lack of joy and even depression when the Fire Element is deficient, and hysteria when it is excessive. People who are manic-depressive often suffer from some kind of Fire imbalance.

The tastes that nourish the Fire Element are bitter and slightly burnt. The Fire Element's color is red and its direction is the south, which means that Fire is strongest nearer the equator.

The Fire Element is nourished by the Wood Element (liver and gall bladder), and in turn nourishes the Earth Element (stomach and spleen). When the liver is blocked, due to cirrhosis, for example, the small intestine and heart will suffer, and heart disease is likely. Such people tend to eat more fiery foods (spices, tomatoes, slightly burned steak) to compensate for the deficient qi being sent to the Fire organs from the liver. These people will have fiery red faces, due to the expanded capillaries in the skin, and equally fiery dispositions.

Fire is controlled by the Water Element (the kidneys and bladder). Indeed, as we will see in the discussion of the heart, the kidneys are implicated in many heart conditions. The Fire Element controls the Metal Element (lungs and large intestine).

The Chinese maintain that the stomach and spleen work in coordination with the small intestine. The stomach passes the food's raw material, its nutrients, to the small intestine, while the spleen passes the pure qi, or life force, to the small intestine.

There is a kind of reciprocal relationship among the small intestine, stomach, and spleen. Imbalances in the small intestine will prevent the smooth transfer of life energy from the spleen to the small intestine. Small intestine disturbances will also prevent the organ from accepting chyme from the stomach. In this way, small intestine imbalances upset both stomach and spleen functions. In the same way, imbalances in the stomach and spleen upset the small intestine.

Which, then, is the superior or ruling organ in digestion? The Chinese say the spleen.

On the Five Element schematic, the spleen provides qi to the large intestine (the Earth Element nourishes the Metal Element) and small intestine. Therefore, all digestive problems are seen as related to spleen imbalances.

It's important to keep in mind that small intestine problems are directly related to stomach and spleen imbalances. Therefore, treatment of the small intestine includes the care and treatment of these organs, as well.

Like all traditional healing systems, Chinese medicine is based on the fundamental principle that the body can heal itself, if given the right conditions. Those conditions are arrived at, first, by eliminating the poisons that are causing the illness in the first place; second, by employing acupuncture, foods, and herbs that support the optimal flow of qi to the organ; third, by maintaining daily activities that support healing; fourth, by addressing the underlying psychological and spiritual issues that may be involved in the cause of disease.

All traditional medicine treats illnesses in this way, including those of the small intestine.

Foods that are considered healing to the small intestine include the following:

- *Grain:* Corn on the cob, whole corn, and glutinous millet.
- *Seeds:* Sunflower and sesame seeds (both in small amounts).
- *Vegetables:* Brussels sprouts, asparagus, endive, okra, scallion, dandelion, and chicory.
- *Fruit:* Apricots, raspberries, strawberries, and raisins.
- *Beans:* Red lentils.
- *Medicinal soups:* Miso or tamari broths, with small amounts of wakame seaweed (about one tablespoon-size shard of seaweed per cup of soup), and vegetables. Miso and tamari create alkaline broths that sooth and tonify the small intestine, stomach, and spleen. They contain digestive bacteria and enzymes that assist digestion. For indigestion, chronic stomach and small intestine problems, a light miso soup (one-quarter teaspoon of miso per cup of soup) in the morning will help to alleviate stomach and digestive problems.
- *Animal foods:* Shrimp.
- *Fibrous foods:* To cleanse and strengthen the small intestine, be sure that the diet is composed chiefly of whole grains,

fresh vegetables, and fruits. These foods are rich in fiber and assist in cleansing the small intestine of fat deposits and undigested waste.

Strengthen the spleen by including Earth Element foods in the diet. (See chapter on spleen.)

Avoid the following foods until small intestine symptoms disappear:

- Red meat and all fatty animal foods. Fat requires greater quantities of bile acids (see section on the large intestine, below), which create and exacerbate ulcers and any inflammation.
- Spices, especially hot spices, which irritate the intestinal lining and cause greater acid reactions in the stomach. Hot spices are fire foods, but clearly too much fire to create a balanced condition in the small intestine and heart.
- Highly acidic foods, such as peppers, eggplants, and tomatoes, until symptoms abate.

(See large intestine and spleen for related illnesses of the digestive system.)

Lifestyle considerations for improving small intestine function: Chew every mouthful of food at least thirty-five times each. Chewing breaks down food and makes it easier on the stomach and small intestine to digest food. Saliva assists in the digestion of carbohydrates. Saliva also makes the food more alkaline, which creates less gas. (Gas is experienced in the stomach and intestine, of course, but it is caused by spleen imbalances, according to the Chinese.)

Walk daily, weather permitting. Walking increases oxygen intake and circulation, which improves small intestine function. Aerobic exercise is good for the Fire Element; it strengthens and helps to cleanse organs of waste.

Laughing is healing to the small intestine—to say nothing of the rest of our lives. Laughter concentrates life force in the small intestine region. As an experiment, focus on your solar plexus region the next time you laugh. You'll notice that laughter is concentrated in this part of the body—especially a really good "belly laugh." Laugh, and your small intestine laughs with you.

THE SEAT OF PITTA

Of the three doshas (vata, pitta, and kapha), the one most closely related to the small intestine is the pitta dosha. Pitta mediates between the state of kinetic energy (vata) and potential energy (kapha). Vata is associated with the nervous system, the realm of activity and movement. Kapha is associated with physical stability and the lubrication of the body. Pitta is associated with digestion and metabolism—the fire within.

The small intestine is said to be the "seat of pitta," meaning that, like the Chinese system, Ayur-Veda closely associates the small intestine with the Fire Element. It is here that the raw materials of life (nutrition) are converted and made accessible to the body. The small intestine is the crucible of the body. Small intestine problems, therefore, reveal a weakness in the pitta dosha.

The following foods and tastes will balance and strengthen pitta energy:

- *Grains:* Barley, oats, rice (including basmati rice), and wheat.
- *Vegetables:* Asparagus, broccoli, brussels sprouts, cauliflower, celery, daikon, green beans, leafy greens, lettuce, mushrooms, okra, peas, parsley, sprouts.
- *Beans:* Lentils, chickpeas, mung beans, tofu.
- *Fruit:* Apples, apricots, pears, avocado, melons, oranges, plums, prunes, raisins.
- *Animal foods:* Shrimp and small amounts of chicken, without the fat.
- *Tastes:* Avoid excesses of sour, salty, pungent, and hot spices. Eat small amounts of sweet, bitter, and astringent foods.

Naturopaths recommend a whole-food diet to deal with digestive problems. Whole grains, fresh vegetables, beans, and fruit are emphasized as part of the healing regimen. Also among the most frequently recommended foods are kelp and other seaweeds. Foods rich in the following vitamins are recommended for digestive problems:

- *Beta carotene, or the vegetable source of vitamin A:* Squash, collard greens, broccoli, carrots, and brussels sprouts.

- *B Vitamins:* Whole grains, leafy greens, sea vegetables, peas, and beans.
- *Vitamin B12:* Present in all animal foods, including fish. Include white fish as part of your regular diet (at least once per week). Cod, haddock, flounder, sole, and halibut are among the fish lowest in fat and richest in nutrition, including B12.
- *Vitamin C:* Present in broccoli, sauerkraut, sprouted beans, cabbage, squash, tart fruits such as strawberries, and citrus fruit.
- *Vitamin E:* In whole grains, especially wheat, wheat germ, and dried beans.

(If a person has been on a particularly unhealthy diet for many years, supplementation of these vitamins may be necessary for a short period. See a naturopath for specific recommendations.)

Herbs that aid digestion include: Chamomile tea (soothes and heals), dandelion tea (cleanses blood of toxins), ginger root tea (stimulates digestion and circulation), goldenseal (tea or infusion; heals and cleans blood), and slippery elm (tea or infusion; heals and cleans blood). One or two of these teas can be used, alternating them every two days.

For ulcers, drink chamomile tea, three times per day.

Like so many other parts or of the body, the small intestine is an organ we typically take for granted, at least until it causes us trouble. Yet, its health is among the easiest to maintain. So, the next time you're having a shrimp dinner, or a little chamomile tea, think of your small intestine, with gratitude.

The Large Intestine

The large intestine is about six feet long, and two inches wide. It is shaped like an inverted horseshoe, and frames the many coils of the small intestine. There are no villi within the large intestine wall, only small pores that absorb mostly water.

The organ is made up of four sections: an ascending colon, which joins with the small intestine at the cecum, a bulblike structure within which the ileocecal valve is located; the transverse colon, which travels latterly just below the diaphragm; the descending colon, which is the downward leg of the organ that brings waste material to the pelvic portion, called the sigmoid colon. The sigmoid colon is an "S" shaped tube that, after the last bend in the "S," continues as the rectum, the anal canal, and its opening, the anus. The rectum is lined with a set of thick vertical muscles that narrow to an inner sphincter muscle and, at the anus, an outer sphincter.

At the cecum—where the small and large intestine join—is a small wormlike structure, about three and a half inches long, known as the appendix. According to the American Medical Association, the appendix "has no known function." (Traditional medical systems maintain that there are no unnecessary parts of the body, and that even the appendix serves an important function.) In appearance, the appendix is a miniature intestine. Its interior is basically a replica of the colon, with a concentration of lymph glands within the mucous membrane.

Living inside the large intestine are many trillions of bacteria (the organ is more heavily populated than the small intestine). As with the small intestine, the colon is filled with a variety of healthful and harmful bacteria (described above in the section on the small intestine). As we will show, the health of the large intestine and the effect of its bacteria are greatly influenced by diet.

These bacteria help convert nutrients into essential vitamins, including vitamin K, which are then absorbed by the intestine. They also create gas (methane, hydrogen, and carbon dioxide), through the putrefaction and fermentation of foods.

The primary purpose of the large intestine is to absorb water from the liquid waste of the small intestine, thereby making the waste solid, and efficiently eliminating it from the body. The organ also absorbs some vitamins and minerals not taken up by the small intestine.

L.A. Belly and Other Intestinal Problems

Otherwise known as gastroenteritis, swelling of the stomach and/or intestine is usually caused by viral or bacterial infection. Foreign bacteria can find their way into the intestine via poorly prepared or unclean food, or the consumption of water that contains unfamiliar bacteria (Americans traveling in Mexico often contract diarrhea, commonly called "Montezuma's Revenge";

Mexicans traveling the U.S. sometimes get "L.A. Belly," the same disease with a different name). These bacterial infections usually pass within a few days or a week. Typhoid and cholera are among the serious forms of bacterial infections, and are considered life-threatening.

Single-celled animals such as protozoa, giardia, and amoebas also can cause inflammation of the small and large intestine. Larger parasites, such as tapeworms or pinworms, can give rise to these symptoms, too.

Ulcerative colitis usually affects the descending colon and/or rectum. Like Crohn's disease (see small intestine), colitis causes swelling and ulcers to form in the intestinal wall. Blood and mucus emanating from the ulcers are often discharged in the stools. Other symptoms include abdominal pain, diarrhea, and occasionally fever.

Colitis is most prevalent among young adults. Though the illness may arise from the presence of bacteria, virus, or amoebas, the cause is still unknown, according to the AMA.

Treatment includes antibiotics to deal with infection; corticosteroid drugs to control nutrient absorption; and special diets that include multiple vitamin and mineral supplements. The diets are designed to restrict foods that promote gas and intestinal irritation. The foods commonly avoided are cabbage, beans, spices, milk, alcohol, and drinks that are either excessively cold or hot.

Antibiotics taken for more than two weeks can worsen the symptoms of colitis. Antibiotics upset the bacterial balance within the intestines by killing healthy bacteria and promoting harmful growth. This, of course, can exacerbate the symptoms.

Complications resulting from the illness (such as internal bleeding and fistula) may require surgery. If infection is the cause, the symptoms of colitis usually pass without treatment.

Diverticula are small sacs, or protrusions, in the lining of the intestines. Pressure from within the intestine causes these sacs to form. Often, undigested food gets caught in the sacs and remains there to putrefy and foster the growth of harmful bacteria. The formation of these sacs within the intestine causes that part of the colon to weaken, thus preventing healthy peristalsis and efficient bowel elimination.

Diverticulosis is the presence of diverticula in the intestines. Diverticulitis is a complication of diverticula in which inflammation occurs within the sacs; occasionally, a hole forms in the lining, as well. Symptoms of diverticulosis include bloating, pain, and alternating diarrhea and constipation. There can be bleeding if ulcers or holes form within the intestinal wall.

Both of these conditions are rare in developing countries and those where the diet consists mainly of whole grains, vegetables, and fruits. Fiber is one of the primary means of treatment for the illness, as well as antispasmodic drugs, and bed rest.

Irritable bowel syndrome is the name given to alternating bouts of diarrhea and constipation, often accompanied by diverticula, intestinal bloating, discomfort, and gas.

One of the three common forms of cancer in the Western world (besides breast and prostate cancer), colon cancer is unquestionably caused by a high-fat diet, and specifically the consumption of red meat. In December 1990, *The New England Journal of Medicine* reported the results of the largest study ever conducted on the relationship between diet and colon cancer. For six years, researchers followed 88,751 women between the ages of thirty-four and fifty-nine, recording their dietary habits and health patterns. The results showed that as fat intake and red meat consumption rose, so too did the rates of colon cancer. Those eating the most animal fat were twice as likely to develop colon cancer as those eating the least.

These findings were consistent with an enormous body of evidence that has been showing for decades that dietary fat causes colon cancer. The National Research Council of the National Academy of Sciences said in 1982 that fat—especially saturated fat found in animal foods—has a "causal" relationship with cancer, especially colon cancer. In 1979, the U.S. Surgeon General urged Americans to reduce their overall fat intake to reduce their risk of cancer and heart disease. The Surgeon General recommended specifically that Americans reduce their consumption of red meat.

Dr. Walter Willet, a researcher at the Brigham and Women's Hospital in Boston who directed the most recent study, stated, "If you step back and look at the data, the optimum amount of red meat you eat should be zero."

Scientists believe that fat causes cancer in a number of ways. Increased fat intake causes the liver to produce more bile acids in order to break down the fat in the intestinal tract. These acids act upon carcinogens, already present in the bowel, making them more virulent.

At the same time, fat within the colon increases the population of anaerobic bacteria that secrete estrogens. These estrogens, scientists have found, promote the growth of tumors. So, too, do high blood levels of cholesterol.

These factors—dietary fat and cholesterol, bile acids, estrogens from bacteria, and carcinogens derived from food and other environmental sources—combine to deform the DNA of cells and cause unrestricted growth, or cancer.

While there are dietary constituents that promote tumor growth, there are also foods that prevent intestinal disease. Low fat and cholesterol diets have been shown to reduce the size and the number of tumors in the bowel. Diets high in fiber have been shown to prevent all forms of intestinal problems, especially cancer. Studies dating back to the mid-1970s performed by Drs. Denis Burkitt and Hugh Trowell demonstrated that people living on high-fiber diets have low rates of intestinal disease, including cancer.

As shown in the chapter on the stomach, fat slows digestion and intestinal transit time. Fiber speeds up intestinal transit time and thus diminishes the likelihood of carcinogens remaining in the bowel to promote the growth of tumors.

Former director of the National Cancer Institute Dr. Gio Gori has reported that Japanese who remain in Japan and subsist on their traditional diet show low rates of cancer. However, when they come to the West and adopt the American high-fat diet, their cancer rates—including colon cancer—increase to those of Americans.

Finally, vegetables rich in vitamins A, E, and C—the so-called antioxidants—have been shown to enhance immune function (see chapter on the immune system) and prevent serious disease, including cancer.

THE RIGHT WAY OF LIVING

The Chinese view the large intestine as a yang, or expanded organ. It is regarded as one of the "six bowels"—the others being the stomach, small intestine, bladder, gall bladder, and an organ

The person who is afraid to alter his living habits, and especially his eating and drinking habits, because he is afraid that other persons may regard him as queer, eccentric, or fanatic forgets that the ownership of his body, the responsibility for its well-being, belongs to him, not them.

PAUL BRUNTON

of qi, known as the "Triple Heater." The triple heater is composed of three spheres of life energy that supply qi to the upper, middle, and lower parts of the thorax, coordinating the internal organs, according to the Chinese.

The large intestine is joined by the lungs as a paired set. Together, they form the Metal Element. The Metal Element is associated with dryness (the function of the large intestine is to draw water from food) and the color white.

The large intestine and lungs receive their optimal amounts of healing energy during the autumn months. During the day, the large intestine receives the most qi between the hours of 5 A.M. and 7 A.M. These are ideal months and times to take appropriate measures to heal the large intestine. Conversely, problems associated with the large intestine and lungs tend to manifest during the fall and in the early morning hours.

The food that has the greatest healing effect on the large intestine, according to Chinese medicine, is rice. Orientals revere rice as the "gift of the gods"; it was and still is their central food. Rice, more than any other grain, said the Chinese, strengthens and heals the large intestine.

Today, science understands that fiber from whole grains, vegetables, and fruit promotes intestinal health above all other foods. (See foods that heal the large intestine, below.) Fiber is undigestible vegetable matter. It speeds intestinal transit time; cleanses the colon of accumulated fat and stored-up waste; and treats diverticulosis.

The large intestine meridian begins at the tip of the index finger (large intestine point #1) and proceeds along the top of the hand, up the inner ridge of the arm, to the back of the shoulder, up the neck, and around the mouth. Ted Kaptchuk writes in *The Web That Has No Weaver* that the large intestine meridian has a branch that goes to the lungs and the large intestine, as well.

Problems associated with the shoulders, neck, and around the mouth are all related to disorders of digestion, according to Chinese medicine. So, too, are sinus problems, especially sinus congestion. The Chinese maintain that the large intestine is responsible for moving energy and waste downward and out of the body. When this downward movement is impeded, energy becomes backed up, especially in the upper respiratory tract and sinus areas. Treating sinus problems, therefore, includes treating the large intestine. Once the large intestine becomes unblocked, energy from the lungs and sinuses will flow downward and out once again.

In the same way, clear thinking is also associated with healthy elimination. Anyone who has been constipated knows that one of the first side effects of "irregularity" is a sluggish or "constipated" mind.

Human intestines, which are essentially a single system, some twenty-eight feet in length, perform their duties by moving crude matter (food) a great distance. They do this by virtue of their ability to expand and contract, their peristaltic action. In order for the power and dynamism of this expansion and contraction to endure, there must be considerable energy. As any engineer will tell you, all energy is made possible by the existence of a polarity between opposites, like the north and south poles of a magnet, or the positive and negative ions of an electrical charge.

The Chinese maintain that the long, expansive intestinal system must be balanced by a short or contracted organ in order to maintain a dynamic balance. Hence, the appendix. Unlike modern medicine, the Chinese do not view the appendix as an unnecessary appendage. There are no unnecessary organs; everything exists for a reason. The appendix serves as the intestinal tract's opposite pole, in the same way that the south pole of a magnet serves the north. Together, they create the dynamism that makes movement and function possible.

Removal of the appendix will, therefore, weaken the overall digestive tract. Those who have had the appendix removed should eat foods that provide optimal nutrition and are easy to digest and eliminate.

The Yellow Emperor said that the "lower intestines are like the officials who propagate the right way of living and they generate evolution and change." What he meant was that there is little ambiguity about the colon: we know very well when it is healthy or ill. To live according to the limits and peculiarities of the large intestine is to follow the "right way," because health is sustained in a large measure by our ability to eliminate poisons from the body. To change our behavior when intestinal health changes is to live in harmony with "evolution and change," meaning that to follow the dictates of our intestines ensures health and longevity, say the Chinese.

Evolution often means letting go of the past. The large intestine serves this purpose in the body: it receives the unwanted aspects of food from the small intestine and eliminates what is unneeded. The act of digestion and elimination can be seen as a metaphor for our ability to absorb what is useful from our experiences (a small intestine function) and eliminate what is unnecessary, harmful, or holds us back (a large intestine function).

People with disorders of the large intestine tend to live in the past. They hold onto things that should have been let go of a long time ago. For this reason, their lives are often burdened by sadness and grief. Taking care of the large intestine, say the Chinese, is the first step toward forgiveness and letting go of the past.

It's no coincidence, therefore, that the emotion associated with the large intestine is grief. People with weak intestines often have a weeping tone in their voice; they tend to speak with a hint of sadness. Since the mind and body are one, our psychological efforts at letting go of the past enhance the function of the large intestine.

The entire intestinal tract is regarded as the "roots" of the body. They are lengthy and absorbing. They draw nourishment from the earth in the form of food. When the roots are strong, we can draw the nourishment we need from life. If we are poorly nourished by life, Chinese healing begins by strengthening the intestines.

Our roots also stabilize us against the vicissitudes of life. The old axiom of a person having "guts," or courage, comes from this perception: the roots within the body give us a strong foundation in the face of danger.

FOODS TO KEEP YOUR INTESTINES HAPPY

The following foods and herbs are used in Chinese medicine to strengthen and treat the large intestine.

- *Grain:* Brown rice, sweet rice, mochi (pounded sweet rice).
- *Vegetables:* potato, sweet potato; cabbage, Chinese cabbage, celery, watercress, turnip greens, mustard greens; all roots, including daikon, carrot, lotus root, ginger, turnip, taro root potato.
- *Beans:* navy, soybeans, great northern, tofu, and tempeh.
- *Fish:* Cod, haddock, herring, flounder, halibut, scrod, carp.

- *Fruit:* Pears, peaches, loquat.
- *Herbs:* Garlic, dill, fresh grated ginger, horseradish, nutmeg, Job's tears, cinnamon, basil, fennel, bay leaf, black pepper, coriander, rice bran, cayenne, thyme, licorice.

There are dietary considerations for specific illnesses. Irritable bowel syndrome and diverticulosis can be caused by extremes in lifestyle, diet, and stress. Irregular hours, chaotic behavior, and chaotic relationships all lead to spastic bowel behavior.

When foods that have a contractive effect on the body, such as red meat and other animal foods, are combined with those that are extremely expansive, such as spices, sugar, and alcohol, spastic colon and diverticula are often the result. Individually, these foods represent extremes in qi. The body will try to balance these extreme influences, usually with little success.

The initial effects are indigestion, gas, heartburn, and alternating bouts of diarrhea and constipation. The forceful expansion and contraction will cause alternating tightness and inflation of the intestinal tract.

Finally, the absence of fiber in the diet causes accumulation of waste, especially undigested animal protein, fat, and sinew.

For constipation:

- Boil brown rice with carrots, onions, and grated ginger root. Cook with a pinch of sea salt until rice is soft, usually about forty-five minutes to an hour. Chew well.
- Ginger tea. Grate a tablespoon of fresh ginger in the bottom of a tea cup; pour hot water or kukicha (bancha) tea over grated ginger. Add one or two drops of tamari or shoyu to tea. Drink hot.
- Kuzu and apple juice drink. Kuzu, also known as kudzu, is a hardy root and an excellent herb for the intestines. Boil apple juice. Use two and a half tablespoons of kuzu per cup of juice. Dissolve kuzu in cup of cold water before adding to juice. Stir kuzu into juice, while simmering juice. Liquid will gradually thicken into a gelatin. Turn off flame and allow to cool.

For diarrhea:

- Kuzu and umeboshi plum drink. Dissolve five tablespoons kuzu in two cups of cold water; add an umeboshi plum and bring to a boil. Stir water while simmering until liquid thickens. Eat while hot.

- Pressure-cooked white rice, with a pinch of sea salt; white rice can be mixed with brown rice and pressure-cooked, as well.
- White potato, boiled.

Note: Constipation and diarrhea should subside quickly on a whole-foods diet. If either of these conditions persist, seek appropriate health-care advice. Persistent diarrhea during infancy is a dangerous condition; parents should seek appropriate medical advice immediately. See chapters on the spleen and small intestine for additional information on digestive disorders.

Foods to avoid: Red meat, fried foods, dairy products, especially hard cheeses and milk. If constipated, avoid eggs and all refined foods.

Naturopath Ross Trattler points out that the most common causes of intestinal disorders are diets rich in refined foods and deficient in fiber; excesses of meat, milk products, fried foods, coffee, tea, alcohol, and acid-producing foods; overeating; inactivity; stress; and long-term laxative use. He also includes pregnancy, anemia, and appendectomy among other causes of chronic constipation. Among Trattler's recommendations for constipation are:

- Stew figs and prunes in a small amount of apple juice for fifteen to twenty minutes. Eat and drink broth at night, at least two hours before sleeping, and as the first meal in the morning. This is a very effective treatment that can be used on an ongoing basis for chronic constipation.
- *Herbs:* Cascara sagrada, a natural herbal laxative. Cascara should only be used in conjunction with general improvement in diet and lifestyle. Bowels can become dependent upon any laxatives, including cascara. Small doses of cascara are recommended (fifteen to twenty drops in water).
- Chamomile tea.
- Garlic, either raw or in cooking, in small amounts.
- Aloe vera juice.
- Slippery elm, either as infusion or tea.
- Licorice root tea.
- Psyllium seed.

- Flax seed.
- Hot and cold sitz baths.
- *Avoid the following foods while constipated:* all refined grains, coffee, tea, sugar, spices, alcohol.
- *Lifestyle:* daily exercise. Walking, sit-ups to strengthen abdomen, leg lifts, while lying on your back, to strengthen abdomen.

For diarrhea, Trattler recommends the following:

- Green apples with no skin.
- Banana.
- Barley water (boil barley, making broth very watery).
- Carrot and cabbage juice.
- Toasted white bread (Trattler recommends this for one to two days; use only highly refined bread).

Ayurvedic tradition views the large intestine as the province of the vata dosha, meaning that it is most influenced by the kinetic force within the body. The vata dosha controls bodily movements. When it is depleted or deficient, digestion becomes lethargic and constipation results. When vata is excessive, we are more likely to suffer from diarrhea or ulcers. When efficient elimination is prevented, skin problems arise, according to Ayurvedic medicine. Since the skin is a major organ of elimination, it naturally attempts to compensate for the inability of the intestines to fully eliminate waste and toxins. However, this often results in rashes, blemishes, or acne. Repressed emotions disturb vata and create intestinal imbalances.

Ayur-Veda teaches that we must cultivate detachment from our emotions. During meditation, emotions must be allowed to rise to the surface, be witnessed and experienced fully, and then released. Repression only leads to ill health.

Foods that balance and support the vata dosha are as follows:

- *Grains:* rice, wheat, and oats.
- *Vegetables:* cucumber, cooked vegetables, including leafy greens, okra, onion, potato, radishes, squash, asparagus, beets, carrots.
- *Fruit:* apricots, avocado, berries, cherries, grapefruit, grapes, lemons, melons, oranges, peaches, plums.

- *Herbs:* senna leaf tea, dandelion root, psyllium seed, prunes, bran, flaxseed husk, castor oil, raisins, mango juice, grape juice.
- If suffering from intestinal disorders, avoid raw vegetables, eggplant, white potato, peppers, tomatoes.

A homeopathic remedy for constipation is pulsatilla, especially for women and pregnant women with morning sickness. For those who are addicted to laxatives, take nux vomica a few hours before bed for several days, but not as a permanent substitute for the laxatives. Sulphur is good for those who experience pain while defecating, and byronia for those with hard, dry stools and for children who are constipated, or for those whose constipation is the result of the anticipation of an upcoming professional or social event.

Like the ancients, we are still struggling to achieve intestinal health. It is as important as ever. Fortunately, there is an abundance of information today that we can turn to for help. For the vast majority of those who suffer from intestinal disorders, a cure can be as close as your next meal.

Homeopathic remedies for gas:

CARBO VEGETABLIS: For belching and gas, no matter what you eat.

CHINA: Midsection feels distended. Stomach feels full of gas.

LYCODIUM: Fullness before you finish eating or after a light meal. Belt feels too tight. Rumbling gas.

Homeopathic remedies for hemorrhoids:

ARNICA: Useful for hemorrhoids that develop after childbirth.

SULPHUR: Itching and burning around anus, made worse by bathing.

COLLINSONIA: Feels like there are sticks in rectum. Usually constipated.

NUX VOMICA: Itching that feels better from cool bathing.

CHAPTER 10

THE GALL BLADDER

$\mathcal{T}$HE GALL BLADDER is a pear-shaped organ, about three inches long, and found at the back of the liver, on the right side of the body. It serves as a reservoir for bile, produced by the liver to emulsify fats. Bile flows from the liver to the gall bladder via a small tube, called the cystic duct, which is a branch of the common duct.

The gall bladder is composed of four layers of tissue: an inner lining of mucous membrane; a layer of smooth muscle; a layer of connective tissue; and a covering layer of tissue, called serosa. When food passes from the stomach into the small intestine, hormones stimulate the gall bladder to expel bile into the first stage of small intestine, called the duodenum. Bile breaks down the fats, permitting them to be absorbed by the small intestine.

Bile is a mixture of bile acid (also called bile salts) and cholesterol. The cholesterol acts as a buffering agent, preventing the bile acids from eating away at the gall bladder and small intestine.

To wish to be healthy is a part of being healthy.

SENECA

ILLNESSES AFFECTING THE GALL BLADDER

By far, the most common illness affecting the gall bladder is gall stones. Sixteen million Americans suffer from gall stones, twelve million of whom are women. No one is certain why this disparity between the sexes exists, but it may be due to the dropoff of estrogen levels in postmenopausal women, which is associated with higher cholesterol levels and greater incidence of heart disease.

Each year, 500,000 gall bladder surgeries are performed. The operation is called a cholecystectomy. Gall stones are composed almost entirely of cholesterol.

People who consume high-fat and high-cholesterol diets have higher rates of gall stones than those who consume low-fat and low-cholesterol diets.

Common symptoms of gall stones include pain and tenderness on the right side of the body. Occasionally, the pain can be sharp and severe, causing people to think they are experiencing a heart attack or an appendicitis. Sometimes, stones can be found in the cystic or common ducts, which can cause serious complications. The most common form of treatment is the surgical removal of the gall bladder.

AN UPRIGHT OFFICIAL

"The gall bladder occupies the position of an important and upright official who excels through his decisions and judgment," explained the Yellow Emperor, meaning that the gall bladder plays an important role in our decision-making function. This assertion springs from the Five Element Theory, which states that the liver and gall bladder are responsible for controlling and balancing anger.

All emotions are grounded in various parts of the body. A person with a healthy liver and gall bladder will have a balanced temperament, but one whose liver and gall bladder are troubled will likely suffer outbursts of anger and ill-temper. This, of course, will lead to rash decisions. When the liver and gall bladder are balanced and healthy, decisions are made from emotional equilibrium, a characteristic of a healthy Wood Element. However, when decisions are difficult to make, many Oriental healers will

God heals and the doctor takes the fee.

BENJAMIN FRANKLIN

urge people to eat simply, avoid extremes in emotions, and meditate, so that harmony can be restored throughout the body, and the gall bladder function can assist in making a correct decision.

The gall bladder is the recipient of bile from the liver, which in Chinese medicine is viewed as taking the liver's excess. If the liver becomes excessive and produces too much bile, the gall bladder will suffer, since its capacity to store bile is limited.

The gall bladder is most vulnerable to dietary fat and cholesterol, which are the major causes of gall stones. People who subsist on diets low in fat and cholesterol have a lower incidence of gall stones, as compared to those of Western nations, where fat and cholesterol consumption is higher. Since the liver and gall bladder comprise the Wood Element, the gall bladder is strengthened by the same foods (wheat and leafy greens), tastes (sour), and emotions (avoidance of anger) as those mentioned in the chapter on the liver.

The gall bladder meridian begins at the temples, zigzags along the sides of the head, behind each ear, and then runs down the neck and shoulders. From there, it travels along the sides of the body, and down the outside of each leg. The meridian continues to the fourth toe, next to the little toe. As a diagnostic point, traditional healers will examine the fourth toe to see if a bunion protrudes from it. The presence of such a bunion usually indicates some kind of gall bladder imbalance. (Other factors are examined to corroborate that assessment and make it more detailed.)

Many headaches are caused by liver and gall bladder imbalances. Any disturbance in the liver also will upset the gall bladder, which in turn will create an imbalance of qi along the gall bladder meridian. Such imbalances often will manifest in the form of headaches, since the gall bladder meridian begins at the temples and covers both sides of the head. Sometimes these kinds of headaches are referred to simply as gall bladder headaches. Many people who suffer such headaches will see yellow blotches before their eyes, indicating a disturbance in the bile. They are prevalent in the springtime, when the liver and gall bladder are receiving an increase in qi, and when underlying symptoms may manifest.

Perhaps the clearest and most persuasive insight into our modern epidemic of gall bladder problems was made by Nathan Pritikin, the late scientist and creator of the Pritikin Program for Diet and Exercise. Pritikin pointed out that bile, which is composed of bile salts, cholesterol, and lecithin, is kept in solution by a delicate harmony of these three constituents. The most important is the bile salts-to-cholesterol ratio. The bile salts are acid. Without this acid, the cholesterol would form crystals and stones. So, there must be sufficient bile acids to keep the cholesterol from forming stones in the gall bladder. When the cholesterol in the bile becomes too concentrated, it saturates the bile acids and begins to form crystals and then stones.

In a healthy gall bladder, the cholesterol content is around 350 mg. Most Americans who eat a standard high-fat diet have gall bladder cholesterol levels in excess of 650 mg. This quantity of cholesterol cannot be kept in solution by the available quantity of bile acids, which allows the cholesterol to form stones.

Pritikin maintained that the surest way to cure gall stones is to lower the body's overall cholesterol level. This will reduce the cholesterol in the gall bladder, and thus create a healthy bile-to-cholesterol ratio. Once this ratio is reestablished, the bile acids can dissolve the cholesterol crystals and stones, and restore health to the gall bladder. This can be done, he said, as long as there are no stones in the cystic duct, the canal leading from the gall bladder to the common bile duct. Once stones are in the cystic duct, they can seal off the gall bladder and cause serious problems, for which surgery may be necessary. Ultrasound and X-ray tests can confirm if gall stones exist and where they are located.

Naturopaths and other traditional health counselors can offer dietary programs that include a gall bladder flush. The flush is one of several kinds of drinks that include olive oil and herbs, which together cause the gall bladder to pass the stones into the small intestine and then eliminate them through the feces. This can be a dangerous procedure; the stones can get caught in the cystic duct if they are too large. Before attempting such a flush, people should know the size of the stones and get a variety of opinions.

Some common therapeutic agents for the gall bladder (and liver, too) according to Dr. Ross Trattler:

- Apple juice.
- Beet extract tablets.
- Beet tops and juice.
- Dandelion tea and greens.
- Grapefruit juice.

Herbs for the gall bladder:

CELANDINE: Reduces inflammation of bile ducts.

FRINGE TREE: Increases bile flow.

OREGON GRAPE ROOT and YELLOW DOCK: Stimulate bile.

Six to eight glasses of water a day will help prevent gall stones.

CHAPTER 11

THE LIVER

Indeed, the liver is so crucial biologically that it can be called the balance of the wheel of life.

HAKIM G. M. CHISHTI

*P*OISONING ALWAYS HAS been among the favored methods of assassination, largely because it is efficient, silent, and neat. However, there have been cases when the intended victim refused to succumb, no matter how powerful the poison, or the quantity consumed. Among the more famous of these stubborn victims was the Russian mystic, Rasputin.

During the early part of this century, Rasputin exercised great influence over the ruling Russian family, Nicholas II and his wife Alexandra. His power was particularly strong with the czarina, Alexandra, who regarded him as a spiritual master and the savior of the Russian people. Through Alexandra, Rasputin influenced national policy, disposed of ministers who opposed his power, and appointed people who supported him. By 1916, people were saying he ruled Russia by day and seduced the ladies of the court by night. Some historians credit Rasputin with bringing down the ruling Romonov family, having thoroughly corrupted their morals with his theory that if one wants to be close to God, it is necessary to become the greatest sinner imaginable. To this end Rasputin put considerable effort, especially indulging his passion for the fairer sex. When it became clear that his hold on Alexandra was ironclad, a powerful Russian elite—who disagreed with the direction of their country—decided that Rasputin had to go.

The plot was simple enough: On December 16, 1916, Rasputin was invited to the house of an associate, where he would be fed cakes and wine laced with abundant quantities of potassium cyanide. The conspirators made certain that the dosages of cyanide in a single cake or one glass of wine were sufficient to kill a large elephant.

A short while after arriving at the house, Rasputin was eating and drinking copiously. Apparently, he had taken a liking to the cakes and wine and was presently wondering aloud what time the women—whom the host had promised—would arrive. In a nearby room, a group of conspirators waited for Rasputin to die, but just the opposite happened. The only apparent effect from the food and drink on Rasputin was his unhappiness with the absence of female company.

Frightened by Rasputin's mysterious powers over the poison, the host excused himself from his guest's company and hurried into the nearby room to beg advice from his fellow murderers. Feed him more poison, was their answer. The host complied. But alas, even greater quantities of the cyanide were impotent against Rasputin.

Fed up with the slow way, the murderers produced a gun and shot Rasputin at point-blank range. Now they were certain he was dead, and even began to relax over his body when suddenly Rasputin got up, staggered to the door, and ran out of the house. The central figure in the plot, a V. M. Purishkevich, who recorded the entire event in his diary (published under the title *The Murder of Rasputin*), ran after him, shooting wildly at Rasputin, who miraculously gained speed as he ran.

Eventually, Purishkevich managed to put two bullets in Rasputin, one in his back and another in his head. Now, the men were sure he was dead. But, driven by fear of Rasputin's mysterious powers, one of them began to hit Rasputin on the head with a heavy object. The group was horrified when the mystic opened his eyes and let out a moan. "He's still alive!" they shouted. Shaken but determined, the murderers took Rasputin to a nearby canal and threw his body through a hole in the ice and into the frozen waters. He disappeared and was finally dead. Among the questions that perplexed the killers afterwards: How did Rasputin survive such quantities of poison, to say nothing of three bullets? Each man answered it in his own way, but one thing is certain: Rasputin had a very strong liver.

THE BODY'S LABORATORY

Even the human brain cannot match the liver for its varied and essential functions. The liver is a veritable laboratory, testing and identifying chemicals that enter the system, neutralizing poisons, and creating essential blood, metabolic, and immune constituents.

The liver creates bile, which aids in the digestion of fats, and also serves as the medium by which the organ eliminates waste. In addition, the liver creates a variety of essential elements for the blood, including: albumin, which regulates water exchange between blood and tissues; complement, an immune constituent that protects against infection; coagulant, which produces blood clotting; globulin, which combines with iron to carry oxygen in the blood; and cholesterol, a protein that carries fats throughout the body.

There are two types of cholesterol created by the liver, and each type determines where fat in the bloodstream goes. LDL cholesterol (low density lipoproteins) brings lipids, or fats, to tissues and the walls of blood vessels. When there is too much LDL, atherosclerosis (the formation of cholesterol plaques) occurs within the walls of blood vessels, thus blocking the flow of blood. HDL cholesterol (high density lipoproteins) removes fats and cholesterol from the body, and thus lowers overall blood cholesterol.

The liver creates more than 1,000 different enzymes necessary for digestion and nutrient assimilation. It also creates and regulates some of the body's hormones.

The liver absorbs glucose, or blood sugar, and stores it in the form of glycogen. When the body needs energy or heat, the liver converts the glycogen back into glucose, and releases it into the bloodstream. It assists in the breakdown and metabolism of fats.

It also breaks down proteins into their component parts—amino acids—and then reassembles them into proteins appropriate for your body. The liver helps break down old red blood cells, as well.

Finally, the liver detoxifies the blood by removing drugs and other poisons, and then altering their chemical structure to render them harmless. Even drugs you might consider helpful, such as aspirin or antibiotics, are regarded by the liver as poisonous substances that must be eliminated from the organism. For this reason, physicians give prescribed dosages of drugs, in part to overcome the liver's diligence against all but the most healthful foods and substances.

Once a poison has been rendered harmless, the liver releases it as a water-soluble compound in the bile. From there, it travels to the gall bladder and small intestine. Much of the feces is composed of bile.

Needless to say, you cannot live without a liver.

Your Body's Blood Reservoir

The liver is the body's largest internal organ. In adults, it weighs anywhere from two and a half to four pounds. It is cone-shaped, extending from the left side of the sternum just below the left nipple to the right side of the body, filling much of the upper right abdominal cavity. It is composed of two lobes, a smaller left lobe, and a larger right; these are further divided into smaller sections.

The body's largest internal organ and reservoir of blood, the liver is a remarkable chemical laboratory that plays a major role in digesting foods, eliminating wastes, preventing infection, and producing essential blood elements.

The Liver

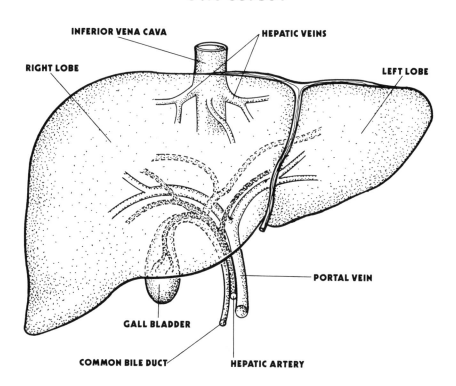

INFERIOR VENA CAVA

HEPATIC VEINS

RIGHT LOBE

LEFT LOBE

PORTAL VEIN

GALL BLADDER

COMMON BILE DUCT

HEPATIC ARTERY

The liver has a remarkable blood supply: it receives oxygenated blood from one vessel, called the hepatic artery, and nutrient-rich blood from another, called the hepatic portal vein. Blood flows through to the liver from the spleen and small intestine. Once it arrives, it passes through the organ via a network of tiny vessels called the "portal tracts," where the blood provides oxygen and nutrition to cells. Here it is purified of poisons, and receives essential blood constituents created by the liver. Eventually, the blood exits the organ via the hepatic vein, found at the back of the liver.

The liver is a great reservoir of blood. About one-quarter of the heart's entire output is held within the liver when the body is at rest. Because the body contains up to five quarts of blood, about one and a quarter quarts are passing through the organ at any moment. Much of that blood is dispersed when you exercise.

The structural unit of the liver is called a lobule, a cylindrically-shaped cell. These lobules arrange themselves in long chainlike structures. Although the liver performs an incredible array of tasks—more than 500 functions already have been counted—they are all done, apparently, by the same type of cell, the lobule.

This lack of specialization may explain, in part, why the liver is so resilient: up to three-quarters of it can be destroyed, yet the organ will continue to perform its tasks. Moreover, the liver can restore itself—much like a salamander can restore its tail—even after half of it has been damaged, if appropriate corrective actions are taken. (See illnesses associated with the liver, below.)

Bile is secreted by the liver through a series of ducts, or tiny tubular canals. Like many tributaries that ultimately join two rivers, these liver ducts link up eventually with two larger tubes, called the hepatic ducts, at the base of the liver. From there, the two form a single, or common, hepatic duct, which brings bile to the gall bladder and then to the duodenum, the first stage of the small intestine.

ILLNESSES OF THE LIVER

There are a variety of serious illnesses affecting the liver, but the most prevalent are hepatitis, cirrhosis, and cancer. Hepatitis, or inflammation of the liver, is caused mostly by the hepatitis virus or cirrhosis. There are two forms of viral hepatitis, designated as A or B. Hepatitis A, sometimes called infectious hepatitis, is spread by consuming infected food or water. Hepatitis B results from blood transfusions, sexual contact with an infected person, or through the use of contaminated intravenous needles. Type B is usually more serious than A; it is often chronic, sometimes lasting years. This, of course, increases the chances of serious liver damage and cirrhosis.

Sometimes medical tests fail to reveal the presence of either hepatitis A or B in people who nonetheless have all the symptoms of hepatitis. Doctors have labeled such forms of hepatitis as non-A and non-B. This form of the illness is often the result of infected blood transfusions, alcohol, or contact with a toxic chemical substance in the environment.

Other causes (besides cirrhosis, which is described below) are drugs and chemical poisons. Some very common chemicals, such as those found in dry-cleaning agents, can cause hepatitis, particularly if there is an underlying liver problem.

Symptoms of hepatitis are usually flulike: fever, nausea, vomiting, sweating, loss of appetite, and pain or tenderness in the upper abdomen; aching muscles; joint pain; and malaise. Sometimes hepatitis can cause jaundice, with its characteristic yellowing of the skin and eyes. This occurs because of the buildup of bile within the system.

There is no known cure for hepatitis and no effective treatment in the arsenal of orthodox medicine. Rest, nutritious diet, and the removal of the causative toxic agent (alcohol, drugs, or some other chemical toxin) are the only reliable therapies. Hepatitis can result in serious liver damage and even death. Yet, most people overcome the illness within several months.

Cirrhosis is the destruction of the liver due to the accumulation of fatty acids that cut off blood flow to the liver cells. The primary cause of cirrhosis is alcohol abuse, though drugs, chemical toxins, and birth defects can cause the disease as well.

The reason fatty acids accumulate in people who consume alcohol is that the liver selects the alcohol as its primary source of fuel. Fatty acids, which would ordinarily be the liver's chosen fuel, are therefore neglected and allowed to build up within the tissues. As fatty acids accumulate, blood supply is cut off and cells

Half of what we have taught you is wrong. Unfortunately, we do not know which half.

DEAN BURWELL

115

die. This causes scar tissue to form, which eventually deforms the liver's normal structure, and reduces its functional size.

The first stage of the illness is called "fatty liver," because of the accumulation of fat within the organ. There may be no symptoms associated with fatty liver or even cirrhosis—that is, until the illness progresses to the acute phase. At this point a variety of dangerous side effects may manifest: high blood pressure (resulting from the destruction of veins leading to the liver); accumulation of fluids in the abdomen, caused by the liver's inability to create albumin; the vomiting of blood, due to the increase in blood pressure and the consequent rupture of veins in the esophagus; and hepatitis. Cirrhosis can be fatal on its own. It also can result in cancer of the liver.

According to the American Medical Association, men who consume an average of four 80-proof ounces of alcohol a day—the equivalent of two double shots of whiskey or four glasses of wine—have a substantial chance of contracting cirrhosis of the liver. Women require only half that amount—the equivalent alcohol intake of about two glasses of wine per day—to suffer from cirrhosis. Abstinence from alcohol can lead to a full recovery, with all or most of the liver function returning to normal.

Malignant tumors can begin in the liver or originate at some other location within the body and migrate to the liver through the blood and lymph. In the U.S., cancers originating at the liver are less common than those occurring there as a secondary site. Usually, cancers that have spread to the liver have originated in the stomach, pancreas, or intestines. Enlargement of the liver is usually the result of leukemias and lymphomas—cancers affecting the white blood cell or the lymph system, respectively.

THE BODY'S COMMANDING GENERAL

The liver attempts to eliminate all the poisons that infiltrate the bloodstream. These include fat, alcohol, drugs (both pharmaceutical and recreational), and artificial colors, flavors, and preservatives. In addition, there is an equally unprecedented array of pollutants in the environment that are ingested through the air we breathe and the water we drink, which ideally should be eliminated by the liver.

Virtually all traditional medicines—that is, Chinese, Ayur-

If I were informed tomorrow that I was in direct communication with my liver, and could now take over, I would become deeply depressed. I'd sooner be told, forty thousand feet over Denver, that the 747 jet in which I had a coach seat was now mine to operate as I pleased; at least I would have the hope of bailing out, if I could find a parachute and discover quickly how to open a door. Nothing would save me and my liver if I were in charge. For I am, to face the facts squarely, considerably less intelligent than my liver.

LEWIS THOMAS

Veda, Greek, and naturopathy—see the liver as having a limited capacity to eliminate poisons from the body. If the toxins from the diet and environment exceed the liver's blood-cleansing limits, the poisons will accumulate within the liver, the blood, and the body at large, creating a toxic internal environment that will add to a decline in liver health and function.

Other blood-cleansing organs, especially the kidneys, will be called upon to rid the body of these foreign substances. If the toxins continue to be ingested, these organs, too, will be exceeded in their capacity to cleanse the blood. Meanwhile, the immune system will be forced to maintain an ongoing war against these harmful substances.

The net effect is an overworked and exhausted immune system, an equally exhausted set of blood-cleansing organs, and an ever-increasing level of toxicity within the body. In short, a breeding ground for disease. Such a toxic condition makes the liver vulnerable to a wide assortment of illnesses, some of which modern medicine does not normally associate with the liver. Among the disorders that arise from liver disease are headaches, chronic fatigue, allergies, fatty liver, anemia, skin problems, toxemia, hepatitis, and immune deficiency. Eventually, even liver cancer can manifest.

These problems cannot occur in a healthy liver, which is simply too strong and too regenerative to be overcome by viruses or small quantities of pollution. Traditional medicine therefore treats the liver by first eliminating, as much as possible, the toxins entering the body, starting with changes in diet and exercise patterns. As we have already seen, the liver has miraculous regenerative powers and can restore health once the offending problems are eliminated. An assortment of additional remedies is offered, depending on the system employed. Let's have a closer look.

The liver is associated with the gall bladder, its paired organ, and the Wood Element. Its season is the spring, when the liver enjoys an increase in qi. This heightened state of life energy can bring about greater healing, if appropriate measures are taken, or it can cause manifestation of underlying symptoms.

Metaphorically, the liver's general condition should be similar to that of spring: light, open, and flowing with energy (as opposed to winter, which is contracted and holding back). The liver suffers most when it becomes hard and stagnant.

The liver is associated with the color green, derived from its "tree nature," and the wind. The Chinese maintain that the "wind creates wood," perhaps in part because the wind spreads seeds. In any case, too much exposure to the wind can injure the liver; the wind is said to enter the body through the neck or throat, and it is here that one should be especially protective in the winter and early spring.

The Chinese regard the liver as the commanding general of the body, coordinating an army of functions that, together, form the human organism. When the body runs smoothly and in a coordinated way, the general is clear, well-ordered, and in command. But if the body is chronically ill, pained, or arthritic, the general suffers. The Chinese ascribe many vital functions to the liver, which are:

- Producing bile and contributing to healthy digestion.
- Detoxifying the blood.
- Providing blood and qi to the muscles, tendons, ligaments, and nails.
- Providing blood and qi to the eyes.
- Influencing the ability to sleep deeply.
- Maintaining stable emotions, especially the emotion of anger.

According to the Five Elements, the Water Element (kidneys and bladder) nourishes Wood (the liver and gall bladder) with qi, while Wood nourishes Fire (the heart and small intestine) with life force. At the same time, the liver controls the stomach and spleen (Wood controls Earth by grasping it and holding on).

Clearly, the liver does support the small intestine function by producing bile, which helps to emulsify fats in the duodenum. It also produces more than 1,000 enzymes, which are essential to good digestion and healthy metabolism. Also, because it receives blood from the spleen, the liver controls the spleen to some extent, since the degree of the organ's receptivity could influence how the spleen functions.

Like Western medical doctors, the Chinese view the liver as a reservoir of blood. The liver ensures that adequate blood and qi are sent to the muscles, tendons, and joints. Muscles, joints, and tendons that are supple and strong reflect a healthy liver. Conversely, tendons, muscles, and ligaments that are tight, stiff, or weak reflect a deficient liver, meaning that the organ is unable to distribute adequate blood, oxygen, and qi to these areas of the body. Even injuries to tendons—such as those suffered by many professional athletes—are regarded as symptomatic of an over-worked or burdened liver.

The liver is said to open into the eyes, meaning that the liver nourishes the eyes with qi (so that they can "see the mystery of Heaven and discover Tao among mankind," said the Yellow Emperor). So, most eye problems have their origin in the liver.

The maintenance of healthy vision depends upon the health of the muscle tissue within the eye itself, and the integrity of the shape of the eye. (See chapter on sight.) The shape of the eye determines where the image is focused within the interior of the eye. In myopia, for example, the light of the image is focused at a point in front of the retina—not directly upon it. The retina is the light-sensitive membrane in back of the eye. Since the retina does not receive the full and clear impact of the light, the image appears to us as blurred.

The liver not only sends qi to the eyes, it also governs the health of all the body's muscles, including the muscles within the eyes. As the liver becomes congested, its ability to send qi to the eyes is diminished, causing the weakening of the eye's muscles and its ability to maintain its original shape. Diminished qi also reduces the eyes' ability to efficiently eliminate waste, thus increasing the likelihood of floaters (cholesterol crystals and cellular waste products) inside the eye and lens.

As the flow of waste from the eye slows, pressure within the eye increases, as well, like a pinched hose or a river that is backed up. This can result in glaucoma, among the most common eye disorders today. Just as the liver influences the health of the eye, the reverse is also true: eye strain or overwork causes the liver to become tired.

Each day, the liver is said to receive optimal amounts of qi between the hours of 1 A.M. and 3 A.M. The gall bladder receives optimal amounts of qi during the hours of 11 P.M. and 1 A.M. These, of course, are prime sleeping hours. During this time, the liver is able to heal itself, as long as we are resting and the organ is not forced to deal with external stimuli. People who party late at night are damaging their livers, probably in more ways than one.

Insomnia usually affects us between the hours of 11 P.M. and 3 A.M., when the liver and gall bladder are being infused with additional qi. If the liver is congested or unhealthy, the increased qi will not flow smoothly through the organ. Instead, the liver will become unsettled, active, and even chaotic. This will give rise to an underlying discomfort, a sense of internal conflict, and excessive thinking that attempts to work through such conflicts. Hence, insomnia.

According to the principles of acupuncture, the liver meridian originates at a point on the rib cage, directly above the liver on the right, and over the spleen on the left. It travels downward along the groin and inside of the leg, over the inner part of the knee, down the calf, over the foot, and to the big toe of each foot.

When the liver becomes congested, qi becomes obstructed along the meridian, causing a diminution of the qi flowing to the sex organs and knees. This reduction of qi along the liver meridian is the main cause of hydrocele in men, or the swelling of one or both of the testicles. Rest and care of the liver (see below) are usually enough to clear up the problem in a few days.

Wherever qi flow is inadequate, problems arise. When qi is insufficient to the knees, tendons and ligaments can deteriorate and become vulnerable to injury. When qi is diminished to the toes, ingrown toenails, bumps, or an often painful turning of the toe can occur.

As the commanding general, the liver maintains both physical and emotional balance of the body. Vertigo is most often a liver disorder, according to the Chinese, and treatment of the liver restores balance.

THE SEAT OF THE SOUL

The liver maintains overall emotional stability, but imbalances reveal themselves as excesses of anger. People who abuse their livers, either through alcohol or junk food, are prone to chronic anger, which also injures the liver. As liver health is restored, anger diminishes.

The liver's role as the body's detoxifier extends metaphorically to our general capacity to maintain a clean and orderly environment. People whose desks or rooms tend to be messy usually suffer from a liver imbalance—perhaps the liver is too "cluttered," too. In the same way, clear and well-ordered thinking tends to reflect a strong and healthy liver.

The relative flexibility of the body—especially the tendons, muscles, and joints—is viewed as a metaphor for the flexibility of one's thinking. Those with strong livers have flexible connective tissues, which is reflected in flexible minds.

Such a philosophy forms the basis for both Indian yoga and Chinese exercises derived from acupuncture. The Chinese maintain that the liver is associated with tears, particularly repressed or unspent tears. When the liver begins to heal itself, anger and grief—which have been stored away within the tissues of the organ—tend to be released in the form of old tears, say the Chinese sages.

Since the liver is associated with the Wood Element, the organ is associated with the metaphor of a tree. A tree reaches upward toward the heavens, and is thus considered highly spiritual, inspirational, and exciting. The liver's natural tendency, therefore, is to restore the spirit, to lift it above the poisoned events of the day into a more pure and rarefied understanding of life. For these and other reasons, many traditional cultures maintain that the liver is the "seat of the soul."

CAUSES OF LIVER DISORDERS

According to Oriental medicine, the source of most liver problems is stagnation of blood and qi, brought about primarily by excessive amounts of fat, sugar (which converts in the liver to fat), alcohol, and a variety of common poisons in the food system and environment.

If the diet is composed primarily of junk foods—specifically fat, sugar, refined grains, and artificial ingredients (but no alcohol)—the liver will likely become overly contracted and deficient (yin). The organ can become tight, congested, and lethargic. Inadequate amounts of blood and qi pass from the organ to those areas that depend upon the liver for nourishment. Gradually, overall liver function will decline.

According to Chinese physiognomy, the face of a person with this type of deficient liver will be pale, drawn, and tight, with dark furrows and indentations. Such a person tends to be stiff in the joints. He or she will likely have very exact ways of doing things and a tendency toward perfectionism and intolerance. This person will likely be impatient, angry, and prone to chronic headaches.

Wherever you see two or a dozen people of ordinary bulk talking together, you know they are talking about their livers. When you first arrive here your new acquaintances seem sad and hard to talk to, but pretty soon you get the lay of the land and the hand of things, and after that you haven't any more trouble. You look into the dreary dull eye and softly say: "Well, how's your liver?" You will see that dim eye flash up with a grateful flame, and you will see that jaw begin to work, and you will recognize that nothing is required of you from this but to listen as long as you remain conscious.

MARK TWAIN

The most common liver problems, however, result from a diet rich in animal foods and alcohol, which combine to make the liver expanded, overactive, and inflamed (yang). This condition reveals itself on a person's face as a reddish complexion, often with the capillaries exposed at the surface. Such people tend to be fiery, and given to extremes of emotion, from anger to jolliness.

Both forms of liver imbalance can give rise to serious illness, but the inflamed liver is more prone to hepatitis, cirrhosis, and cancer.

HEALING THE LIVER

The first step in healing the liver is to eliminate excesses of fat, cholesterol, refined foods, artificial ingredients, drugs, sugar, and alcohol. Ideally, the diet should be composed of mostly low-fat fish, whole grains, vegetables, beans, and fruit. It should contain only small to moderate amounts of vegetable oils.

According to Chinese medicine, the grain that has the most healing effect on the liver is whole wheat.

Sour foods, such as lemon, grapefruit, and sauerkraut, have a medicinal effect, as well. However, the sourness of the food must be balanced. Too much sourness causes astringency, preventing the liver from releasing toxins. A balanced sourness will act as a catalyst to stimulate the liver to produce bile and release stored waste.

The beans that stimulate healing in the liver are limas, green lentils, and split peas.

Many leafy greens have an energetic nature similar to that of a tree—that is, they reach upward and outward toward the heavens. Using the law of like-cures-like, such vegetables have a medicinal effect on the liver, in that they stimulate the organ to open and circulate blood and oxygen. Vegetables that are especially helpful are broccoli, parsley, collards, and a variety of lettuces. Dark lettuces, such as romaine, are richer in nutrients, especially calcium, than iceberg lettuce, and are therefore preferable.

Carrots and carrot juice are among the most effective and widely used liver tonics in all of traditional medicine, including Chinese. They are rich in minerals and beta carotene, an antioxidant that can help prevent free radical formation and the decay of tissues within the organ. Carrots and carrot juice strengthen liver function and promote healing. Seaweeds are commonly recommended because they are rich in minerals, A and B vitamins, all of which are immune-enhancing. All kinds of squash are suggested for their rich concentrations of beta carotene, the vegetable source of vitamin A. Beta carotene is one of the most powerful immune-enhancing nutrients, as well as an antioxidant.

In general, foods should be lightly cooked. Grains should be boiled or pressure-cooked. Fruits can be eaten raw or lightly cooked (as in compotes). But all refined sweeteners should be avoided.

Regular amounts of fermented foods, such as miso, sauerkraut, and pickles, should be added to the diet to promote healthful digestion, assimilation, and elimination. But fermented foods often contain sodium, which should be minimized. So, only small amounts of fermented foods should be used per serving, but can be eaten daily.

Healing fruits include green apple, sour cherry, sour oranges, and lime.

In order to ensure maximum circulation within the organ, blood cholesterol and fat content should be kept low. Therefore, no animal-derived oils are recommended, and only small amounts of vegetable oils should be used by those attempting to restore the liver. Sesame, corn, and olive oils are the most healthful. Olive oil tends to relax the liver and stimulate release of bile and toxins. Research indicates that olive oil is an antioxidant, as well. Oil should be limited to two or three times per week until health is restored.

As with all traditional medicine, only small amounts are necessary to effect healing. Also, too much of a good thing turns into its opposite: poison.

These foods will have a healing effect on the entire Wood Element, meaning that the gall bladder also will be healed by following this same program. (See gall bladder.)

Using the Five Elements, people with liver disease should increase foods associated with the Water, Wood, and Fire Elements, while decreasing Metal foods. Water (kidney and bladder) nourishes liver function. Fire (heart and small intestine) has more than likely been diminished due to the decrease in liver qi, which would ordinarily nourish the Fire Element. Metal foods control the Wood Element, and therefore should be reduced, but not entirely eliminated.

Naturopaths recognize the same disease process within the

Even as the wise physician takes full advantage of the armamentarium available to him, he never misses the opportunity to educate the patient to the truth that drugs aren't always necessary and that the human body is its own best drugstore for most symptoms.

NORMAN COUSINS

liver as that outlined above. The most common healing foods suggested by naturopaths are as follows:

- *Protein:* Low-fat protein foods should be eaten daily to include: fish, a few times per week; tofu, an excellent source of protein and calcium; a wide assortment of beans, rich sources of protein and fiber; and wheat germ, rich in protein and vitamin E, an antioxidant and a medicinal food for the liver.
- *Vegetables:* The diet should include a wide variety of leafy greens, rich in many minerals (such as calcium), vitamin A, and fiber; beets, with tops, rich in iron and fiber; spirulina, a sea vegetable, rich in minerals, B vitamins, and an antioxidant; and garlic, which is antifungal, antibacterial, and an immune-enhancing herb.
- *Fermented foods:* Miso, rich in B vitamins, healthful bacteria, and protein; sauerkraut, rich in bacteria.
- *Supplements:* Vitamin A, an antioxidant and one of the most powerful immune-enhancing vitamins available; B vitamins, immune-enhancing and essential for rebuilding tissue; folic acid, for immune response; and vitamin E, immune-enhancing and an antioxidant.

Herbs that have been used throughout the ages for liver disorders include the following:

- *Dandelion tea:* Perhaps the most commonly used herb for liver disorders since Galen. Dandelion directly neutralizes acids and stimulates the liver to cleanse the blood and eliminate waste via the bile. It also stimulates and strengthens immune response. Dandelion stems, twigs, or leaves can be boiled for ten minutes in water to make a tea. Allow herbs and water to steep for another ten or fifteen minutes and then drink two to three times per day. Use one tablespoon of twigs per cup of water.
- *Dandelion and burdock root tea:* Use twigs and stems from both herbs, boiled and steeped. Burdock is another blood purifier. It directly supports and stimulates the kidneys to cleanse the blood and eliminate waste from those organs. Make one tablespoon of each per cup of water.
- *Garlic:* Use two to four cloves of garlic in cooking daily, until symptoms abate.

• *Other Herbs:* Celandine (as drops in water or as a tea), Culler's root (as tea), goldenseal (as drops in water, or as a tea).

In *The Way of Herbs,* Michael Tierra recommends the following liver tonic, which has been traditionally used to rebuild the organ, restore function, and assist in the "recovery from hepatitis, liver sclerosis and toxicity from a bad diet."

Oregon grape root—1 part
Wild yam root—1 part
Dandelion root, raw—1 part
Licorice—¼ part (demulcent)

Simmer the herbs in distilled water for forty minutes, using three ounces of herbs in one quart of water. Refrigerate. Take two tablespoons, three to four times per day, between meals.

THE KIDNEYS

IN ORIENTAL ART—whether Indian, Chinese, or Japanese— you will see the Buddha depicted with a beautifully serene face and abnormally large ears. The message in the Buddha's face is obvious: it is the picture of bliss—gentle, yet full of vitality and compassion. This, says the artist, is the ultimate human face, the hope and the goal of humanity.

But what are we to make of those huge ears? The ears are like a pair of wings on each side of the Buddha's head. The lobes dangle around his shoulders like heavy pendulums. These are the ears of an elephant on a human being!

The answer lies hidden in the ancient Oriental art of physiognomy, the practice of reading a person's character and health in the face and body structure. Every characteristic on a person's face has meaning to the trained diagnostician, and the ears bear special significance.

To the practiced eye, they reveal, first and foremost, the constitutional or inherited strength of the kidneys. A trained physiognomist also can determine genetic strength of the circulatory, nervous, and digestive systems by examining the curves within the ear. But it is the kidneys with which the ears are most associated.

In the Orient, the kidneys are among the most revered organs because, it is said, the kidneys distribute qi throughout the body and parcel out the gifts of ancestry in the form of individual talents and life's opportunities. Whatever an individual's innate talents may be, they are believed to be housed in the kidneys, awaiting the right moment to be manifested in life. In this way, the kidneys are said to be instrumental in directing the course of a person's life, the maturation and realization of destiny. So, to care for the kidneys is to care for your very soul.

Which brings us back to Oriental art and the Buddha's ears. The Buddha's elephant ears reveal the lofty spiritual development he had attained even before he began his life. They also suggest that he had very strong kidneys.

FILTERING AND BEYOND

The urinary tract is composed of two kidneys, a bladder, two ureters, and a urethra. Each of the two ureters connects a kidney to the bladder. The urethra allows urine to pass out of the body. In the case of men, the urethra serves as a conduit for semen, as well.

We tend to think of the kidneys as the body's filter system, and indeed, that is among their important tasks. But the kidneys also identify everything that is in the blood, and then decide what to do with it. They recognize and separate waste materials from the essential elements in the blood; determine how much of a specific substance the body needs; retain that amount; and then let the rest go. And that is just the beginning.

The primary waste products that the kidneys filter are those resulting from protein metabolism, such as nitrogen, urea, and ammonia. The kidneys also eliminate excess hormones, vitamins, minerals, and foreign substances, such as food additives and drugs.

They regulate electrolyte balance, retaining more or less of the blood's supply of sodium, potassium, hydrogen, magnesium, calcium, bicarbonate, phosphate, and chloride. The quantities of these elements that are retained by the kidneys depend on the body's overall needs.

They also convert vitamin D into a usable state, a hormone. They maintain the body's acid-alkaline balance, too, by altering the acidity or alkalinity of the urine.

Blood pressure is controlled by the kidneys, as well. Depending upon the body's current blood pressure, the organs will secrete varying amounts of the enzyme renin, which converts in the blood to angiotensin. Angiotensin causes blood vessels to constrict, and thereby increase pressure. It also alerts the kidneys to retain more sodium and excrete more potassium. Sodium increases the volume of water within the body—including that within the blood—and thereby increases blood pressure.

The kidneys also produce another hormone, erythropoietin, which stimulates the body to produce more red blood cells.

When excess water is consumed, the kidneys release it; when the body needs more water they retain it. In short, the kidneys are constantly monitoring the body's overall needs, and adjusting fluid and mineral balances to meet those needs.

Remarkably, the method the kidneys use to filter the blood is not as simple as you might think. The kidneys remove the blood's constituents, separate the essential ingredients from the waste, and then reassimilate the essential parts back into the blood. The process is analogous to emptying an entire room and then putting back only what is needed.

Once it is thoroughly filtered and cleansed, the blood is collected in a holding area, called the medulla, and then allowed to continue on its journey throughout the body. The kidneys perform this task with a miraculous efficiency. About two and a half pints of blood pass through the kidneys every minute, or about 450 gallons per day.

Although we possess two kidneys, only one is necessary for life.

ANATOMY

Each kidney is about four to five inches long and weighs approximately six ounces. They stand parallel to the spine, well above the waist (not in the small of the back, as is usually believed), just behind the twelfth rib. The right kidney is below the liver, the left below the spleen; the left kidney is slightly higher than the right.

They are oval-shaped, with a slight indentation on the inside (or spinal side). Here, blood vessels, lymph glands, and nerves enter the organs. This indentation, called a hilius, is also the place from which the ureter emerges—a thin tube that allows urine to pass from the kidneys to the bladder.

Each kidney is embedded in a mass of fat, called perirenal fat, which helps support them and acts as a shock absorber. Each is kept in place by sheets of connective tissue. The kidneys touch the diaphragm and therefore move while you breathe, that is, with the expansion and contraction of the diaphragm. A tough fibrous tissue surrounds the kidneys, further protecting them from shock.

Inside, the actual filtering unit of the kidneys is called a nephron, which consists of two primary parts: The first is called a glomerulus (glomeruli is the plural), and the second a tubule. The

The Kidneys and Bladder

INFERIOR VENA CAVA

RIGHT ADRENAL

RIGHT KIDNEY

RIGHT RENAL ARTERY
AND VEIN

RIGHT URETER

MEDULLA

RENAL PELVIS

LEFT KIDNEY

LEFT RENAL ARTERY
AND VEIN

ABDOMINAL AORTA

LEFT URETER

URINARY BLADDER

URETHRA

The two kidneys, the urinary bladder, two ureters, and the urethra make up the urinary tract, filtering liquid nutrients and passing the waste out of the body.

129

glomerulus is a bulblike structure. The tubule is a long, wavy tentacle. The tubule surrounds the bulblike glomerulus and extends beyond it. Together they look like an octopus with a single long and wavy arm.

Capillaries form a complex net that intersects at various places with the tubule, allowing blood to flow back into the capillary system after it's been cleansed in the tubule.

During youth, there are more than 1 million nephrons in each kidney, but that number decreases with age. By the time you are, say, seventy, each kidney contains fewer than 250,000 nephrons, or about a quarter of its original filtering capacity. Aging, dietary poisons, and stress—with its consequent wear and tear—destroy nephrons.

The arteries that provide blood to the kidneys flow directly from the aorta, the primary artery of the body carrying oxygenated blood directly from the heart. From there it flows into the kidney's capillary system that leads to the glomeruli, where the first stage of filtration takes place.

Once inside a glomerulus, the blood is cleansed of its larger waste products. Then it passes onto the next stage of filtration, the long and looping tubules, which removes virtually everything from the blood, and decides what to put back in, and what to eliminate as urine. Most of what is reinstated to the blood is water (about 99 percent of it), amino acids, glucose, minerals, and vitamins.

Urine is composed mostly of water (about 95 percent) and about 5 percent solids, including urea (a by-product of protein metabolism, which makes up about 20 percent of solids); a variety of minerals, including chloride, sodium, potassium, phosphate, and sulfate; creatine, a naturally-occurring chemical; and a very small amount of uric acid. The presence of glucose (blood sugar) or protein in the urine indicates some form of disease. (See kidney-related illnesses, below. Also, see the chapter on the bladder.)

Once the blood is cleansed, it is temporarily held in the medulla, and then allowed to pass to the renal vein, which is the exit vessel leading to other parts of the body.

Meanwhile, the urine is sent from the tubules to the renal pelvis, which is a collecting point for urine. The renal pelvis empties into the ureter and then to the bladder.

The kidneys are vulnerable to a wide variety of disorders, including cancer, cysts, stones, impairment of the blood supply, infection, and autoimmune disorders. The kidneys also are affected when a person suffers from diabetes mellitus. Finally, the kidneys are highly vulnerable to stress, which, if chronic, can cause kidney damage and even death.

The most common form of kidney cancer is renal cell carcinoma, which affects people over the age of forty. Among the common symptoms are blood in the urine, swelling in the abdomen, fever, and weight loss. Another cancer is transitional cell carcinoma, which develops in the renal pelvis; it is most common among smokers and people who have taken painkillers for many years.

About half of the population over fifty has noncancerous fluid-filled cysts within the kidneys. Usually, these do not present any symptoms, and there is no medically known cause. Medical treatment includes draining the cysts or surgically removing them.

Kidney stones, also known as calculi, are caused by a precipitation of substances found in urine. About 70 percent of the stones found in the kidney or ureter—the most common sites—are made of calcium oxalate and/or phosphate. These are salts derived from calcium and oxalic acids.

Scientists do not know the cause of such stones, but believe that they may be due to a diet rich in oxalic acid. Foods such as spinach, rhubarb, sesame seeds, and coffee contain high amounts of oxalic acid. Scientists also speculate that such stones may be due to dehydration because they are most common in the summer months, when people tend to sweat more, lose more water, and have more concentrated urine.

Sometimes stones contain calcium, which is often a symptom of metabolic disorders and hyperparathyroidism, an illness affecting the parathyroid gland (see endocrine system). A small percentage of stones occur from chronic kidney infections; these are usually composed of calcium, magnesium, ammonium phosphate, and other minerals.

In poorer countries, where the diet is low in protein and phosphate, bladder stones are common. In developed countries, bladder stones are largely the result of urinary tract infections or an enlarged prostate gland, which prevents adequate elimination of urine. If a stone blocks the flow of urine, a severe infection can result and can cause kidney damage.

He is the best physician who is the most ingenious inspirer of hope.

SAMUEL TAYLOR
COLERIDGE

Stones are diagnosed by X rays, ultrasound, blood and urine analysis. The latter two tests may show infection; sometimes urine will reveal red blood cells—perhaps the result of some tissue damage done by the stones—or tiny crystals, which may indicate the presence of stones.

The passage of stones can be painful. Treatment includes bed rest, pain relievers, and increased liquid intake in order to encourage the stone to pass through the urinary tract. Since the majority of stones are less than one-fifth of an inch in diameter, they are usually passed easily. Larger stones may require surgery, however.

Once a stone enters the ureter or bladder, it can sometimes be removed by the insertion of a crushing device and a viewing tube. Other methods include the use of shock-wave treatments, which can disintegrate stones in the kidneys.

There are two kinds of stress: eustress, which is considered a healthful and enthusiastic response to a challenge, and distress, which is a response characterized by fear, mounting dread, and the anticipation of defeat or disaster. Distress causes a wide variety of physiological changes in the body. Among the most significant are changes in respiration; elevation of blood pressure and blood cholesterol levels; and hormonal imbalance, including the elevation of cortisol and epinephrine (adrenaline), all of which combine to have detrimental and sometimes destructive effects on the heart and kidneys. As blood pressure and cholesterol levels increase, the likelihood of glomeruli and tubule damage rises significantly. Also hormonal imbalance requires the kidneys to work harder and faster, thus putting added stress on these organs.

Doctors recommend a variety of medical therapies for stress, including high blood pressure medication; drugs to lower cholesterol; diets lower in fat and cholesterol; and relaxation techniques.

Often, depression sets in following extended stressful periods, in which case antidepressive medication and/or psychotherapy may be prescribed.

More than 90,000 people each year undergo kidney transplant surgery in which a donated kidney is used to replace a failed kidney. And more than 50,000 Americans have their blood filtered by artificial kidney machines each day.

THE SITE OF THE WILL

According to practitioners of traditional Chinese medicine, the kidneys and bladder are the paired organs that make up the Water Element and govern the body's fluid content.

The kidneys are associated with the winter months, December 21 through March 21. Though they receive optimal amounts of healing energy during this season, they are injured by too much cold. The idea is that life energy descends into the earth during winter, but bursts forth in the spring. Qi does the same thing within the human body: it descends into the lower organs during winter—the kidneys, bladder, and sex organs—but rises into the liver and eventually into the heart during spring and summer.

As in all traditional medicine, balance is the key, even for those things that have potential healing and strengthening properties. Cold weather, which is contracting, directs the energy down into the kidneys, but too much cold can injure them.

As contracted organs (they are referred to in the Yellow Emperor's Classic as "lesser yin"), the kidneys can easily become too contracted and tense, thus preventing adequate blood, qi, and fluids from flowing.

"Those who disobey the laws of Winter will suffer an injury to the kidneys," stated the Yellow Emperor. "For them Spring will bring impotence, and they will produce little." In other words, they will not be able to expand and flower in the spring.

The Yellow Emperor used the word "impotence" both literally and figuratively, for the kidneys govern the sex organs and the body's overall sexual energy. The Yellow Emperor warns that too much sexual intercourse will harm the kidneys, weaken the sex drive, and reduce the overall vitality of the body. All types of sexual dysfunction originate from kidney/bladder imbalances. Deficient kidney energy can cause a variety of sex-related disorders—from premature ejaculation to infertility and sterility. Excessive kidney energy, on the other hand, can cause excessive sex drive and obsession with sex.

While qi flows through the body, the kidneys are said to be the source of the body's overall vitality. Weakness, lethargy, and lack of endurance comes from deficient kidney energy.

The emotion most associated with the kidneys and bladder is

Traditional
Chinese
Meridians

經 腎 陰 少 足

左右五十四穴

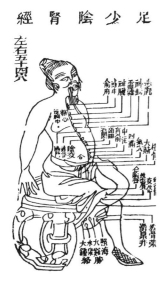

fear. People with weak kidneys will experience more fear than those with strong kidneys. Also, fear damages the kidneys and can ultimately destroy their ability to function.

The Chinese maintain that the kidneys are the site of the human will. Our ability to focus on a goal and see it through, come what may, is derived from the strength of our kidneys. If the kidneys are weak, the will is weak. Conversely, a person with strong kidneys will feel an intuitive connection with certain goals that will help him or her persevere through difficulties to see the goal's realization.

"The kidneys are like the officials who do energetic work and they excel through their ability," said the Yellow Emperor.

A person's drive to succeed is said to emanate from the kidneys. People who wish to strengthen their ambition, drive, and will are encouraged to heal their kidneys.

The kidneys draw in the breath deeply into the body. They are called the root of the breath. Interestingly, studies have shown that people who are shallow breathers are more prone to nervous tension, anxiety, and fear. Those who breathe deeply tend to be more relaxed. A Chinese healer would concur, pointing out that weak kidneys would make a person more anxiety-prone and less able to draw breath deeply into the body. Conversely, those who wish to strengthen their kidneys are advised to make a habit of deep breathing, which effectively draws qi into the kidneys, bladder, and sex organs.

Oriental healers maintain that many respiratory problems, including asthma, begin with kidney imbalance. When the kidneys are unable to draw the breath deeply into the lungs, or exhale deeply, stagnation within the lungs increases and eventually gives rise to illness.

The kidneys also rule and nourish the bones, keeping them vital, flexible, and resilient. Weak, brittle, or broken bones are, at their root, a kidney imbalance, usually resulting from deficient kidney energy or qi.

The taste associated with the kidneys and bladder is salty flavor, and the kidneys crave it. Light to moderate amounts of salt stimulate and strengthen the kidneys and bladder. Too much salt, however, can injure the kidneys, causing them to become too contracted and leading to high blood pressure.

The Yellow Emperor also warns that too much salt will cause

despondency. The Chinese maintain that excessively salty diets—or contracted life conditions—can lead to chronic depression.

Kidney energy opens into the ears, said the Yellow Emperor, meaning that kidney qi nourishes the hearing mechanism. All hearing problems, including ear infections (common in children) and hearing loss, originate from kidney imbalances (see the section on healing the kidneys, below). When kidney energy is deficient, blood and qi will be inadequate to maintain the health and vitality of the hearing mechanism. Kidney imbalance, either excess or deficient qi, can also cause ringing in the ears.

The kidneys rule the body hair. Strong, luxurious hair is a sign of strong kidneys. Conversely, split ends, broken hair, and baldness are signs of weak and (usually) deficient kidney energy. Since the kidneys rule the sex organs, unhealthy hair, especially split ends, is a sign of weak or degenerating sex organs.

Baldness occurs when the kidneys are unable to maintain proper water balance within the body. Each hair is rooted in a follicle that contains oil and water. The kidneys control the amount of water present in tissues throughout the body. When excessive amounts of water infiltrate the scalp, the hair follicles swell, allowing the hair to uproot and fall out. Hence, baldness. Hair care begins with treating the kidneys well, say the Chinese.

The kidney meridian runs upward from a point at the bottom of the foot, in the soft tissue below the ball; from there, it runs along the arch of the foot; up inside the calf and thigh; across the groin; over the stomach and the middle of the chest; to the clavicle bone. (All acupuncture meridians run in pairs, on opposite sides of the body, and are mirror images of each other.)

People with overworked and tired kidneys often suffer from weak or heavy legs. The weakness is usually perceived most acutely in the thighs.

Kidneys provide qi to the lower back area. Lower back problems, therefore, are related to kidney and bladder issues (see chapter on the bladder).

The kidneys and liver are the body's main blood-cleansing organs. When the kidneys are overworked, due to high levels of toxicity in the diet or environment, their capacity to filter the blood can be exceeded. When this occurs, the body attempts to eliminate excess waste through the skin in the form of rashes,

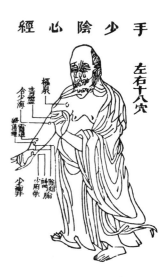

Antique Chinese drawings from Ling Shu Su Wen Chieh Yao, *a medical text compiled during the Ch'ing dynasty (1644–1912), show, left, the twenty-nine points of the kidney "vessel" or meridian and, right, the nine points of the heart meridian.*

135

pimples, and acne. As toxicity lowers to a level that the kidneys can handle, such rashes and blemishes disappear.

The kidneys receive optimal amounts of qi energy between 5 P.M. and 7 P.M. The bladder receives its peak qi from 3 P.M. to 5 P.M. Weakness or fatigue at these hours can indicate a kidney imbalance.

THE GIFT OF THE ANCESTORS

The kidneys are said to contain the gift of the ancestors, meaning that from the kidneys your life and spiritual path unfold. The kidneys possess the talents, abilities, and special gifts with which you entered the world. Your unique purpose is locked within the spiritual qi of these organs, awaiting the right moment to manifest. In this way, the kidneys are said to be responsible for maturation.

Interestingly, this corresponds with many Western and Eastern spiritual traditions, which have maintained that the true gift of heaven comes not from above, but from below. In Kundalini yoga, for example, the divine and primary energy flows upward from the base of the spine (from the area of the kidneys) to the brain, where the person receives self-knowledge, or illumination. The Gnostic traditions are founded upon a similar understanding that spiritual awakenings emerge from deep within, rather than from outside the self.

Our ability to focus on a goal and see it through to its completion determines, to a great extent, the degree of success we experience in life. Completion is not only the foundation of success, but the basis for healthy psychological and spiritual development. The kidneys play a vital role in this process, and therefore were revered among Orientals throughout the East.

HEALING THE KIDNEYS

Generally speaking, there are three essential kidney conditions: overly contracted and excessive; overly expanded and deficient; and balanced.

Foods that cause the contraction of the kidneys are salt and fatty foods, especially hard fats from red meat and hard cheese.

Eggs also cause the kidneys to contract and become excessive. So, too, does chronic fear or stress. Such foods and life conditions cause the capillaries, glomeruli, and tubules to contract. This prevents adequate blood, oxygen, and qi from flowing through the organs and causes accumulation of toxins and the degeneration of tissues. Stagnation and accumulation can lead to urinary tract infections, which, in the case of the kidneys, can be very dangerous.

Before such problems arise, however, a variety of less severe symptoms emerge. These include excessive sex drive, restless sleep, and grinding of teeth while asleep. Children often grind their teeth at night as a result of excessive kidney energy, which manifests during the day as frustration. Contracted kidneys also give rise to poor blood circulation, and cold hands and feet.

Eventually, these conditions will turn into their opposite: they will exhaust the kidneys and create deficient kidney energy. This is particularly true of stress, which, if not dealt with properly, can lead to chronic fatigue, despondency, and depression. In short, the loss of will.

Weak or expanded kidneys are the cause of another set of problems: excessive fear, anxiety, and depression; weak sex drive or no sex drive at all; poor circulation, including cold hands and feet; lack of will, ambition, or drive; inability to complete things and a general lack of direction. Deficient kidney energy can cause ringing in the ears, ear infections, and bedwetting in children.

Adequate water intake is important to healthy kidneys. There is no rule that can be followed by everyone for appropriate daily liquid intake. In general, we should drink when thirsty. However, we also should be aware of the body's need for clean, pure water, which is commonly forgotten by most of us today. The body's reaction to the first few sips of water is subtle, but revealing. Often, the body responds with such enthusiasm for pure water that we are suddenly awakened to its need, which we may have been unaware of before. This reveals the necessity of being conscious of our own physical needs, for which there is no hard rule that can substitute. We should consciously drink small amounts of clean water daily; the amount is up to you. Let your body guide you by its reaction to the water, and the frequency of urination, to determine how much water you need.

In Chinese medicine, beans are the most effective healing food for the kidneys. Beans strengthen and support kidney function and promote healing. Common beans include: aduki, black beans, chickpeas, green and red lentils, navy beans, mung beans, limas, and split peas.

Small amounts of salt tonify the kidneys, but too much salt can cause kidney damage. Use only a pinch of salt in cooking—usually the tip of a teaspoon (less than one-eighth teaspoon) is necessary to cook two to three cups of grain. Also, avoid adding salt at the table. Salt is essential in cooking grain because it opens the grain and makes it digestible.

The grain that promotes kidney function and healing most is barley.

Small amounts of salted fermented foods, such as pickles, miso, tamari, shoyu, and sauerkraut, enhance kidney function and promote healing. But these foods can also cause the kidneys to contract and stagnate if used excessively. (About one-quarter teaspoon of miso is all that is necessary for a single serving of miso soup.) Tamari and shoyu should be used only in cooking, not added to foods at the table.

For excessively contracted kidneys, watermelon and watermelon tea promote urination and elimination of waste. Watermelon relaxes the kidneys. Watermelon tea can be made by grinding dried watermelon seeds, boiling them in water, and steeping them.

Other fruits that are helpful to the kidneys include grapes (to promote urination), blackberries, blueberries, and cranberries.

According to traditional medicine, kidney stones form for several reasons:

- Overly contracted kidneys, due primarily to excess salt, fat, and cholesterol.
- Insufficient amounts of liquid intake, especially pure water.
- Excessive intake of foods rich in oxalic acid, particularly spinach, rhubarb, Swiss chard, beet tops, chocolate, and coffee.
- Refined flour and sugar, low in B vitamins, calcium, and other minerals, but rich in fat.
- Chronic stress.
- Chronic overwork, which can cause kidney fatigue and exhaustion, preventing adequate elimination of toxins.

To heal the kidneys, Oriental medicine advocates a diet low in fat and cholesterol, with only small or moderate amounts of salt.

The diet should include regular amounts of barley (two to three times per week); daily portions of beans; small amounts of sea vegetables; a variety of vegetables daily; fish; fruit; and pure water. In addition, the following foods, drinks, and preparations are recommended for kidney and bladder problems.

- *Daikon root:* This long, white radish is reputed to melt fat deposits and stones and help to eliminate stagnation from tissues throughout the body. There are two daikon drinks that serve different functions.

  To encourage urination and elimination, grate two to three tablespoons of fresh daikon into a cheesecloth sack; squeeze the sack so that daikon juice falls into a cup. Pour boiled water into the cup; add one to two drops of shoyu or tamari. Drink twice a day. Another drink is prepared as follows: Grate one to two tablespoons of daikon radish into a cup; pour hot water into the cup; add two drops of tamari or shoyu. Drink once or twice a day. This drink is reputed to dissolve blockages and stones in kidneys.

- *Burdock root:* A hardy, medicinal food, revered by Chinese, European, and American healers for many centuries. Considered one of the strongest blood purifiers in the entire herb kingdom, burdock is used for a wide variety of disorders, but is generally recognized as one of the best herbs for breaking down and eliminating waste products from metabolism. In Chinese medicine, it is regarded as a strengthening herb for the entire urinary tract and sex organs. Pressure-cook sliced burdock for fifteen minutes with sliced carrots and kombu seaweed in about one and a half inches of water.

- *Burdock tea:* Detoxifies the blood; stimulates and tonifies kidneys and bladder; and eliminates waste and stagnation within kidneys. Boil one to two tablespoons of stems, twigs, and leaves in one cup of water; steep for ten minutes and drink two to three times per day.

- *Basil:* This herb can be used in cooking and boiled in water to make a tea; it strengthens the kidneys.

In *The Way of Herbs,* Michael Tierra recommends the following herbal remedy for kidney stones.

Gravel root—2 parts
Parsley root—2 parts
Marshmallow root—2 parts
Lobelia—$\frac{1}{2}$ part
Ginger root—$\frac{1}{2}$ part

"Simmer two ounces [of these herbs] per quart of water for about an hour until the liquid is reduced by half," writes Tierra. "Add an equal volume of vegetable glycerin [about two ounces] to preserve."

In addition to the above-mentioned recommendations, naturopaths also suggest the following herbs and supplements for kidney and bladder disorders, including stones.

- *Vitamins:* A; B complex; B6; C and E.
- *Minerals:* Magnesium.
- *Herbs:* Bearberry tea, to ease passage of stones; chamomile tea, to dissolve stones; yarrow tea, also to dissolve stones; hydrangea decoction (bark of herb boiled for an hour in water), reputed to dissolve stones; nettle, leaves and roots infusion (add nettle leaves to water that's already been boiled and then allow it to steep for about twenty minutes; tightly cover pot top while steeping). Nettle, one of the most revered herbs in Europe and the Middle East, contains a variety of minerals and vitamins, all of which combine to strengthen immune function. Nettle is reputed to dissolve stones and eliminate blockages.

CHAPTER 13

THE BLADDER

THE BLADDER HOLDS URINE, the liquid waste of the body, and releases it when it's full. Most people's bladders can hold up to a pint of urine, which is produced in the kidneys and flows downward through two tubes, called ureters. The average person urinates from three to eight times per day. Greater frequency can suggest any one of several possible problems, including excessive intake of fluids, urinary infection, or diabetes.

Up to the age of three to four, children have no control over their bladders. When a child's bladder is full, nerves within the walls of the bladder send a signal to the spinal cord, which relays a message back to urinate. Maturity brings with it development of the nervous system, which allows the brain to intercede in this process. When the bladder signals that it is full, the brain can tell the bladder to wait. Hence, the familiar sense of discomfort, without an untimely elimination.

The bladder is a muscular, spherically shaped sac, located in the lower part of the body directly behind the pubic bone, within the pelvis. The bladder is lined with a mucous membrane and has walls composed of three layers of tough muscle. These muscles give the bladder its ability to expand as it is filled and contract dur-

Human beings seem less capable of being healthy the more they believe they have to be healthy.

ALFRED J. ZIEGLER

141

ing elimination. At the back wall of the bladder are the entrances of the two ureters from the kidneys. Each ureter opening is covered with valvelike folds of skin, which prevent urine from flowing back into the ureters.

The bladder narrows at the bottom. There, at its base, is the entrance to the urethra, the tube from which the urine flows outside the body. There are circular sphincter muscles located inside and outside the area where the urethra joins the bladder. In men, the urethra passes through the prostate, which sits directly below the bladder. The prostate produces seminal fluid, which is expelled during ejaculation. Inside the prostate, the urethra has two ducts that open to the prostate, allowing semen to flow from the prostate, down along the urethra and out the penis. During urination, of course, these ducts are closed. The urethra is approximately eight to nine inches long in men, and about an inch and a half long in women.

As the bladder fills with urine, the walls expand and send nerves impulses to the brain, via the spinal cord, alerting you to the need to urinate. If you give the okay, nervous impulses from the brain order the smooth muscles surrounding the urethra to relax, allowing it to open. Next, the external sphincter is ordered to relax. Then the internal sphincter gets the same message, while the muscles within the bladder walls are ordered to contract. The bladder will continue to contract until all the urine has been expelled. It is common to hold the breath when urinating, while at the same time pushing down with the diaphragm and contracting the abdomen muscles. This puts more pressure on the bladder to eliminate.

The bladder and urethra are held in place by a group of muscles called the pelvic floor that extend from the pubis to the tail bone. The pelvic floor includes the sphincter muscles of the anus. In women, these muscles also control the vagina and support the developing fetus during pregnancy.

Illnesses of the Bladder

The most common illnesses affecting the bladder are urinary tract infections, incontinence, and stones. In men, bladder problems also arise with disorders of the prostate. Urinary tract illnesses can involve any of the urinary organs, including the kidneys, ureters, bladder, or urethra, but most often affect the bladder (an infection called cystitis) or the urethra (called urethritis). Bacteria, which are normally present in small quantities in both the urethra and the bladder, can increase and cause infections.

Women tend to suffer urinary tract infections far more frequently than men because their urethras are shorter than mens'. The shorter urethra makes it easier for bacteria to travel up into the bladder and multiply. Also, it is easier for bacteria to pass from the intestines to the urethra in women because of the close proximity of the anus.

There are numerous other causes of urinary tract infections. In general, anything that prevents full elimination of urine from the bladder and urethra will increase the likelihood of bacterial buildup and infection. Common causes include injury to the urethra or bladder, causing inflammation, which can impair full elimination of urine; swelling of the urethra from sexual intercourse (most common in women); kidney or urethra stones; pregnancy; irritants present in bubble baths, douches, feminine sprays, or diaphragms; vaginitis; congenital abnormalities of the urethra or some other part of the urinary tract; prostate enlargement or inflammation; psychological stress; and the use of a catheter during medical tests or surgery. If the infection spreads to the kidneys, serious illness can result.

Symptoms of urinary tract infection include frequent urination, with only small amounts of urine being expelled; burning or stinging pain during urination; fever; and discomfort in the lower abdomen. Occasionally, there are chills or a foul smell to the urine.

One of the few dietary treatments that doctors will recommend is to encourage patients with urinary tract infections to drink cranberry juice, which makes the urine more acidic and thus less supportive of bacteria. Doctors also may tell patients to consume large quantities of liquids. This causes frequent urination, which will help flush bacteria from the urinary tract. Of course, frequently doctors also will prescribe antibiotics to kill bacteria and stop infection.

There are several types of incontinence, but the most common is stress incontinence, suffered mostly by women past their childbearing years. Stress incontinence occurs when small amounts of urine are released while coughing, laughing, or lifting a heavy object. Other forms of incontinence include urge in-

In the final analysis, the survival and health of the individual and [the] species may depend not so much on further developments in technology as on the collective application of common sense.

S. BRYAN FURNASS

continence, in which the need to urinate is accompanied by the inability to withhold urine, or when changes in sitting positions trigger a sudden release; and total incontinence, which is the complete inability to prevent elimination. Women far outnumber men in incidence of incontinence.

There are a variety of causes of incontinence, including nervous system disorders, such as multiple sclerosis; injury to the nervous system, brain, bladder, or pelvis; urinary infection; stones; and anger, stress, or anxiety. By far, the most common cause is weakened sphincter and pelvic floor muscles, which occurs in many women after pregnancy and childbirth. During pregnancy, the growing baby puts pressure on the pelvic floor muscles. If prenatal and postnatal exercises are not performed, these muscles can become stretched and weakened, causing the pelvic floor to sag. This allows the bladder and urethra to reposition themselves inappropriately, preventing adequate control of the bladder. Being overweight can further weaken the pelvic floor and contribute to incontinence. After menopause, hormonal changes can cause these and other muscles to degenerate, thus further exacerbating the problem and causing incontinence in older women.

Dr. Arnold Kegel, a professor of obstetrics and gynecology at UCLA, created a set of exercises for preventing and treating incontinence. They're now widely taught at childbirth classes and have helped millions of women to regain control of the muscles that control urination. Here are the basic steps:

1. Practice controlling the bladder by slowing urine flow and then stopping it. When you are able to stop the flow, hold it one or two seconds. Do this six or eight times as you urinate. You may have to do this exercise numerous times before you are able to stop the flow entirely, but eventually you will be able to control the flow without leakage. Practice relaxing and contracting the pelvic floor muscles, as well.

2. Practice relaxing and contracting the same muscles used in exercise 1 throughout the day. Hold the contraction for several seconds and then relax. Do this exercise anywhere from fifty to 100 times per day, and repeat exercise 1 when urinating.

3. Contract the pelvic floor during love-making.

In general, exercises that strengthen the abdomen will help to restore strength and control to the pelvic floor, as well.

FEAR, STRESS, AND CONTRACTION

Like the kidneys, the bladder is associated with the winter months in Chinese medicine. It is said to store the overflow of the kidneys, meaning that it stores the urine. The bladder responds to the same Water Element foods and herbs as those mentioned for the kidneys, including beans, barley, and a mild salty flavor. In the same way, the bladder is easily affected by fear and stress. Thus, maintaining calm and centeredness in difficult situations strengthens bladder function.

In general, bladder problems arise from an excess of contraction. In men, the prostate can become inflamed or contracted, causing the contraction of the urethra, which prevents full elimination of the bladder. Too much salt can cause bladder and kidney problems in both sexes, and thus prevent adequate elimination of urine.

The bladder meridian is long and complex, beginning at the inside corner of the eye and running down along the spine and the back of the leg to the foot. Since it provides qi to the spinal column, back problems are said to be related to the health of the bladder and its meridians. When the kidneys and bladder are strong, the spinal column is also strong and healthy. Back problems emerge, however, when bladder and kidney function are troubled. Given that stress powerfully affects the Water Element organs, Chinese healers say that no one should be surprised that back problems are so prevalent in modern society.

The placement of the bladder meridian is interesting because it is exposed and stretched somewhat whenever you sit down on the toilet, thus positioning the body so that the downward motion of qi will enhance the act of elimination. All rashes, blemishes, or skin eruptions along the bladder meridian are associated with the inefficient elimination of waste from the kidneys and bladder.

Urine can be a useful diagnostic tool to help determine whether you are drinking too much fluid or eating too much salt. Ideally, urine should be pale yellow in color, with only a mild

Health is the normal and harmonious vibration of the elements and forces composing the human entity on the physical, mental and moral (emotional) planes of being, in conformity with the constructive principle (great law of life) in nature.

HENRY LINDLAHR

odor. In general, the more liquid and expansive foods one consumes (such as fruits, sugar, and alcohol), the more clear the urine will be. Conversely, the more salt, fat, and animal foods you consume, the darker the urine will be. The kidneys must work harder to eliminate these waste products from the blood. Because they are emerging in sufficient quantities to color the urine, they suggest a greater possibility of kidney and bladder stone formation. For this reason, people with dark urine should drastically reduce salt and animal foods.

Healing the bladder calls for increasing Water Element foods, such as those good for the kidneys, as well as Metal and Wood. Especially helpful to the bladder are aduki beans, burdock, barley, and buckwheat. Consume only pure water or mild teas. Aromatic teas are highly expansive and tend to require more effort from the kidneys to eliminate. Also increase mineral-rich foods, such as leafy green vegetables, carrots, and other roots. Particularly helpful are small amounts of sea vegetables (one to two tablespoon servings per day) such as kelp, nori, wakame, and arame. Useful fruits include watermelon, blueberry, blackberry, cranberry, and grapes (all in moderation).

Kidney and bladder infections are caused by a decrease in circulation and elimination, often due to a diet rich in fat, sugar, and cholesterol. To heal bladder infections, avoid fatty foods and those rich in cholesterol, sugar, and artificial ingredients. Increase foods rich in beta carotene, such as carrots, broccoli, squash, and collard greens. Also increase foods rich in vitamin E, such as whole grains (especially whole wheat), and vitamin C, such as tangerines and broccoli. Increase foods rich in minerals, especially zinc (grains and seafoods). Mineral-rich foods include all leafy greens, sea vegetables, grains, and fish.

The following teas can help to strengthen the bladder and immune system to ward off infection:

Boil one to two tablespoons of burdock stems, twigs, and leaves in two cups of water and drink two or three times per day.

Boil one to two tablespoons of echinacea twigs in two cups of water and drink two times per day. Or take fifteen to thirty drops of echinacea in water or kukicha tea, two times daily until infection is eliminated. Echinacea is among the most powerful natural antibiotics in the plant kingdom.

CHAPTER 14

THE HEART

No ORGAN HAS been the focus of more emotion, mythology, and technological wizardry than the human heart. We have given it credit for our greatest achievements, and blamed it for our darkest deeds. No other organ has been invested with so much meaning. It has been said that the heart is the inspiration for poetry, sacrifice, war, and peace. It is the source of love and hate, good and evil, courage and cowardice. The heart is the king of the body, the most human of all our parts.

It has always been so. The Bible asserts that the heart is the seat of the psyche, the place in which our true nature exists. "For God sees not as man sees, for man looks at the outward appearance, but the Lord looks at the heart" (1 Samuel 16:7).

It is the source of feeling, tenderness, and love. A broken heart is perhaps the saddest of all human experiences, with the possible exception of death. In fact, the former often precedes the latter. Wrote one rabbi in the Talmud: "I can tolerate any illness, any pain, but not heart pain . . ."

Even today, we consider the heart the place of truth. "He spoke from his heart," we often report when someone says something sincere and honest. The list goes on: an open heart, a deceit-

With what words will you describe this heart, so as not to fill a book . . . ?

LEONARDO DA VINCI

ful heart, a cruel heart, a tender heart, my heart is heavy, I love you with all my heart. These are just a few of the common expressions used to describe something deep and true about human experience. Words are clues to the psyche. Clearly, the heart has come to symbolize the truest part of our being.

The physical workings of the heart have been studied since antiquity, beginning with the ancient Egyptians, whom the early Christians believed had discovered all the secrets of anatomy. In fact, none of the earlier anatomists, including Aristotle, Galen, Avicenna, and Hippocrates, fully understood the workings of the heart. All of them maintained that the heart had only two chambers, and no one understood how blood got from the right chamber to the left. Galen said that it passed through tiny holes in the septum, the muscular barrier that separates the two sides of the heart.

In the sixteenth century, Michael Servetus, a philosopher and anatomist, wrote *The Seven Books of Mistaken Conception of the Trinity,* in which he correctly described how blood travels from the right side of the heart to the lungs, and then from the lungs to the left side of the heart. Unfortunately, his book included certain heretical statements about the unity of God and the oneness of creation. Thinking he might be able to influence Christian doctrine, Servetus sealed his own fate by sending the treatise to John Calvin, the religious zealot who, after reading the work, had Servetus tracked down, arrested, and then sentenced to death.

Upon hearing the court order him to be burned at the stake, Servetus did not plead for his life, but for the life of his convictions. "I fear that through excess of suffering I may prove faithless to myself and belie the convictions of my life," he told Calvin and the court. "If I have erred, it was in ignorance; I am so constituted mentally and morally to desire the glory of God."

Calvin tried to have every copy of Servetus's book burned with him, but three or four survived, one of which is in the National Library of Paris. Servetus's death, which occurred on October 27, 1553, put science back another seventy-five years, for it would not be until 1628 that the truth would surface again, this time in England, thanks to one of the giants of medical history.

That year William Harvey, a British doctor, published a book entitled *On the Motion of the Heart and Blood,* in which he accurately described the workings of the heart and circulation of the blood. Harvey's book revealed some of the difficulties of un-covering coronary circulation, which he studied by vivisection, and why the heart remained a mystery so long. "I found the task [of studying the heart] so truly arduous," wrote Harvey, "so full of difficulties, that I was almost tempted to think . . . that the motion of the heart was only to be comprehended by God. For I could neither rightly perceive at first when the systole and when the diastole took place, nor when and where dilation and contrac-tion occurred, by reason of the rapidity of the motion, which in many animals is accomplished in the twinkling of an eye, coming and going like a flash of lightning; so that the systole presented itself to me now from this point, now from that; the diastole the same; and then everything reversed . . ."

No one was sure why the blood went to the lungs in the first place. Galen had said that the blood derived "air" and "natural spirits" from the lungs, which was as far as anyone had come to explaining oxygen. It wasn't until the seventeenth century that oxygen was discovered (it was called "dephlogisticated air") and not until the eighteenth century that it was named oxygen by French chemist and doctor Antonie Laurent Lavoisier.

And then there was the question of the heart's sounds. The ac-tual beating of the heart appeared to physicians as a mysterious and indecipherable language. No one knew what to make of that familiar "lubb, dubb" until 1816, when Rene Theophile Laennec, a French physician, made a serendipitous discovery while exam-ining an overweight woman who was suffering from tubercu-losis. Modesty prevented him from placing his ear against the woman's breast, so Laennec rolled up a piece of paper and placed it near the woman's heart. "I was surprised and gratified," he later wrote, "to find that I could thereby perceive the action of the heart in a manner much more clear and distinct than I had ever been able to do by the immediate application of the ear."

Laennec, of course, had invented the stethoscope, albeit a pa-per one. He then produced a series of more elaborate wooden tubes, and began to study the sounds of the heart and their meaning. His masterwork, *Del'Auscultation,* which appeared in 1819, described the diagnostic meaning of various heart sounds, as well as the percussive sounds heard when a physician taps on a patient's back.

Laennec, who suffered from tuberculosis and eventually died

The Heart

A fist-sized double-pump that's also cited as the seat of the soul, the heart is truly a marvel of marvels that is still only partially understood after decades of close scientific study.

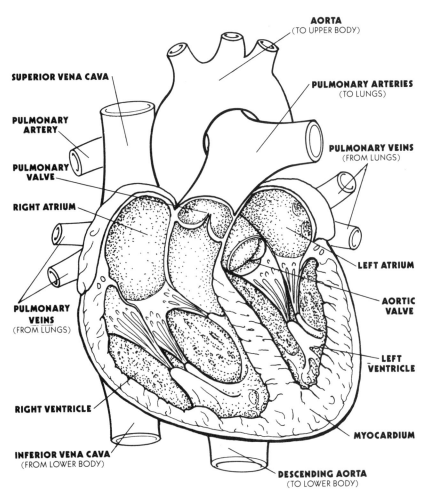

AORTA
(TO UPPER BODY)

SUPERIOR VENA CAVA

PULMONARY ARTERIES
(TO LUNGS)

PULMONARY ARTERY

PULMONARY VEINS
(FROM LUNGS)

PULMONARY VALVE

RIGHT ATRIUM

LEFT ATRIUM

AORTIC VALVE

PULMONARY VEINS
(FROM LUNGS)

LEFT VENTRICLE

RIGHT VENTRICLE

MYOCARDIUM

INFERIOR VENA CAVA
(FROM LOWER BODY)

DESCENDING AORTA
(TO LOWER BODY)

from the disease, gave the world its first heart instrument, as well as the word "stethoscope," which he derived from the Greek words *stethos,* meaning chest, and *scope,* to examine. Today electrocardiograms measure the electrical impulses coming from the heart (see anatomy and physiology of the heart, below); angiography, in which a radioactive dye is inserted into the coronary arteries and the heart itself, determines the extent to which the vessels are closed by cholesterol plaque; heart valves can be replaced; machines can take over the functions of the heart and lungs, pumping and oxygenating blood during surgery; and hearts can be transplanted from one person to another. All of this attention testifies to the value we place on this essential organ.

Meanwhile, research goes on. The Jarvik 7 mechanical heart, which was first used in humans in 1985, is a steel and plastic device that has proven a failure as a replacement for the real thing, though it has been used to keep people alive for short periods while they await a donor heart. Heart transplantation was first attempted in humans in 1967 by South African physician Dr. Christiaan Barnard. The early patients died shortly after the operations, but in 1984, a team of Stanford University physicians, led by Dr. Norman Shumway, showed that more than half of those who received heart transplants could survive up to a year.

There are a number of problems that have prevented heart transplants from becoming more widely used. The first, of course, is the tremendous difficulty of providing live hearts. Another is that the human body's immune system recognizes the new heart as a foreign object and attacks it, thus preventing the organ from surviving inside the body. Scientists point out that many cardiac patients are in need of a donated heart because coronary heart disease, the leading cause of death in the Western world, has destroyed their own. That illness is often caused by a high-fat and cholesterol diet, the typical regimen consumed in the West. In other words, it is entirely preventable by adopting the low-fat and low-cholesterol diet traditionally consumed by humans.

This brings us full circle, historically speaking. We know a lot more about the heart than the ancients did, but they probably took better care of their hearts than we do today. Indeed, many of the ancient ways of eating and living are proving to be the best medicine the heart can get.

NOT ONE BUT TWO PUMPS

The heart beats between sixty and eighty times per minute in most of us, or about 100,000 times a day. Assuming that you are in good health and will live to be sixty-five or seventy, your heart will beat some 2.5 billion times during the course of your life.

While your body is at rest, your heart pumps about a sixth of a pint of blood per beat, or about twelve pints per minute. While exercising, it will race at about 200 beats per minute and pump a

*In the midst of this machine
we call a body, nothing is more
orderly and reliable than the
heart. Its complex workings
have challenged brilliant medical minds for four hundred
years. But like every other
part of the body, the heart is
just empty space when you get
down to it. The "real" heart
is not this tough bundle of
twitching muscles that beats
3 billion times before it expires
but the organizing power that
pulls it together, that creates a
thing out of nothingness.*

DEEPAK CHOPRA

half pint per beat, or 100 pints per minute. Your entire blood supply passes through your heart every sixty seconds. The left and
right sides of the heart pump blood in two different directions.
During the average day, each side pumps approximately 2,000
gallons, or 50 million gallons in a lifetime.

To say that the heart is a marvel of marvels would be to describe this wondrous organ in understatement. No other part of
the body is more appreciated by us all. Yet, our appreciation is
meager in comparison to wonders performed by this miraculous
organ.

The heart is about the size of a man's fist. It is shaped like an
inverted cone, at the top of which is a network of blood vessels
that allows blood to flow to and from the heart. It is located in the
center of the chest, just behind the sternum, and tilts slightly to
the left.

Most of us think of the heart as a pump, but in fact it is two
pumps, a left and a right, that work in a precisely coordinated
fashion. Each pump sends blood to different parts of the body.
Yet, both must act in complete harmony in order for us to go on
living.

Another common misconception about the heart is that it has
only two phases—diastole (expansion) and systole (contraction).
In fact, the heart has three phases: The first is diastole—the moment it relaxes and allows blood to enter the upper chambers, or
both atria; the second is atrial systole, when both upper chambers
contract, sending blood into the lower chambers, or ventricles;
and the third is ventricle systole, when the lower chambers contract, sending blood to its respective destinations.

Blood enters the right atrium through the superior vena cava,
a large vessel that brings blood from all over the body, and a
smaller vessel called the coronary sinus, which brings blood back
to the heart from the heart muscle itself. The blood that enters the
right atrium is filled with carbon dioxide, having already ex-
changed its oxygen for carbon dioxide with cells throughout
the body.

After the blood enters the right ventricle, it is pumped to the
lungs via the pulmonary artery. Once in the lungs, the blood surrenders its carbon dioxide load and receives a new infusion of oxygen. We breathe out that carbon dioxide and inhale more oxygen.

Thanks to the heart's relentless beat—which forces blood to

move continuously through the body—the blood passes out of the lungs and onward to the left side of the heart, where it enters the left atrium during expansion phase (diastole), and the left ventricle during atrial systole.

From here, it is pumped into the aorta, the main highway for oxygenated blood leaving the heart. Now it is on its way to your cells.

Pumping blood through the lungs is easier than pumping it through the body's general circulation because there is more resistance in the circulatory system than there is through the lungs. Consequently, the left side of the heart is stronger and more heavily muscled than the right.

Despite the fact that the left and right sides of the heart have distinctly different tasks—one requiring greater effort than the other—the two must work in complete coordination, filling and contracting simultaneously, otherwise there would be chaos and death.

The beating of the heart is life itself. How it manages this miraculous feat is only partly understood. As far as science can ascertain, there are four main factors responsible for the heart beat: the first is the heart's unique cells which, by design, contract and expand; the second is electrical stimulation; the third is the body's nervous system; and the fourth is chemical or hormonal. Other factors, such as body heat, play a role, but these four are the primary influences.

The nature of the cardiac muscle is to expand and contract, and it is inherent in its smallest part, the cells themselves. This is true in humans and in many animals: if you remove the heart of a frog or a turtle and keep it in a saline solution, it will continue to beat, despite the fact that it is no longer connected to the body. In a human fetus, the heart begins to contract and expand before it is connected to the nervous system. Even heart cells, when grown in test-tube cultures, will carry on their own primordial dance, contracting and expanding rhythmically to a music only they can hear.

Indeed, the heart is the ultimate dancer. Unlike other muscles within the body—which can go into sustained contraction, causing cramps or spasms—the heart muscle does not go out of rhythm, unless it is changed by electric shock, trauma, or lack of oxygen.

The heart is an electrical pump, or as we said earlier, two electrical pumps working together. Electrical impulses are conducted by a series of muscle fibers. These impulses are initiated by the Sinoatrial node (SA), which sits above the right atrium, near the entrance of the superior vena cava. The SA node, which is also called the pacemaker, fires a charge that flows through the atria and down to the septum. There, another node, called the Atrioventrical node (AV), fires a second charge, which passes through a bundle of fibers (called the bundle of His) that branch through the two ventricles, thus causing them to contract.

The impulses occur with precise timing. The SA node causes the atria to contract, thus sending blood to the ventricles. At the moment the atria contract, the ventricles must be relaxed and open to receive the blood. Thus, there must be a time lapse between the firing of the SA node and the AV node, to allow ventricles to pause and remain open. Once the ventricles are filled, the AV node sends an impulse to the ventricles to contract and expel blood.

Heart rate is also controlled by a part of the nervous system called the cardiac center, located in the lower part of the brain (called the medulla oblongata). For the most part, heart rate is automatic, as described above, but nerve impulses will decrease or increase the heart rate, depending on whether we are resting or in a state of excitation.

When resting, the cardiac center will send a signal over the vagus nerve to inhibit the heart beat, thus slowing it down. When we are about to exercise, and then during exercise, the cardiac center will prevent vagus-inhibition, and instead signal acceleration of the heart beat. This occurs because muscles throughout the body need more blood and oxygen to function during exercise.

The nervous system also will increase heart rate when we are afraid (the so-called flight or fight reaction), angry, sexually aroused, or experiencing some other highly charged emotional state.

The final method of controlling heart beat is hormonal or chemical. When emotionally or physically excited, the adrenal glands will pump out norepinephrine and epinephrine, increasing heart speed; the thyroid will secrete thyroxine, which speeds metabolism and heart rate; and the nervous system will release norepinephrine. When the state of excitement has passed, the cardiac center stimulates the vagus nerve to slow down the heart rate. The nervous system will secrete acetylcholine, which inhibits the speed of the beat.

Emotions and the Heart

One of the great ironies of heart research is that modern science is proving just how closely connected the emotions are to the health and function of the heart. An emerging science, called psycho-neuroimmunology, demonstrates that emotional states dramatically change heart rate and function, the health of our arteries, and our immune response.

The heart is the root of life.

The Yellow Emperor

Science is proving that the Biblical axiom, "A merry heart doeth good like a medicine," is more than folk wisdom. Laughter and joy are among the most powerful means of preventing heart attacks and other serious illnesses. The heart is particularly susceptible to stress and depression. Stress elevates cholesterol level, which causes atherosclerosis, a disease in which cholesterol plaque builds within the arteries—especially the coronary arteries—and blocks blood flow to the heart. Stress also changes hormonal balance, increasing norepinephrine and other hormones that increase heart rate, causing the heart muscle to require greater amounts of oxygen. By increasing cholesterol plaque, which blocks blood flow and oxygen to the heart, and creating greater demands for oxygen, stress can lead to heart attack. In short, our emotions affect our hearts directly and dramatically.

But the reverse is also true. Studies have shown that people who undergo coronary bypass surgery experience a marked decline in memory, ability to reason, and emotional life. Depression and mood changes are common among those who undergo bypass surgery, even more than a year after the surgery has been performed, according to a team of European and American scientists led by Dr. Allan Willner, of Jewish Medical Center at Long Island, New York. Scientists are baffled by this phenomenon, but theorize that perhaps some changes in brain chemistry take place during or after heart surgery.

When we consider the heart's remarkable ability to react to differing degrees of stress; the fact that the left and right sides of the heart must perform entirely different chores, requiring different degrees of torque behind the blood; and that the whole job is performed over a lifetime, we can only marvel at this organ.

HEARTACHES AND PAIN

There are a variety of illnesses that afflict the heart, but most of them manifest in a relatively small number of people. Among the less common forms of heart disease are the following:

- Birth defect, in which a structural abnormality occurs during gestation; this is usually dealt with by surgery.
- Endocarditis, or infection of the heart, afflicting some drug addicts and a minority of those who have had rheumatic fever.
- Cardiomyopathy, in which the heart muscle becomes increasingly weak, due to infection, alcohol abuse, chemical toxicity, autoimmune disorders, or a deficiency of minerals and vitamins, especially B1.
- Alcohol abuse, which can cause the heart muscle to swell and result in heart failure.
- Obesity, which can give rise to a number of heart-related illnesses, including high blood pressure, diabetes, and atherosclerosis.

Most of these are treated by removing the toxic agent, such as alcohol or chemical poisons, or by antibiotics.

Serious as these illnesses are, they are not the most common form of heart disease. That distinction is reserved for one illness above all the rest: atherosclerosis. Approximately 60 million Americans suffer from cardiovascular disease, or illnesses of the heart and arteries. These illnesses include heart attack, stroke, and high blood pressure. The underlying cause of most cardiovascular disease is atherosclerosis, a disease in which cholesterol plaque clogs the arteries leading to the heart and other organs. If the plaque becomes large enough, it can prevent adequate amounts of blood and oxygen from getting to tissues, including the heart and brain, and thereby cause a heart attack or stroke, either of which can be fatal.

Atherosclerosis is responsible for approximately 800,000 deaths per year in the U.S., and is the leading cause of death in the Western world. Bypass surgery is among the most common surgical procedures performed in the United States. More than 350,000 heart bypasses are conducted each year.

Cholesterol is a waxy substance, classified as a lipid, which is used by the body to make hormones and various cell components.

It is also a constituent of bile. All cells make cholesterol, but the liver produces most of it. The body makes cholesterol from fat and/or cholesterol that comes from your diet.

We often hear about two kinds of cholesterol: LDL, for low-density lipoprotein; and HDL, for high-density lipoprotein. Actually, LDL and HDL are not cholesterol, but proteins that carry cholesterol to different places in the body. LDL brings cholesterol to the walls of arteries, where it forms cholesterol plaque. This plaque resembles a boil growing inside the blood vessel. It is often capped by a hard, fibrous surface. Eventually, the boil can become so large as to block the flow of blood to organs, such as the heart or brain. When part of the heart does not receive adequate blood and oxygen, it suffocates and dies, an event typically referred to as a heart attack. When a part of the brain is deprived of oxygen, brain tissue dies, causing a stroke.

HDL brings cholesterol into the large intestines and out of the body. Consequently, HDL is often referred to as "good cholesterol," because it reduces the amount of cholesterol in your body.

Atherosclerosis is a leading cause of high blood pressure, or hypertension, as well. As plaque builds within the walls of blood vessels, the passageway for blood is narrowed, thus causing pressure to build within the circulatory system. Also, cholesterol plaque accumulates inside the kidneys, specifically in the glomeruli and tubules, causing blood flow within the kidneys to be reduced. This causes more pressure to build within the circulation. High blood pressure is a leading risk factor in heart attack and stroke.

Atherosclerosis in the coronary arteries of the heart is also the most common cause of angina pectoris and arrythmia, or irregular heartbeat. Angina is the characteristic pain that usually appears in the center of the chest and sometimes streaks down the left arm. It is caused when insufficient oxygen gets to the heart. Cool evenings, cold weather, or excessive demands placed upon the heart, such as too much exercise or stress, cause the heart to beat more rapidly. This increases the heart's need for oxygen. Since the coronary arteries are blocked from atherosclerosis, the oxygen demand cannot be met, resulting in pain. If the demand continues to increase, the person can suffer a heart attack.

Arrythmia is caused when the electrical system of the heart is disturbed. Cholesterol plaque inside the coronary arteries prevents adequate oxygen from getting to parts of the heart. This can damage conductive fibers within the heart muscle, thus preventing the electrical impulses from spreading evenly throughout the heart, which causes an irregular heartbeat.

The amount of cholesterol found in the blood is measured in milligrams per deciliter of blood, or as mg/dl. The average American's blood cholesterol level is approximately 220 mg/dl. Numerous scientific studies have shown that cholesterol levels above 160 mg/dl. are atherogenic, meaning that they are causing atherosclerosis in the body's major arteries, including the heart and brain. A cholesterol level below 160 mg/dl. causes the elimination or discharge of plaque from the arteries, and the reversal of atherosclerosis.

The U.S. Surgeon General has repeatedly advised Americans to reduce the level of fat and cholesterol in their diets to prevent the most common forms of cardiovascular disease.

BUILDING THE HEART MUSCLE

People with coronary heart disease should not engage in competitive sports. Competition causes us to forget our limits and increases the likelihood of overstressing the heart. The best exercise for people with heart disease is walking. Walk for twenty minutes at a mild pace, increasing the pace as your stamina increases. Rest and then continue. Do not get too far from home or from public places. Work your way up to a brisk pace over time. Walking is the safest of all exercises and can be done by everyone (except those suffering from physical handicap). For those whose hearts are in better shape, bicycle riding, tennis, or some other sports pursuit can be enjoyed. People should see their doctors before engaging in any regular exercise program.

Exercise raises HDL cholesterol, thus lowering blood cholesterol. It also stimulates the body to grow new blood vessels, which increases blood flow throughout the body, especially to the heart.

THE FIERY HEART

According to traditional Chinese medicine, the heart is joined with the small intestine to form the Fire Element. It is associated

[Although there are] vague descriptions of chest pains in the medical literature of the ancient Egyptians and Greeks [it was not until 1912 that] a classification of coronary obstructions was published in the United States . . . A condition that only the most erudite specialists could have identified as recently as 1930 is so common now that it can be diagnosed by the average person.

JEAN MAYER

with the summer months—June 21 to mid-August—and the hours of 11 A.M. to 1 P.M. During these months and hours the heart receives its optimal amounts of qi. These are also the periods in which underlying problems associated with the heart tend to surface. Fatigue at midday suggests heart trouble, according to Chinese medicine. And many people suffer heart attacks during the summer months.

Too much heat in summer injures the heart, just as too much cold in winter injures the kidneys and bladder. Moderate warmth of summer is healing.

Naturally, the heart is associated with the arteries, blood vessels, blood, and the pulse. The pulse is among the important tools of diagnosis used in Chinese medicine. (See chapter on Chinese medicine.)

The heart pumps blood throughout the body. In this way, it brings what is essential to every part of the body. It accomplishes this service through its capacity to expand and contract. The heart is, therefore, the clearest expression of yin and yang in the body. The heart functions, say the Chinese, because it follows the Tao. It is in harmony with yin and yang and therefore everything within the body—the microcosmic universe—receives what is needed and is enriched.

In the Five Element system, the heart is controlled by the kidneys (Fire controls Water). This is easily understood by the fact that if blood flows smoothly through the kidneys, blood pressure is normal and balanced. Healthy kidneys serve as a mild form of resistance to the flow of the blood, causing appropriate blood pressure to exist throughout the system.

But if the kidneys are too contracted, blood pressure increases and the heart is unduly stressed. As blood pressure increases, so, too, does resistance within the circulation, causing ever-increasing stress upon the heart. As any physician will tell you, hypertension is a leading risk factor in heart attack and stroke. Since salt is a kidney contractor in Chinese medicine, its intake must be closely monitored. Salt should be used minimally in cooking and never used as a condiment on foods. Processed foods that contain salt should be avoided.

Conversely, if the kidney energy is weak or expanded, there will be low blood pressure and thus the heart will have to work

*As to diseases, make a habit of
two things: to help or at least
to do no harm.*

HIPPOCRATES

harder to pump blood. Low blood pressure—though not as severe a problem as high—can be unhealthy, as well.

The heart is also associated with the sweat, especially the kind of sweat created by nervous tension. Sweaty palms, for example, are a symptom of an overworked and excited heart.

The heart controls the tongue and speech. All speech problems, such as stuttering or poor enunciation, are heart related. Stuttering is said to be caused by weak heart qi, perhaps caused by excessive kidney qi. The kidneys may be overactive from too much salt and liquids; this can cause the kidneys to restrict heart energy and thus prevent adequate life force from flowing from the heart to the tongue. Without an adequate supply of heart qi, the tongue is hesitant, redundant, and has trouble shaping words.

Murmurs, palpitations, excessively high or low blood pressure will all affect the way a person speaks. The Chinese treat speech problems by balancing and harmonizing heart energy.

The tongue is also one of the most direct ways of diagnosing the heart. If the tongue is deeply red to purple, heart qi is excessive; the heart is overworked and struggling for greater amounts of oxygen. There is probably suffering from atherosclerosis. Such a person will be driven, overly aggressive, and prone to violent outbursts of temper. If the tongue is pale or whitish pink, heart qi is deficient. The heart is weak and lethargic. The person may be suffering from anemia. (A coated or whitish tongue indicates digestive problems, especially stagnation throughout the intestinal tract. The body is attempting to eliminate waste in any way it can, including through the mouth, as indicated by the excess coating on the tongue.)

The grains that provide the greatest qi to the heart are corn and millet. The tastes that nourish the heart most are bitter and slightly burnt tastes.

The heart is associated with joy. Interestingly, joy is not considered an emotion so much as a state of inner tranquility. For the Chinese, joy rises from within when we do what we love. At that moment, we are attuned to our essential nature, our true inner being. Joy is, therefore, a kind of compass, a guide, to the nature of the soul.

From this state comes such well-known phrases as "follow your heart" and "follow your bliss," the latter made familiar by mythologist Joseph Campbell to describe the true path of the soul.

When heart qi is excessive, the emotional reaction tends to be hysteria. The heart and the breath are the most obvious rhythms of our bodies. Both are largely involuntary (though the breath easily comes under voluntary control), and both are a reflection of our current state of being. A person with an easily excited heart tends to react emotionally to changes in his or her environment. He or she quickly loses perspective, seeing life as extremes of success and crisis.

The heart is associated with laughter in Chinese medicine. Laughter lightens the heart, and also heals it, just as singing is said to be therapeutic to the spleen.

The color associated with the heart is red. An excessively red complexion, especially when capillaries are visible at the surface of the skin, indicates a swollen and overworked heart. Red-colored clothing—a red tie, for example, or a red dress—can stimulate heart energy and all its associated characteristics in one's life. It connotes passion, initiative, leadership, aggression.

The Yellow Emperor states that the heart controls the spirit, the part of us that fights for what we believe in. In both East and West, the heart has long been associated with courage. "He showed real heart" or "She has the heart of a lion" are common phrases used to describe people who persevere in the face of great adversity. "Weak-hearted" or "the faint of heart" suggests a weak spirit or a fearful person.

Using the Five Elements again, we can see that joy is restricted or limited by fear, the emotion associated with the Water Element. The more we are ruled by fear, the less chance we have of following our true inner natures. So, fear keeps us from experiencing joy.

Fear or stress (another word for fear) causes heart disease. Fear changes heart rate and respiration, elevates cholesterol level, and creates hormonal imbalances. Fear can destroy the heart. For those with heart disease, it is essential to limit stress or fear, either by removing oneself from stressful situations, or acting more courageously, or both. At the same time, more emphasis should be placed upon doing what one truly enjoys. By encouraging joy, laughter, and spontaneity—all of which are the opposites of fear—we encourage heart qi and thus strengthen the heart. The heart is associated with beginning a great adventure—"taking heart"—and setting out on our journey.

161

So, it is important to begin things that we have been postponing for one reason or another. Begin, initiate, show courage—these are the characteristics of a strong and healthy heart.

Avoid foods rich in fat and cholesterol, especially red meat, whole dairy products, eggs, and poultry. Also, consumption of oils should be reduced, especially oils that are composed of saturated fats, such as palm kernel, coconut, and peanut oils.

It is also important to limit or avoid alcohol, which weakens the heart muscle.

Foods such as coffee, chocolate, colas (which contain caffeine), hard liquors, beer, and wine all stimulate the heart. Continuous use of the more extreme of these foods, such as liquors, coffee, chocolate, and wine, tend to have a weakening effect on the heart in the long run, however. This, say the Chinese, conforms with the law of yin and yang. Those things that excite and overly stimulate the organ (or the entire body) leave it exhausted in the end. Moderation is the key.

The following foods are used in Chinese medicine to strengthen the heart.

- *Grain:* corn, including whole corn and corn on the cob; glutinous millet; amaranth.
- *Vegetables:* asparagus, brussels sprouts, chives, dandelion, endive, scallions.
- *Beans:* azuki, red lentils, mung beans.
- *Fruit:* apricot, raspberry, persimmon, strawberry, watermelon.
- *Fish:* shrimp, in small to moderate amounts.
- *Herbs:* In general, herbs and spices should be mild. All fiery herbs overly stimulate the heart and thus tax the organ. Herbs that are beneficial to the heart include cinnamon (warms and improves circulation), cloves (warming), coriander, ginger (usually used for intestines, but also improves circulation), daikon radish cut up and steamed or boiled (said to break up fat deposits throughout the body and improve circulation).

To improve the health of the heart, exercise is also recommended. Walking, tai chi chuan, and dance are among the best exercises because they are mild, aerobic, and do not overly tax the heart.

[The heart is] a creature of some internal, unknown majesty.

THOMAS THOMPSON

162

Other foods that heal the heart are any whole grains that contain water-soluble fiber that binds with cholesterol and eliminates it from the body. Although oat bran has received the most publicity, the fibrous grain that is most effective at reducing cholesterol is brown rice.

Fiber also improves bowel function, which is the body's most efficient means of eliminating cholesterol. (Up to 100 milligrams of dietary cholesterol can be eliminated through the feces in a single bowel movement. This will prevent a great deal of cholesterol from getting into the blood.)

Use small to moderate amounts of polyunsaturated oils, such as sesame, corn, and safflower oil. Also use olive oil, which is a monounsaturated oil, but is highly effective at lowering cholesterol.

Excessive use of polyunsaturated oils has been linked to cancer. Therefore, moderation in the use of all oil is recommended.

Salmon, cod, haddock, scrod, and other cold-water fish contain omega 3 polyunsaturated oils, which studies show reduce blood cholesterol level.

Vitamin E is an antioxidant, meaning that it prevents tissue decay from fatty acids turning rancid within the body. Vitamin E is available in whole grains, leafy green vegetables, and sea foods.

Limit red meat, dairy foods, eggs, the skin of poultry (which is higher in fat), coconuts, avocado, and olives, all of which contain high levels of fat.

Reduce blood cholesterol level to below 160 mg/dl, which will gradually eliminate cholesterol plaque from arteries and tissues throughout the body.

According to Ayurvedic healers, the heart is most influenced by the vata dosha, or the force of kinetic energy. Foods that balance the vata dosha include the following:

- *Grains:* Rice, wheat, oats.
- *Vegetables:* All cooked vegetables, especially asparagus, beets, carrots, cucumber, onion, okra, garlic, potato, zucchini.
- *Beans:* Mung beans, tofu, black and red lentils.
- *Fruit:* Apricots, berries, cherries, figs, grapefruit, oranges, plums.
- *Tastes:* Pungent increases vata and pitta; is warming, light, and dry. Bitter increases vata, tones, and increases appetite.

163

Science continues to search for ways of improving the health of the heart through drugs and surgery, but the best medicine remains food, herbs, exercise, and joy. Therefore, have a good meal and put a smile on your face. It may be the best first step to a healthy heart.

Herbs for the heart:

BLACK COHOSH: For angina.

CACTUS: For angina with irregular heartbeats.

ALFALFA: Lowers cholesterol.

HAWTHORNE BERRIES: For cardiac problems, high blood pressure.

CHAPTER 15

THE LUNGS

"OH, EAST IS EAST, and West is West, and never the twain shall meet," said Kipling. But lately the "twain" has been inching closer and closer. Sometimes, there are even magical moments of understanding that seem to unify the two worldviews, like a bridge suddenly thrown across the chasm. A journey into the world of the lungs offers a glimpse of this unifying perspective.

Many of us think of the lungs as balloons of air. We know that the body needs oxygen, but how many of us realize why we need it? The short answer is energy. Oxygen is essential in the process by which blood sugar is burned as fuel. Without oxygen, cells are deprived of energy and consequently die.

In the West, we think of food as energy, not oxygen. But food would be useless as a fuel without oxygen. It would be inert. Oxygen brings it to life; it makes the fuels that are derived from food reactive and life-sustaining (see respiration, below). In short, both food and oxygen are essential in the process by which energy is created.

Our need to get food has defined the American highway. But in fact, we need more oxygen than we do food, and we need it a

If we cultivate the habit of keeping the air pure and of breathing only fresh air, we can save ourselves from many a terrible disease.

MAHATMA GANDHI

Most of the muscles of the respiratory system are connected to the cervical and lumbar vertebrae and breathing therefore affects the stability and posture of the spine, while conversely the position of the spine will affect the quality and speed of breathing. Good breathing therefore also means good posture, just as good posture means good breathing.

MOSHE FELDENKRAIS

whole lot faster. People have fasted for up to sixty days and lived to tell about it. But if you suddenly hold your breath, your body will demand that you resume breathing in less than sixty seconds. The brain can last about four minutes without oxygen before it is damaged, but it can last as many as fifteen minutes without glucose, or blood sugar, before damage occurs. Without oxygen, cells die and organs stop.

On the hierarchy of needs, oxygen is first. The reason is simple: Oxygen is energy, and energy is life.

Oriental culture elevated this understanding into a realm in which science and religion become one. In the East, energy is understood in religious terms. In India, it's called prana, or the vital life force. According to Swami Rama, coauthor of the book *Science of Breath* with Drs. Rudolph Ballentine and Alan Hymes, the word *prana* is derived from the syllables *pra,* meaning the first unit, and *na,* meaning energy. Prana is the original cosmic energy that has brought everything else into being.

"All the diverse forms of this universe are sustained by the energy of prana," says Swami Rama. This energy is available to all. And it can be understood and controlled for human development. "One who has learned to control prana has learned to control all the energies of this universe—physical and mental," writes Swami Rama. "He has also learned to control his body and his mind."

Swami Rama was the first Indian Yogi to demonstrate under scientific conditions the ability to control various involuntary functions, including stopping his heart and emitting various brain waves at will. Many of these experiments were conducted at the Menninger Foundation in Topeka, Kansas. Swami Rama, who is the recipient of the Martin Buber award for service to humanity, has been among the most influential figures to demonstrate the authenticity of yoga to Western science.

According to the yogic tradition, the breath is the vehicle of prana. Prana enters the body when we inhale. How we breathe—whether it is shallow or deep, hurried or slow—controls how prana affects the body, that is, how it influences the body and mind. Indian yogis have long taught that to control the breath means to control the universal energy within, which is to say, to control the physical health and state of mind.

Studies have shown that people who breathe in a shallow and hurried way tend to be nervous and emotional, while those who

The Lungs

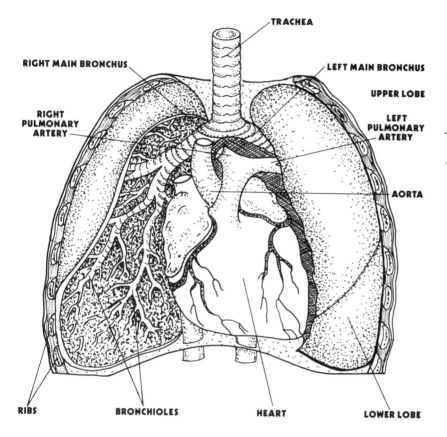

TRACHEA

RIGHT MAIN BRONCHUS

LEFT MAIN BRONCHUS

UPPER LOBE

RIGHT PULMONARY ARTERY

LEFT PULMONARY ARTERY

AORTA

RIBS

BRONCHIOLES

HEART

LOWER LOBE

The body's main organs of respiration, the lungs work closely with the heart and blood to take in energy in the form of oxygen and eliminate waste in the form of carbon dioxide.

breathe rhythmically and deeply—into the abdomen—tend to be more emotionally balanced, centered, and less affected by changes in their environment.

"All breathing exercises—advanced or basic—enable the student to control his mind through understanding prana," says Swami Rama.

One of the unique properties of breathing is that it is both an involuntary and a voluntary action. Breathing is normally controlled by the respiratory center of the brain, but it is brought under voluntary control at will. According to yogic tradition, the breath is a gateway to the deeper physical and psychological recesses of our being. The reason it has such powers of influence is

167

because the nervous system works in both directions: If you are breathing unconsciously, the state of your mind will control your breathing, which will serve to reinforce your current attitudes and belief system. But if you begin to control your breath by making it deeper and more rhythmic, the opposite effect takes place: this deeper rhythm and greater abundance of life force re-shapes your attitudes and strengthens your health. Thus, the breath is a gateway to the involuntary systems and the deeper recesses of your nature.

But this is just the beginning. Yogic breathing techniques are not only designed to influence various parts of the body, but to awaken levels of consciousness, to illuminate the soul. Thus, breath is regarded as more than a gateway to the inner being; it is a door to the divine within each of us. In the East, the science of breath is ultimately a religious path. "The human body is sustained by the same prana that sustains the universe," said Swami Rama. It is entering each of us between ten and fourteen times per minute.

To a Westerner who breaths an average of 20,000 times per day, perhaps without considering a single breath, such speculation about oxygen, life energy, and the divine must surely represent final proof that "never the twain shall meet."

But at this very moment, deep within each of us, trillions of tiny cells are embracing an equal number of tiny atoms of oxygen, each one bearing the gift of life.

THE PATH OF AIR

The lungs are the main organs of respiration. They supply the body with oxygen, which is essential for energy. The lungs also eliminate carbon dioxide waste. There are two lungs, one on each side of the thorax; together they weigh about two and a half pounds and stretch from the bottom rib to just below the collar bone. In childhood, they are pink, but for most adults they become gray. In men and women who smoke or are exposed to highly polluted air, the lungs often turn black.

Each lung is surrounded by a protective, double-membraned sack called a pleura. It allows the lungs to expand and contract inside the chest wall.

The respiratory system begins in the mouth and nose, where

we take in and exhale air. From there, it travels down the trachea, or windpipe, a long tube that divides into two smaller tubes, called bronchi, which enter the lungs. Once inside the lungs, the bronchi further divide into many smaller branches called bronchiolies, which lead to tiny grapelike air sacs called alveoli.

Most of the air we breathe is nitrogen (about 78 percent); the rest is oxygen (21 percent), with minute quantities of carbon dioxide (CO_2), trace gases, and water vapor. Once the air is inside the alveoli, the oxygen separates from the other gases and diffuses along the walls of these tiny sacs. There it seeps through the alveoli and into surrounding capillaries, and makes its way into the bloodstream. At the same time, the carbon dioxide inside the blood seeps into the alveoli, from which it is breathed out when we exhale.

Once oxygen is inside the blood, it binds with hemoglobin, the iron-rich part of the red blood cell. The blood is then pumped to the left side of the heart, and then on to tissues throughout the body.

Each quantity of oxygen-rich blood eventually reaches a part of the body where it surrenders its load of O_2 and receives the carbon dioxide waste from the cells. Onward it flows, back to the right side of the heart, which pumps the carbon-dioxide-rich blood into the lungs and down into the tiny alveoli.

There the CO_2 seeps past the walls of the capillaries and into the tiny alveoli, which expel the CO_2 when we exhale. In exchange for the CO_2, the blood receives oxygen.

The act of breathing requires a well-coordinated effort among the muscles of the rib cage and the diaphragm, a dome-shaped muscle system located between the thorax and the abdomen. The diaphragm pulls downward, while muscles within the rib cage expand. This causes the lungs themselves to expand and open. During relaxed breathing, the downward movement of the diaphragm is about two-thirds of an inch, which only minimally opens the lungs. But during deep breathing the diaphragm will descend as much as three inches.

Our experience of breathing is actually an illusion. It seems as if we are drawing or sucking air inside us, but in fact the air is being forced into us. It works like this: The lungs are in contact with the air outside the body through the nose, mouth, trachea, and bronchial tubes. As long as the pressure inside the lungs is

He lives most life whoever breathes most air.

ELIZABETH BARRETT
BROWNING

169

According to natural medical philosophers, breath is not the lungs as such or the air moved by them but a divine emanation of potentiality, carrying the essence of every human faculty at its beginning and making it manifest in the various physical organs as it circulates through the body.

HAKIM G. M. CHISHTI

equal to that outside, there will be no movement of air between the lungs and the outer atmosphere. The balance is analogous to putting your palms together and maintaining equal pressure in both arms; the hands will remain stationary.

By expanding our lungs, we have caused the air molecules already inside the lungs to be spread out over a larger area. This causes the relative pressure within the lungs to drop.

Outside the body, molecules of air are packed together much more densely than they are now inside the lungs. So, the relative air pressure is greater outside the lungs than inside, which causes the high-pressure air to rush through the nose (or mouth) and down into the low-pressure zone of the lungs.

To go back to the metaphor of the two hands pressed against each other, the act of expanding the lungs is like reducing the pressure in one hand; the other hand suddenly advances.

When we breathe out, the reverse takes place: the diaphragm pushes upward and the rib cage collapses, thus applying pressure to the lungs that forces air outside of us.

The amount of air breathed into the lungs depends upon the oxygen demands of the body. During relaxation, an adult breathes in about ten to fourteen times per minute. Each breath takes about four to six seconds and draws into the lungs about nine to twelve pints of air per minute. During exercise, that same adult breathes at a rate of about one breath per minute, and takes in about twenty gallons of air per minute. An adult breathes in about 3,300 gallons of air per day, on the average.

The brain will signal changes in respiration due to a variety of conditions, including the following:

- Higher concentrations of carbon dioxide in the blood will increase the rate of our breathing. Conversely, lower concentrations of oxygen, such as when traveling at higher altitudes, will cause an increase in the rate of breathing.
- Higher body temperatures, such as fever, increase the respiration rate; lower temperatures reduce it. High blood pressure reduces the rate of breathing, while lower blood pressure increases it.
- Exercise increases the rate of breathing to meet the body's demands for oxygen, while resting and sleeping causes a reduction in the rate of breathing.

At any moment, we can voluntarily control our breathing, causing it to become deeper or shallow. However, if our oxygen demands do not go up, and we force more oxygen into the body (a condition typically called hyperventilation), the brain will usually compensate for the additional oxygen by slowing the breath or stopping it for a period of forty to sixty seconds in order to re-establish the oxygen and carbon dioxide balance in the bloodstream.

We tend to think of respiration as limited to breathing in and out, but the act of respiration includes the burning of fuel, which is the reason we breathe at all. Once the oxygen reaches the cells, it is combined with blood sugar, or glucose, to cause tiny combustion reactions within the cells. These reactions cause the release of energy which the cells use to maintain life. We might reasonably ask ourselves why we don't burn up in this combustion process, or why we don't breathe out smoke. The reason, in a nutshell, is that our internal combustion is slow and small.

According to Alan Hymes, M.D., coauthor of *Science of Breath,* "All living organisms can be thought of as meeting their energy needs from a slow-burning furnace. This furnace releases energy from a constant supply of fuel by slowly combining it with oxygen."

Hymes points out that in rapidly burning systems, intense heat and light are released, along with carbon dioxide and water vapor. The amount of light and heat released during combustion depends upon the speed with which the fuel is burned. A fire burns fuel at a rate fast enough to emit a visible light and palpable heat; an explosion consumes fuel at an even faster rate, and thus emits even greater amounts of light and heat.

However, if the burning of fuel occurs at a very slow rate, there may be no visible light at all, says Hynes. "Biological systems (i.e., all living organisms) are essentially burning fuel at a very slow rate."

Through a very complex chain reaction, this combination of blood sugar and oxygen oxidizes within a particular part of the cell, called the mitochondria. From there, the energy is stored in a molecule called adenosine triphosphate, or ATP, which is found in living systems throughout nature. When energy is needed, ATP has the capacity to provide it to the cell.

As with other forms of combustion, carbon dioxide and heat

are given off. This heat contributes to a normal body temperature of 98.6 degrees Fahrenheit. The carbon dioxide is released into the blood in exchange for oxygen.

This brings us to why we breathe: energy. The lungs and the digestive tract (which provide carbohydrates) provide the body with the raw materials of combustion, which produces energy. With that energy, the cells can do their work, which is to keep the body alive.

ILLNESSES OF THE LUNGS

Asthma may occur when the muscles wrapping the bronchial tubes contract, or when the membranes that line the tubes' interior expand, or when excess mucus is secreted by the mucous glands inside the bronchial walls. These actions prevent air from passing freely to and from the lungs. Asthma is often brought on by an allergic reaction to pollens, fungus, animal dander, and other substances. Standard medical treatment usually includes the use of such drugs as epinephrine, ephedrine, and atropine, which cause the autonomic nervous system to relax the muscles within the bronchial tubes, allowing the air passages to open. Like all drugs, these pharmaceuticals have side effects.

Infections of the lungs include:

- *Bronchitis:* swelling of the bronchial tubes caused by infectious organisms (bacteria), or chemical agents.
- *Croup:* Usually found in children, croup is caused by infectious organisms. Antibiotics are usually administered as treatment.
- *Pneumonia:* inflammation of the lungs, including the bronchial tubes, bronchioles, and alveoli. Numerous agents can cause the infection, including bacteria, viruses, and fungi. Treatment includes antibiotics.

Lung cancer causes more deaths among men in the U.S. than any other killer disease. It is the second leading cause of death among women, topped only by breast cancer. The principal cause is cigarette smoking. Remarkably, the number of people afflicted with lung cancer continues to increase, despite the fact that, overall, fewer people smoke cigarettes today than a decade ago. Passive or secondary smoking, that is, breathing the fumes from someone else's cigarette, has been shown to cause lung cancers as well. Other causes include highly polluted air, especially air filled with car exhaust fumes.

Emphysema results when the walls of the alveoli begin to break down, thus reducing the area in which oxygen can be passed to the blood. Those with emphysema always seem to be struggling for breath because more breaths are needed to fulfill the body's oxygen requirements. Emphysema can be caused by chronic asthma, bronchitis, or cigarette smoking.

BREATHING IN THE LIFE FORCE

The lungs and the large intestine form the Metal Element in the Five Element Theory. They are associated with the fall, when the seasons provide the lungs with their maximum quantity of energy or life force. It is during the period from late September to December 21 that the lungs can be healed of many problems—or conversely, manifest disease, particularly if they have been abused in the past. During the day, the lungs receive their optimal amounts of qi between the hours of 3 A.M. and 5 A.M. Insomnia during these hours tends to be a symptom of lung imbalances.

As in all of Oriental medicine, the lungs are considered the recipients of the life force, or qi. The rhythm and depth of a person's breathing shapes the qi; the breathing gives the qi definition and behavior which in turn influences the body. If the breath is nervous, shallow and rapid, that same quality of energy will move like an erratic electrical current through the entire body. The personality, shaped by that person's own physical vibration, will be shallow, nervous, and weak. He or she will feel a greater sense of personal frailty, insecurity, and weakness.

On the other hand, if the breath is deep, rhythmic, and strong, the quality of the qi will have the same depth and vitality when it moves through the system. Consequently, a person's life will be rich, deep, and orderly. That person will experience a greater sense of personal security and calm.

In the Five Element schematic, the lungs pass qi onto the kidneys and bladder; control the qi in the liver; and receive qi from the spleen and stomach. They are controlled themselves by the heart and small intestine. While all of these relationships are important in healing, the relationship between the heart and lungs is key.

The heart is regarded as the Fire Element. A balanced heart is associated with joy, while an imbalanced Fire Element is associated with hysteria. The Chinese maintain that if the heart becomes imbalanced, the Fire Element will control the Metal Element excessively. Whenever our emotions go out of control, such as during hysterical moments, the lungs react with wild and irregular breathing. The heart can be seen as controlling the lungs. The lungs therefore take in qi and send it through the body in wild and chaotic waves. In this way, the heart's imbalance influences every system within the body by controlling the lungs and the qi energy they take in.

The system that is immediately affected is the kidneys. The imbalanced and erratic qi passed from the lungs to the kidneys, or Water Element, will inspire fear and a loss of will. Consequently, the Oriental teachers counseled that the way to control the mind and heart (or emotional nature) was to maintain control of the breath in all situations. When highly emotional, angry, or afraid, breathe deeply and rhythmically. The breath acts as a tether on the emotional and psychological realm, say the sages, much as a leash controls an animal.

The kidneys are responsible for drawing the breath deeply into the body. Weak kidneys are associated with chronic stress, nervousness, and shallow breathing. Strengthening the kidneys will deepen the breath and improve the lungs.

The lungs and large intestine are associated with the emotions of sadness and grief. People who hold on to sadness and grief often suffer from lung imbalances. This holding on will weaken lung energy. Conversely, weak lungs will have a tendency to maintain a condition of sadness and grief. Those who have strong lungs will release the past and maintain a balanced emotional perspective.

The Chinese maintain that the lungs control the animal spirit within humanity. This is illustrated best by the lung's relationship with the liver. The liver, or Wood Element, is the ruler of anger. If anger is allowed to run its course, it will become abusive and violent—in short, animalistic. Grief controls anger. A person grieves a loss of control. If the lungs are strong enough, grief will act in advance to limit a person's anger, and thus act as a governor on the animal nature. If the lungs are weak and the liver excessive, however, the lower nature will dominate and anger will have no limit.

The lungs are associated with mucus, and lung imbalances usually result in increased mucus production. The lungs also nourish the skin and hair; they give it luster and brilliance. You can observe strong lung qi as healthy, pinkish skin, while weak lungs can be seen in pale skin. Caucasians with weak lungs can easily be identified by their excessively pale or white faces, often with drawn and hollow cheeks. Such people often appear to radiate a sense of grief or sadness, as if they were carrying a great emotional burden.

The lung meridian runs from a point on the chest, two inches above the nipple, down the inside of the arm and wrist, over the great muscle of the thumb, to the end of the thumb.

The lungs can be injured by too much cold. Therefore, during winter, the chest must be well protected, say the Chinese.

The Chinese heal the lungs in part by treating the large intestine. Problems affecting the large intestine also will affect the lungs. Mucus increases if the lungs are irritated by the presence of toxins or excessive lung qi. Poisons not eliminated by the intestinal tract will remain in the bloodstream and infiltrate the lungs. Poor elimination or constipation will often manifest in the lungs as chronic mucus discharge. Poor intestinal health also can be a contributing cause of asthma. Whenever lung problems emerge, the Metal Element in general is troubled and both organs must be treated, say the Chinese. (See chapter on the large intestine.)

As described above, the lungs are a dense network of capillaries, which are often smaller than the red blood cells. Red cells pass through the capillaries by bending and folding in half. When you consume high-fat foods, however, microns of fat (called chylomicra) infiltrate the bloodstream and adhere to the red cells, causing them to stick together like rolls of coins. These sticky rolls of cells prevent individual cells from absorbing and carrying oxygen. They also prevent the cells from folding and passing through the tiny capillaries. So less oxygen enters the bloodstream, and the lungs become sites of cholesterol plaque, or atherosclerosis.

We must therefore understand that when we administer medicine, we administer the whole world: that is, all the virtue of heaven and earth, air and water. Because if there is sickness in the body, all the healthy organs must fight against it, not only one, but all. For one sickness can be death to them all.

PARACELSUS

Many lung problems quickly clear up when people eliminate dairy foods, eggs, and high-fat meats from their diets.

The spleen and Earth Element provide qi to the Metal Element or lungs. Excess sugar can weaken the spleen and therefore diminish the qi flowing to the lungs. When the lungs are troubled, all refined sugars, spicy and acidic foods should be avoided until the symptoms pass. Sing loudly to strengthen spleen and lungs! (See chapter on the spleen.)

To strengthen the lungs, the grain that has the strongest herbal effect on the lungs is rice. The taste that stimulates lung qi is pungent. In general, leafy green vegetables have a strong healing effect on the lungs.

The following foods and herbs are considered healing to the Metal Element.

- *Grains:* Brown rice and sweet brown rice.
- *Vegetables:* Mustard greens, turnip greens, celery, daikon, carrot, lotus root, onion, turnip, watercress, cabbage, cauliflower, Chinese cabbage, cucumber.
- *Animal foods:* Cod, haddock, scrod, flounder, halibut.
- *Herbs:* ginger, garlic, horseradish, dill, cinnamon, coriander, licorice, fennel, nutmeg, basil, black pepper, bay leaf, and cardamom.
- *Fruit:* pears, tangerines.

As a physical stimulant for the lungs, massage acupuncture point Lung 1. To find acupuncture point Lung 1, move your hand to the clavicle bone on the front of the chest, right where the bone bends forward, directly below the front of the neck. Drop down an inch and find a sensitive point in the muscle tissue, about two inches from the sternum bone in the center of the chest. By pressing this point in a circular manner, you can stimulate lung energy. Lung 1 is used to treat a variety of lung ailments, including colds, coughs, and asthma.

Ayurvedic healers say that the lungs are most influenced by the vata dosha, which is strengthened by eating the following foods and herbs:

- *Grains:* Oats, rice, and wheat.
- *Vegetables:* Cooked green leafy vegetables, asparagus, beets, carrots, cucumber, green beans, okra, onion, radishes.

- *Fruit:* Apricots, avocado, cherries, berries, grapefruit, plums, lemons.
- *Herbs:* Garlic, ginger.

Naturopaths say that chronic lung problems, such as asthma, are associated most often with hypoglycemia, or low blood sugar, and a variety of food allergies. Asthmatics tend to consume excess sweets and dairy products, and often overeat. They are often overweight or have high fat-to-muscle ratios. They may have allergies to milk, wheat, and/or chemical toxins in the home, such as from rugs, paints, or sealants.

Foods to eat include whole grains, a wide variety of vegetables, especially carrots, yellow squash, broccoli, and leafy greens, fruit, especially stewed fruits, and seaweeds, especially kelp. Supplements:

- Liquid chlorophyll, to strengthen lungs and immune system.
- Calcium and magnesium supplements, for immune system.
- Zinc, for immune system.
- B complex, for immune system.
- Vitamin A, for immune system.
- Herbs: garlic tablets, licorice root, coltsfoot.

Herbs for the lungs:

OREGANO and MARJORAM: To promote perspiration and treat colds, flu, and fevers. Can be used in baths and inhalations to clear the lungs and bronchial passages.

REED GRASS: Used for inflammation of lungs with acute symptoms of yellow phlegm, cough, expectoration, gastritis, belching, and vomiting.

EUCALYPTUS: For the treatment of coughs, colds, flu, croup, pneumonia, and asthma. Combine with olive and sesame oil to make an ointment to rub on the chest or make a tea from the leaves and drink it.

CHAPTER 16

THE SKIN

Health is a temporary, dynamic state of balance that has to break down periodically in order to reform as conditions change.

ANDREW WEIL

ERHAPS THE MOST famous skin problem belonged to Job, whose flesh was covered from head to foot with sores and worms, which was probably universal eczema. Others have been equally afflicted, but anyone who has suffered from acne knows the existential pain behind Job's lament: "My flesh is covered with worms and a crust of dirt; my skin hardens and runs."

While some skin disorders can indeed be life-threatening, most are merely ego-bruising. Even the occasional blemish or outbreak of acne exacts a seemingly disproportionate emotional toll, which is all the proof we need to show how important the skin is in our lives.

THE LARGEST ORGAN

The skin is the body's largest organ, responsible for an array of essential bodily functions, including breathing oxygen; eliminating carbon dioxide and other forms of waste; acting as a shield against toxins from outside the body; and helping to maintain body temperature. The skin is continually repairing and renewing itself. It responds almost instantly to sudden changes in emotions. It is also the body's main organ of sexual attraction, showing shape, texture, and allure.

The skin is composed of two layers: an outer epidermis, and a lower dermis, which includes even deeper tissue that some think of as a third layer. The epidermis, or upper layer, is covered with a thin sheath of dead cells, called the stratum corneum, which are continually being pushed up to the surface from below. If the dead cells are not removed, they can mitigate against the skin's effort to breathe and eliminate waste.

At the surface lies a slightly acidic coating of oil, called the "acid mantle," which can protect the skin against some bacteria. This mantle varies in acidity, though typically it has a pH of about 5. (pH, or potential hydrogen, measures the relative acidity of a substance. On the pH spectrum, 7 is balanced; anything above 7 is alkaline, anything below 7 is acidic.)

Below the epidermis is the dermis, a complex of sweat and oil glands, hair follicles, blood vessels, nerves, and muscle tissue. These are held together by a tough connective tissue called collagen, which runs in strands or fibers. The relative health of your collagen determines the contour of your skin, how wrinkled and lined it is. Healthy collagen is often called "soluble collagen," because it can absorb and hold moisture.

Diagram of the Skin

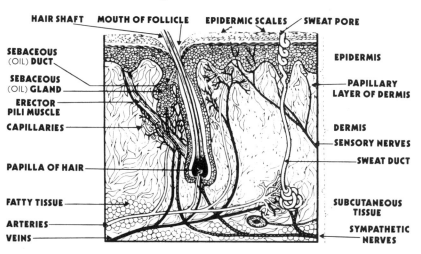

HAIR SHAFT **MOUTH OF FOLLICLE** **EPIDERMIC SCALES** **SWEAT PORE**

SEBACEOUS (OIL) **DUCT**

SEBACEOUS (OIL) **GLAND**

ERECTOR PILI MUSCLE

CAPILLARIES

PAPILLA OF HAIR

FATTY TISSUE

ARTERIES

VEINS

EPIDERMIS

PAPILLARY LAYER OF DERMIS

DERMIS

SENSORY NERVES

SWEAT DUCT

SUBCUTANEOUS TISSUE

SYMPATHETIC NERVES

The body's largest and in some ways most diverse organ, the skin takes in oxygen, eliminates carbon dioxide and other forms of waste, shields the body from toxins, helps to maintain body temperature, manufactures vitamin D, and constantly renews and repairs itself, among various other functions.

179

Below the collagen is a layer of fat and muscle, which also provides some contour and acts as a cushion and an insulating layer.

Aging of the skin occurs when collagen becomes hard and crosslinked with neighboring collagen fibers. This prevents it from holding water and plumping up. Instead, it collapses on itself, binds with other collagen fibers, and forms a kind of fish net below the surface of the skin, which we perceive as wrinkles.

The cause of this crosslinking is a process called oxidation or "free radical formation." What actually happens is the atoms of human tissue begin to decay, or lose electrons. Once an electron is lost, the atom attempts to regain its electrical balance by stealing one or more electrons from neighboring atoms. This stealing creates a chain reaction in which atoms are changing their structures and forming bonds that would not otherwise occur. The net effect is a chaos of crosslinking collagen fibers, revealed on the skin's surface as wrinkles.

Studies have shown that certain nutrients can stop free radical formation. Foods rich in beta carotene (the vegetable source of vitamin A) and vitamins E and C donate electrons to imbalanced atoms, thus restoring health and harmony to tissues throughout the body. Conversely, diets rich in fat, artificial ingredients, and chemical pollutants stimulate free radical formation, and thus contribute to aging and illness.

Natural cosmetic companies place an abundance of these nutrients, called antioxidants, in many of their skin care products, including cleansers, toners, and moisturizers. Skin specialists report that the depths that such products penetrate vary widely, depending on the size of the molecule, the temperature of the skin, and other factors.

Science has established that these nutrients do indeed stop free radical formation—whether they are taken in the diet or applied directly to the skin. But scientists are quick to point out that if people really want to take good care of their skin and slow the aging process, they will watch what they eat. Diets rich in antioxidants provide these substances to the bloodstream, thus getting to tissues throughout the body, including the deeper reaches of the skin. Most agree, therefore, that both diet and appropriate skin care are essential.

Acne occurs when oil, called sebum, blocks the pores and hair follicles at the skin's surface, thus preventing the skin from eliminating oil and waste. This, of course, causes waste to accumulate in the pores, resulting in pockets of infection that manifest as red sores, boils, and pimples. Acne does not occur when the pores remain unblocked.

Adolescents get more acne than adults because they experience a rapid increase in the production of the male hormone androgen—present in both sexes, but more abundant in males. Androgen causes the body to produce more sebum, which results in a greater number of blocked pores and blemishes.

CARING FOR THE SKIN

Skin care specialists maintain that before using any specific product for aging or acne, everyone should follow three skin care steps. The first is to properly clean the skin. Most of us have grown up using ordinary soap to wash with, but the skin experts recommend that we avoid soap because of its high pH, which dries skin and diminishes its life expectancy.

A healthful skin cleanser should be composed of vegetable oils; it should also have a balanced pH, and contain no animal fats, or mineral oils. Skin cleansers, also known as sufectants, can contain a number of different vegetable oils, including coconut, sesame, or palm oils. These are safe and effective cleansers and have a relatively low or balanced pH. Stearic acid, used in some natural skin care products to provide a pearly firmness, is a fatty acid derived from vegetable oils. These cleansers will dissolve sebum; water will dissolve and rinse away dirt.

Seaweeds are increasingly used as skin cleansers, as well. Their high mineral content stimulates circulation, helps eliminate toxins imbedded in the skin, and leaves the skin feeling smooth. Seaweeds can, to some extent, remineralize the skin, thus strengthening its immune and healing functions.

The next step in thoroughly cleaning the skin, especially if your skin tends to be oily, is to wash it regularly with a facial scrub that contains a mild abrasive. These abrasives vary in coarseness, ranging from a very mild base of oatmeal or ground almonds, to coarser materials, such as silica (a finely ground sand) or the shells of almonds or walnuts.

Studies have shown that men's skin tends to be smoother and less blemished than women's. The reason, say scientists, is that men exfoliate their skin every day by shaving. That is, they take off the top layer of dead cells with their razors, allowing their skin to breathe and eliminate waste much more efficiently. Skin care specialists recommend that women use a mild abrasive, such as a skin scrub made of crushed almond or walnut shells. Such exfoliants are widely available in natural foods stores.

While it is considered manly to slap alcohol on your face after shaving, alcohol dries the skin and thus harms the soluble collagen below.

Witch hazel turns up in a lot of natural skin care products, especially toners. Witch hazel has a strong astringent effect, but can dry out the skin somewhat if it is used in high quantities. Most natural cosmetics companies use only small amounts of witch hazel and combine it with moisturizing herbs—such as vitamin E, geranium, or honey—that balance its drying effects. Other common herbs in toners are lemon, ivy, sage, nettle, and burdock.

The third step that most skin care specialists advise is to use a moisturizer on your face after you've washed it thoroughly. Moisturizers, also known as humectants, attract moisture to the skin's surface and hold it there; moisturizers make the skin softer and prevent it from drying and chapping, thus slow the aging process.

Effective and widely used humectants include jojoba oil, vitamins A and E, sorbitol (derived from plants), honey, aloe vera, and iris.

Aloe vera is one of those plants that seems to have been designed by nature to treat human skin. Since ancient times, it has been used effectively to treat everything from dry skin, burns, and insect bites, to skin irritations, acne, cuts, and abrasions. Like many of the herbs mentioned in this article, aloe is surrounded by a great folklore that goes back to ancient Egypt, and a lot of research still needs to be done to investigate all its properties.

Iris is another plant that has remarkable moisture-controlling properties. Despite the fact that the iris grows in hot, dry climates, the plant itself is surprisingly moist, even watery. The secret seems to lie in the rhizome's ability to store water and release it in quantities that balance the prevailing atmospheric conditions.

Avoid moisturizers that include mineral oils, however. Mineral oil, used in many mass market skin care products, including the most popular cosmetic on the market, Oil of Olay, is a petrochemical that can dry the skin, block pores, and prevent it from breathing and eliminating waste.

SKIN CANCER

The number of new cases of skin cancer is more than 600,000 a year, according to the American Cancer Society (ACS). That figure is so high that the ACS does not include it in its annual cancer totals, which the Society now says is more than one million new cases per year.

Skin cancers are now reaching epidemic proportions, according to a study published in an October 1989 issue of the *Journal of the American Medical Association.* Since the 1960s, malignant melanoma has increased 3.5 times in men and 4.6 times in women.

Scientists tell us that the vast majority of skin cancers are caused by the sun's ultraviolet rays. Today, the amount of ultraviolet radiation being showered down upon all of us is increasing dramatically because the ozone layer is growing thinner each year. The ozone layer is a thin, protective covering of ozone gas in the upper atmosphere of the earth. It was formed more than three billion years ago by algae that, among other things, were capable of breathing carbon dioxide and releasing oxygen. Those tiny plants filled the earth's atmosphere with oxygen. Gradually, the oxygen rose into the stratosphere and interacted with the sun's UV light, causing a chemical reaction that formed the ozone molecule, composed of three oxygen atoms.

The ozone layer made advanced life on earth possible. Without it, those first marine animals that crawled up on the shore would have died of skin cancer, a fact we may be relearning today.

As the ozone layer becomes thinner and more diffuse, greater amounts of ultraviolet radiation make their way down to your skin. These ultraviolet rays are highly toxic to you, as well as to animal and marine life. Consequently, skin cancer rates are expected to continue to climb rapidly.

UV light also causes cataracts and harms the immune system, which makes a variety of cancers more likely. Dr. Darrell Spencer Rigel of New York University, who has studied the effects of

The placebo is the doctor who resides within.

NORMAN COUSINS

ultraviolet rays on skin, reported recently that it is particularly important to protect children and young people under the age of twenty from sunburn.

Young people are far more sensitive to cell aberrations caused by overexposure to UV radiation. "Our studies have shown that the twenty-year-old break point is critical," said Rigel. "There's no such thing as a safe tan, and there's no good thing about sunburn. But sunburn is much worse under the age of twenty."

Rigel reports that there are several other risk factors involved that offer clues to who gets skin cancer. Those risk factors include the following:

- Being blond or red-headed;
- Having abundant freckles on the upper back;
- Having a tendency to develop a red, bumpy rash called actinic keratosis after exposure to the sun;
- Having at least three blistering sunburns before the age of twenty;
- Having at least one relative with malignant melanoma.

Common suggestions for protecting against skin cancer include the following:

- Protect children from overexposure from the sun by using a hat, protective clothing, and a good sunscreen. Adults also should use an effective sun block, especially if they are planning to spend any length of time in the sun's direct rays.
- Avoid commercial skin lotions or moisturizers, especially those containing mineral oils, a substance that dries the skin, blocks pores, and causes the skin to heat up in the sun or indirect light. That heat is actually cooking the skin, causing cell aberrations and possible skin disease.
- Use a vegetable-based skin cleanser that will not dry the skin, or block pores. Soaps are highly alkaline; they dry the skin and cause it to age faster. Gentle cleansers will leave the skin moist and the pores open, allowing oils and blood to circulate freely.
- Eat foods rich in antioxidants: beta carotene, and vitamins E and C. Rich sources of beta carotene are carrots, squash, broccoli, and collard greens. Vitamin E is abundant in whole grains and seafoods. C can be found in leafy greens and fruit.

Those foods prevent free-radical formation (the basis of most cancers, including those of the skin, as well as aging) and restore health to tissues throughout the body.

- Reduce fat in the diet. Fat causes free radicals to increase throughout the body, including the skin, which raises the likelihood of cancer and other illnesses.
- Eat foods low on the food chain and rich in nutrition, such as whole grains, vegetables, beans, seaweeds, and fish, which are abundant in nutrients that support the immune system. Cancer is an immune deficiency disease, too. A healthy immune system can deal with the sun and toxins in the environment, as long as we're not poisoning ourselves every day with our food.

Sweating therapy can be used for restoring circulation. It will raise body heat and metabolism, burn off toxins, and relieve congestion.

Herbs for the skin:

SASSAFRAS TEA: Excellent for most kinds of skin eruptions.

PLANETARY BITTERS TEA: Helps chronic skin problems.

CHAPTER 17

THE BRAIN

THE BRAIN IS a vast and mysterious frontier, a universe within a hardened shell. The great constellations of that universe are marked by names that, for most of us, are vaguely familiar: cerebellum, cerebrum, cerebral cortex, frontal lobe, limbic system, and hypothalamus. Even if we know the function of these regions, they nevertheless stir in us wonder and awe.

To paraphrase F. Scott Fitzgerald, the brain is not like other organs. There is something about it that is beyond biology, indeed, beyond science. It is the altar of the body, the root of the mind. It is the place where the visible and invisible meet, where flesh and blood mingle with thoughts, emotions, instinct, and spirit.

Buried deep within lie the secrets of our souls, a record of our days, any one of which can be called forth unexpectedly by the right odor—a stroll past the local bakery, for example; the right face, even a stranger's; a piece of music; a pair of well-thumbed theater tickets.

In our reductionist age, it's tempting to think of the brain as a computer, and a person's worth as measured by the size of his or her brain. Mary Shelley's *Frankenstein: The Modern Prometheus*

(1817) offered up an answer to such thinking when her character, Dr. Frankenstein, installed a dead man's brain inside the head of a cadaver and then jumpstarted the beast with a streak of lightning. When Frankenstein's creation turned out to be a monster, Shelley provided an object lesson that grows more relevant with every passing decade: It takes more than gray matter and electricity to make a human being.

Opening the skull to cure headaches and other ailments, including brain tumors, dates back some four thousand years before Christ. The leading practitioners of cranial surgery were the ancient Peruvians, who successfully conducted hundreds of such operations as far back as the Stone Age. Researchers have proven that many of the patients survived these operations, as evidenced by the fact that bone tissue had clearly mended the original wound. Ancient skulls with plum-sized openings and saw-blade markings have been found throughout Europe, Asia, and North Africa.

In 500 B.C., a Greek living in Italy named Alcmaeon stated that intelligence is associated with the brain. His more famous contemporary, Empedocles, rejected the notion and taught that intelligence was found in the blood. Empedocles's teachings carried the day. Gradually, the brain would be associated with the intellect, but it remained an untouched mystery well into the modern age.

The first real breakthrough in understanding the brain came in 1861, when Dr. Paul Broca performed an autopsy on a man who, while living, could not speak in whole sentences. Broca, a Frenchman, discovered that a section of the left hemisphere of the man's brain was shriveled up in scar tissue. Broca named this part of the brain the speech center.

Broca's discovery stimulated further research on animals. Researchers used electric probes to stimulate parts of the brain, which in turn triggered distinct physical reactions. Gradually, a map of the brain was established showing where many specialized centers of learning and physical capabilities were located.

In the 1970s and 1980s, Dr. Roger Sperry pioneered the study of the left and right hemispheres of the brain. Sperry studied a group of epileptics who had undergone a radical form of surgery that involved severing the corpus callosum, the thick band of nerve fibers that connect the left and right hemispheres. Despite earlier research, many scientists still believed that the brain was largely an undifferentiated mass in which the entire organ was responsible for many specialized tasks. The corpus callosum, they believed, was a useless bundle of nerves.

Sperry discovered that the left and right hemispheres have distinct functions: the left side specializes in speech, analytical, sequential, and logical thinking; the right in spatial relationships, holistic, artistic, and intuitive thinking. The corpus callosum mediates between the two hemispheres, like a traffic cop at a busy corner. Without it, the two sides of the brain perceive life independently, and the person perceives himself as having two minds.

Today, we know that the right side of the brain controls the left side of the body, and vice versa. Interestingly, the left side of the brain is dominant in the Western world, and right-handedness is more abundant than left. This preference is evidenced in our language. The Latin word for left is *sinistra,* from which "sinister" is derived; the Celtic word for left meant "weak," and the French means "gawky" (*gauche*). Meanwhile, the words for the right side mean "dextrous" (Latin), "strong" and "straight" (Celtic), and "law" (French).

There is a growing body of evidence showing that left-handed people do not live as long as right-handers. A study done by researchers at the California State University at San Bernardino and the University of British Columbia found that left-handed baseball players, on the average, died nine months sooner than right-handed players. Other research examining non-baseball players has consistently supported the finding that left-handers experience more accidents and illness and die sooner than righties.

Interestingly, the population of left-handers exhibits greater extremes in intelligence: There are higher percentages of retardation and intellectual giftedness among lefties than among righties, who tend to gravitate toward the middle ranges of intellectual ability. Left-handers also may experience greater communication between the brain's hemispheres than right-handed people do. Theories abound as to why we culturally prefer right-handedness, and why differences in mortality rates exist. But science is still mystified.

During the late '70s and early '80s, researchers started to recognize the differences between the brains of men and women. Like other significant parts of the body, the sexes are different here, too. Scientists discovered that while men tend to have larger brains overall, women usually have larger corpus callosums than men do. This has led to speculation that women enjoy greater communication between the left and right hemispheres, a trait that might explain why women tend to score better on verbal and linguistic tests. Scientists also note that women often are better able to put their emotions into words, perhaps another benefit of the larger corpus callosum. Men, on the other hand, usually score better on tests that require perception of spatial relationships. Researchers speculate that the smaller corpus callosum may encourage greater specialization of the brain among men, more reliance upon the right hemisphere, and a comparatively weaker ability to put their intuitions and feelings into words.

Still, scientists are quick to point out that no one knows for sure what these differences in brain structure mean, if anything, and that the variances between the sexes may be more socially regulated than biological.

It's instructive to remember that most of us use only a tiny percentage of our brain's capacity, no matter which sex we are. In fact, scientists maintain that the brain's six capabilities reach far beyond our current usage, prompting the late author Arthur Koestler to say, "In creating the human brain, evolution has wildly overshot the mark."

Indeed, the brain remains more mysterious than understood. Take memory, for example. Scientists still cannot figure out where it is located in the brain—if at all—and by what mechanism we are able to recall information at will. No one knows what the basis of feelings and thoughts are; how we are able to discern and appreciate musical harmony from chaotic sound; how artistic ability, proven synchronistic events, and extrasensory perception are mediated by the brain; and how relatively tiny parts of the brain, such as the hypothalamus, are involved in so many complex and varied tasks.

Sages and poets make convincing arguments for the unity of body, mind, and spirit. The body, they say, is the physical manifestation of mind and spirit. Humanness, with all its marvelous capabilities, resides as much in the ether that surrounds and permeates the body, as it does in the organism itself. If science ever discovers that unity among the mind, body, and spirit, it will likely come from its explorations of this wondrous organ.

The probability that human consciousness and our infinitely complex universe could have come into existence through the random interactions of inert matter has aptly been compared to that of a tornado blowing through a junkyard and accidentally assembling a 747 jumbo jet.

STANISLAV GROF

189

THE MULTIPURPOSE ORGAN

The brain has six general functions, as follows:

1. It is the regulating center of the body. The brain receives a continual stream of information from the body in the form of sensory impulses. It evaluates this information, and provides an integrated biological response by activating or inhibiting an array of functions, including the endocrine system, muscles, heartbeat, and respiration, as well as conscious and unconscious thought processes. Most of these functions go on unconsciously, that is, without our being aware of them.

2. It is the center of consciousness. Consciousness, as defined by Edwin B. Steen and Ashley Montagu in *Anatomy and Physiology, Vol. 2,* "is the state of awareness of time, place, person, and, in greater or lesser degree, the activities of the body."

3. It is the receiver and interpreter of the senses. It receives and interprets sensory impulses from every point within the body, and from sensory organs that perceive information coming from outside the body. Our capacities for sight, sound, smell, taste, and touch originate at points distant from the brain, but must be processed by the brain before we experience such information. (See chapters on individual senses, Part Three.)

4. It initiates voluntary action. Every conscious act is initiated, coordinated, and processed by the brain.

5. It is the mediating organ for all emotion, urges, drives, and instincts. These emotional responses are processed and dealt with in the brain.

6. It is the seat of all intellectual activity, and the organ of intelligence. Perception, recognition, judgment, reasoning, memory, and learning are the basis for intelligence, and all are processed in the brain.

The brain, located in the cranium, is the main organ of the central nervous system. The spinal cord is its counterpart. (See chapter on the nervous system.) In the average adult, the brain can weigh anywhere from just over two pounds to just under four. Brain size and weight tends to vary between the sexes: the average man's brain is slightly larger than the average woman's—2.9 pounds for men compared to 2.6 for women. No one knows what, if anything, these differences mean. The size of the brain is one of the indicators of overall intelligence, but not the only one. Scientists point out that the largest brains found in humans tend to be those of retarded adults. Nevertheless, as Steen and Montagu state, "In general, the weight of the brain of persons of eminence tends to be slightly above the average."

The basic cellular unit of the brain is the neuron, a microscopic cell shaped like an octopus, with one particularly long tendril, called an axon. The axon terminates on other neurons and in this way makes it possible for nerve signals to travel from one cell to the next. When a nerve impulse is generated from the center of the neuron and then travels to the tip of the axon, it causes the release of a chemical called a neurotransmitter. That neurotransmitter is released from the axon into the spaces between neurons; once it touches the neighboring neuron, it causes the nerve to fire an impulse along its own axon, thus causing another neurotransmitter to be released, which in turns sets off another nerve impulse in the adjacent neuron. In short, neurons communicate with one another according to a basic bucket-brigade strategy. And just like the bucket brigade, healthy brain function depends upon the brain having sufficient chemical neurotransmitters. This, as we will see later, has become a growing problem, particularly among people suffering from Parkinson's disease.

There are different chemical neurotransmitters, and each one causes different reactions inside the brain. Serotonin gives rise to feelings of well-being and relaxation. It enhances our ability to focus our thoughts, and causes deeper and more restful sleep. Dopamine encourages greater alertness and aggression. It is often secreted by the brain when we face some difficulty and need a heightened sense of awareness. Acetylcholine, another transmitter, helps the brain to maintain coordinated motor activity. When acetylcholine levels diminish, a person can suffer from jerky, uncoordinated movements that, when acute, can be crippling.

As we will see later, the availability of these neurotransmitters is highly sensitive to the foods we eat. According to Dr. John D. Fernstrom of the Massachusetts Institute of Technology, "It is becoming increasingly clear that brain chemistry and function can be influenced by a single meal."

The Brain

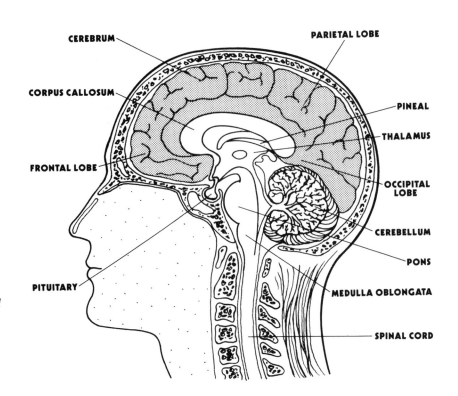

Despite recent medical and scientific advances, the brain remains more mysterious than understood. It stores memory, receives and evaluates a continual stream of sensory input, acts as the center of consciousness, initiates and coordinates voluntary action, mediates emotions, urges, drives, and instincts, and serves as the seat of all intellectual activity, including perception, recognition, judgment, reasoning, and learning. It does this all in a manner and with a speed that transcend any imaginable computer model.

A Marvel of Integrated Circuitry

While the brain is highly specialized, it is also fundamentally interdependent. Nerve impulses fire across the brain in fractions of an instant, linking and coordinating the relatively distant and disparate brain structures so that the body can function properly. In short, the brain is a marvel of integrated circuitry. It is also a supreme paradox in that it is highly specialized, but at the same time awesomely unified.

The brain can be divided into three main structures: the brain stem and cerebellum—the two oldest parts of the brain, in evolutionary terms—and the cerebrum, the most recent and most highly developed aspect of the organ. Within the cerebrum are four main lobes, or regions, in which specific functions take place.

Located in the base of the brain, the brain stem forms a tube-like structure that connects the spinal cord with the corpus callosum and the cerebrum. In general, the brain stem is responsible for connecting the higher and lower centers of the brain. It assists in involuntary movement, communicates sense information, and helps sustain physical balance. The specific functions of the brain stem reside in its four parts. The medulla oblongata controls the heartbeat, breathing, and blood pressure. The pons, an oval-shaped bulb that connects the medulla to the upper parts of the brain, contains sensory and motor nerves that communicate physical movement commands and sense information back and forth from the higher centers in the brain to the spinal cord. The midbrain, which helps maintain equilibrium, is responsible for many reflex actions, receives nerve impulses from the retina and other sense organs, and passes them along to the higher parts of the brain. The hypothalamus is a tiny organ, weighing only four grams—about three-thousandths of the brain's total weight—but its responsibilities are mind-boggling. Through nerve impulses and secretion of hormones, the hypothalamus acts like a great railway engineer, sending signals throughout the body's systems, like trains along various tracks, which in turn set other effects in motion. The hypothalamus performs the following tasks:

1. Controls involuntary organs, such as the heart and intestines, through the autonomic nervous system, over which we have no conscious control.

2. Controls many general involuntary functions, such as body temperature, appetite, thirst, and sex drive.

3. Controls the emotions, including feelings of pleasure, pain, fear, and anger, through creating endorphins, which are morphinelike substances that stimulate moods and provide pain relief.

4. Translates emotional states into physical symptoms, or so-called psychosomatic illnesses. Stress or fear affect hypothalamic function, which in turns influences the nervous, endocrine, immune, cardiovascular, and respiratory systems, and the gastrointestinal tract. If adversely influenced, these systems can manifest an array of symptoms, anything from nervous tension or indigestion, to heart attack or tumors.

All you have to do is rest. Nature herself, when we let her, will take care of everything else. It's our impatience that spoils things. Most men die of their cures, and not of their diseases.

JEAN MOLIÈRE

193

5. Coordinates the nervous and endocrine systems by releasing hormones that stimulate production of other hormones. The nervous system acts with hormones to affect blood pressure, heartbeat, and respiration. This occurs during times of acute stress, such as the moment you see a bear in the woods, or pleasure, such as when you are playing a game or are sexually excited.

6. Controls sleep. The hypothalamus activates parts of the brain that bring about the transition from sleep to wakefulness, and suppresses these brain capabilities when fatigue requires you to go to sleep.

(Other glands found in the brain, such as the pineal and the pituitary, are described in the chapter on the endocrine system.)

The cerebellum, which sits above the brain stem and extends behind it, is composed of two lobes that are striated with many small folds. The cerebellum is the old brain, the primitive part of the nervous system that is responsible for many instinctual and highly complex involuntary movements.

To perform these complex movements, the cerebellum has built-in programs that coordinate an array of muscles, nerves, and bones. For example, the simple act of raising your hand to your face requires the coordination of more than fifty muscles moving thirty bones in the arm and hand alone. You experience this motion as a smooth flow, yet it requires a complex orchestration of events, each with its own job and duration.

The cerebellum also helps to maintain posture, equilibrium, and muscle tone. It is essential to all motor activity, especially complex and instantaneous movements, such as those performed by athletes and performing artists, such as dancers.

The cerebrum is what you think of when you picture a brain: a large, spongy mushroom cap that is permeated with soft folds and fissures, called gyri and sulci, respectively. These folds and indentations give the brain a surface area of approximately 400 square inches. The cerebrum represents five-sixths of the total brain. It is divided from front to back into two hemispheres. It is further divided into lobes, described below.

The surface area, called the cerebral cortex, varies in thickness but averages about an eighth of an inch. Composed of the celebrated "gray matter," associated with intelligence, the cerebral cortex is where many highly advanced intellectual activities occur. These functions are rooted within the four main lobes of the cerebral cortex: the frontal, parietal, temporal, and occipital lobes.

The frontal lobe is the largest lobe, extending from the middle of the brain and emanating forward like a giant outcropping or cliff, to form the entire frontal area. In a band that stretches laterally over the very top of the lobe, or the top of the head, is the motor cortex, which is responsible for controlling all muscle movements of the body. The muscles that control everything from the mouth, tongue, face, eyes, arms, fingers, legs, and toes are controlled by this center.

In a small area in the left hemisphere of the frontal lobe is the word-meaning center, the part of the brain that deciphers word sounds. The frontal lobe also houses your ability to plan and create mental imagery.

However, much of what is in front of the motor center—the largest part of the brain—remains a mystery to scientists. In his book *The Body,* Anthony Smith reports that great portions of this area have been cut away by surgeons, yet patients emerge with only minor changes in behavior. They are highly sensitive to criticism, show little drive, and lack the concentration they enjoyed before. Otherwise they seem fine. However, if you scratch the motor area of the brain, paralysis will result.

The parietal lobe is located behind the frontal lobe. It is responsible for controlling all sensations, such as touch, pressure, temperature, and body position.

The temporal lobe is located on the sides of the brain, near what would be the area of the ears. It is responsible for hearing and discerning the origin of sounds. The left side of the temporal lobe controls the left ear, the right oversees the right ear. The temporal lobe is also the site of the part of the brain that helps us sound out words before we speak them.

Smith points out that the area involved in hearing is quite small, causing scientists to wonder what the rest of the temporal lobe is up to. Some believe it is involved in memory.

The occipital lobe, located in the back of the brain, is responsible for controlling sight. Like the temporal lobe, vision for the right eye is controlled by the right hemisphere's occipital lobe, while the left hemisphere controls the left eye. In the occipital lobe is located the word-reading center, the part of us that discerns

Our bodies are not made up of organ systems presided over by an authoritarian brain that is separate from our hearts, emotions, and spirits. We are instead a complex physical manifestation of our thoughts, dietary choices, relationships, parents, communities, hopes, and dreams.

CHRISTIANE
NORTHRUP

words and then sends the information forward to be interpreted by the frontal lobe.

The limbic system, among the most primitive parts of the brain, is located at the back of the brain stem and plays an important role in experiencing emotions. An emotion involves a two-fold reaction: first, an internal subjective feeling, and second, a response to that feeling, some kind of judgment about the emotion—whether we like it or not—and associations with it. Both of these reactions take place within the limbic system.

The limbic system is also closely associated with the ability to smell. The experience of smell is very much tied up with your associations to stimulating odors or fragrances. Consequently, smell is closely linked with memory (see chapter on smell). Those with injuries to the limbic system exhibit marked changes in emotion, either the diminution or extremes of fear, anger, aggression, passivity, pain, pleasure, and sexual drive.

BRAIN ACTIVITY AND FOOD CHOICES

Researchers at the Massachusetts Institute of Technology have discovered that brain chemistry and function are greatly influenced by dietary choices. According to MIT's Dr. Judith Wurtman, a leader in this research, three groups of foods seem to cause relatively quick and impressive changes in brain activity:

- Carbohydrates (found in whole grains, vegetables, and refined sugars) promote calm, reduce anxiety and stress, and help the mind focus better;
- Proteins (found especially in animal foods) promote brain chemicals that stimulate and energize the body;
- Caffeine has an effect similar to protein foods.

Consumption of whole grains, such as brown rice, corn, barley, buckwheat, and oatmeal (including whole wheat bread and pasta) and vegetables will increase blood and brain levels of an amino acid called tryptophan, says Wurtman. Tryptophan will, in turn, stimulate production of a brain neurotransmitter called serotonin, which produces a heightened sense of calm, reduces stress and anxiety, and aids in inducing sleep.

"Those who eat calming foods consistently report feeling more relaxed, more focused, less stressed, less distracted after their meal," says Wurtman. "Tests confirm the volunteers' subjective assessments of their moods."

The stimulating agent in grains and sugar is glucose. Once in the body, the glucose found in carbohydrates is converted to blood glucose when it interacts with insulin, a hormone produced by the pancreas during digestion. Fruit sugar, which contains fructose, is gradually converted to glucose in the blood. But, according to Wurtman, the process is too slow to produce noticeable changes in brain chemistry and mood.

Further research at MIT has shown that some obese people use sugar as a sedative and to maintain a sense of well-being. When the sugar wears off, however, anxiety returns. The use of sugar—simple carbohydrate, as compared to the long chains of complex carbohydrates found in whole grains—may be counterproductive in the long run. Sugar causes wild swings in blood sugar levels, which may result in lower levels of glucose in the brain. Depleted brain levels of glucose may cause brain fatigue and diminished function. This condition, known as hypoglycemia, is associated with lower levels of blood sugar, cravings for sweets, wide mood swings, depression, and anxiety.

Protein foods, on the other hand, stimulate production of the neurotransmitters dopamine and norepinephrine. These cause people to "think more quickly, react more rapidly to stimuli, and feel more attentive, motivated, and mentally energetic," says Wurtman. "Problems, even big ones, often seem more manageable because of heightened 'brain power.'"

Wurtman counsels people to avoid high-fat sources of protein because fat diminishes the alertness response from protein and also causes an array of other serious illnesses. "It is important to choose protein foods that contain only small amounts of fats and/or carbohydrates when you want to shift quickly into a more alert, energetic, and motivated state," she says.

Caffeinated beverages, such as tea and coffee, stimulate the production of dopamine and norepinephrine. Performance tests on volunteers have shown consistently that reaction times, vigilance, and mental alertness are all enhanced after one or two cups of coffee. Wurtman recommends that people do not exceed two cups.

Illnesses of the Brain

Brain disorders can be grouped into various categories, including congenital defects, injury, tumors, infections, and impaired blood supply.

Genetic disorders: These include a wide variety of disorders that arise during gestation and manifest before or after birth. They include Tay-Sachs disease, a progressive illness associated with blindness, brain deterioration, and death, usually during childhood, and Down's Syndrome, a genetic defect causing mental handicap and characteristic facial features which usually causes death between teenage years and middle age.

Infections: Encephalitis, which is a brain infection, is usually caused by viruses, the most common of which are rabies and herpes simplex. Meningitis, which affects the membranes or meninges surrounding the brain, is caused by bacterial infection.

Degeneration: Multiple sclerosis is an illness in which the myelin sheaths of nerves are gradually destroyed. (See nervous system.)

Alzheimer's disease is characterized by a progressive degeneration or shrinking of brain tissue. People with Alzheimer's disease gradually lose brain function and body control. The illness is responsible for more than 75 percent of all dementia among adults sixty-five and older. At present, scientists do not know the exact cause of the disease. Many believe that aluminum poisoning may play a role in the onset of Alzheimer's. There is no known cure.

Parkinson's disease is a degenerative illness affecting part of the motor function of the brain, located in the basal ganglia. It causes muscle tremors, trembling, rigid posture, and imbalanced walking. It too has no known cure.

Cerebrovascular disease: A diet rich in fat and cholesterol causes atherosclerosis, or cholesterol plaques, to form in the arteries leading to the brain. As the plaque grows larger, the artery passage narrows, thus diminishing the brain's supply of blood, oxygen, and glucose. Eventually, this illness can cut off blood and oxygen to the brain, thus suffocating a part of the organ and causing a stroke. Strokes can be fatal or disabling, depending on where they take place and which parts of the brain are affected.

Before such an event takes place, however, the diminished blood and oxygen to the brain can reduce brain efficiency, vitality, alertness and overall function. Oxygen can be reduced to the brain by progressive atherosclerosis and by reducing the blood's ability to carry oxygen. This occurs when dietary fat and cholesterol causes red blood cells to adhere to one another, thus preventing efficient oxygen carrying. (See circulatory system and rouleaux effect.) Consequently, the brain becomes fatigued. Eventually, atherosclerosis can cause senile dementia.

For many years, Nathan Pritikin, a pioneer of a low-fat, low-cholesterol, high-complex-carbohydrate diet, maintained that brain function is enhanced by avoiding foods rich in fat and cholesterol. Pritikin pointed out that the brain's demands for oxygen and glucose are so sensitive that diminished quantities of either oxygen or glucose will reduce brain efficiency dramatically.

To prove his point, Pritikin conducted before-and-after performance tests on people coming to his Pritikin Longevity Center in Santa Monica, California. The tests consisted of elementary arithmetic problems conducted during a two-minute period. Pritikin found that people scored far higher after they had been at the center more than two weeks—during which they were eating a low-fat diet and exercising daily, thus promoting optimal circulation to the brain.

Though we knew the connections of every tickling thread of every single axon and dendrite in every species that ever existed, together with all its neurotransmitters and how they varied in its billions of synapses of every brain that ever existed, we could still never—not ever—from a knowledge of the brain alone, know if that brain contained a consciousness like our own.

JULIAN JAYNES

"A CURIOUS ORGAN"

The Chinese regard the brain as one of the "curious" organs, the others being the bone marrow, uterus, blood vessels, bones, and gall bladder. Except for the gall bladder, there are no specific approaches to the curious organs, per se. Rather, the Chinese understand the brain in terms of how other organs influence its function. They also view it from the general standpoint of yin and yang.

The brain can be seen as a command center, but other organs in the body provide it with raw data, specific abilities, and even emotions, according to the Chinese. In order for the brain to function properly, the body must be healthy and balanced. The brain responds to general bodily states, according to Eastern medicine, rather than initiating them.

For example, clear and focused thinking, viewed in the West as a function of the brain, is seen as dependent upon healthy intes-

[The brain is a] great ravelled knot.

SIR CHARLES
SHERRINGTON

tinal function in the East. Constipation causes blocked or dull thinking—the inability to move thoughts freely—while diarrhea causes scattered, disjointed, or "spaced out" thinking. Spastic colon causes extremes in behavior—mood swings, rapid insights alternating with blocked thinking. Consistent intestinal health results in clearheadedness.

Good memory depends upon healthy liver function, while a weak liver will diminish one's recall. This may be related to the liver's role in purifying the blood and maintaining immune function. The liver must "remember" the antidotes to many thousands of toxins, bacteria, and viruses that enter the body, and come up with a remedy for each. Also, the liver is associated with the eyes and with sight. Being able to identify what is seen is, in part, a function of memory, and is therefore assisted by a well-working liver.

"The liver has the function of a military planner who excels in his strategic planning," says the Yellow Emperor. So the brain's ability to plan or strategize is dependent upon the liver. Those who have trouble planning ahead have weak livers, say the Chinese. This is probably related to the fact that the liver holds so much blood at any one time, which might be regarded as an enormous resource, and which must be treated carefully and parceled out appropriately.

As we have already seen, emotions and various mental states have their original source in specific organs. Joy and hysteria are related to the heart and small intestine; understanding and sympathy to the spleen and stomach; sadness and grief to the lungs and large intestine; fear and will to the kidneys and bladder; anger to the liver and gall bladder. When these organs are strong and the overall system is balanced, emotional and psychological harmony is maintained, say the Chinese. When these organs are balanced, the mind is balanced and emotional life is more stable. When these organs are imbalanced or in turmoil, the emotional and psychological life is also in turmoil.

Therefore, treatment for mental clarity and many psychological problems is focused on the body, which can be seen as the soil of the brain. Also, many physical problems related to the head and brain are seen as having their origin in the body's various organs.

Serious illnesses associated with the brain, such as stroke, are related to other organ systems, as well. In the case of stroke, the cause lies in the cardiovascular system and the development of atherosclerosis, in which cholesterol plaque builds within the arteries. Ultimately, such plaque can cut off blood and oxygen to the brain, which causes a stroke by killing part of the brain. The underlying cause of both stroke and heart attack is atherosclerosis. However, the place where the illness manifests most acutely depends upon an imbalance between yin and yang. Let's have a look.

The head and brain region can be seen as relatively yang in comparison to the rest of the body. They occupy the upper part of the body, which corresponds with heaven. The feet, on the other hand, can be seen as yin, or the lower part of the body, and correspond with the earth.

The Meridian Origin of Headaches

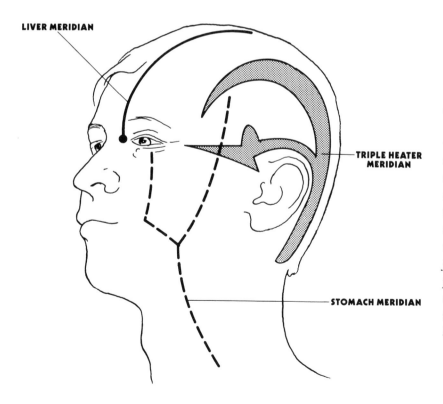

LIVER MERIDIAN

TRIPLE HEATER MERIDIAN

STOMACH MERIDIAN

Where a headache is located may indicate the origin of the imbalance, according to traditional Chinese healers. They diagnose headaches by whether the pain is along the triple heater meridian (which runs in an arc just above each ear and then to the temple), the stomach meridian (which begins at a point just below each eye and runs down to the jawline and then back up to a point just above the temples), or the liver meridian (which runs behind the eyes to the back of the neck).

201

In general, too many expansive foods, drinks, and activities will manifest as problems in the head region, because their influences naturally flow upward and outward, affecting the head. For example, alcohol, which is very expansive, has a profound effect on brain function. Drugs, which are even more expansive—sometimes referred to as mind-expanding—have an extreme effect on brain function. Drugs disorient and change our perception of reality. Foods such as sugar and spices, both less extreme than alcohol and drugs, also influence brain function. Sugar increases the level of serotonin in the brain, making the mind more relaxed, focused, while enhancing one's sense of well-being.

From either perspective, East or West, the brain is still the most mysterious of organs. Yet, experience tells us that it is also the one most dependent upon the rest of the body. If you haven't had enough sleep, enough to eat, or you're feeling ill, the brain's acuity is diminished. This prompted Orientals to offer sage advice: take good care of the body, and the mind will function well.

PART THREE

The Senses

THOSE OF US who have been brought up in the West have been trained to think of our senses as essentially objective sources of information. Indeed, even our sciences are based upon what can be *observed* in a laboratory. We Westerners use the senses to inform us of what is happening *outside* the body. The eyes see the world; the ears hear it; the tongue tastes it; the nose smells it; the skin touches it. We then take this information and quantify it—that is, we break it up into measured units, such as inches, ounces, decibels, or atoms. The result is that we see reality as more or less constant. We use the senses to deliver that outer world to our inner selves. If reality were not objective, a Westerner would argue, life would be reduced to chaos. We couldn't drive down the street without killing each other; we couldn't communicate; we couldn't observe and respect laws. Society would collapse.

In the Orient, the tables are turned. The most important aspects of reality are inward and subjective. Of course, an Oriental healer would agree that the senses deliver information from the outer environment, but your capacity to perceive what is truly happening around you depends entirely upon your inner state. Ten people can witness the same event and report ten very different experiences, as expressed so eloquently in the film *Rashomon*. Experience, in the end, is a subjective reality, say the Orientals.

Even more, the senses can be used to change the inner world, and thereby alter your ability to perceive more information. For example, certain smells can trigger memories and alter moods; certain colors can awaken sensitivities and heighten alertness; certain tastes can be used to strengthen or weaken individual organs; sound, as everyone knows, can transform us.

The senses alter the body and mind. They play with the soul. What you perceive in any moment powerfully affects your inner state, and thereby enhances or diminishes your capacity to further perceive that event. You may walk in a forest or along a beach and experience a tremendous heightening of awareness. Or you may be shocked by terrible violence and experience a state of dull apprehension. In both cases, your ability to sense is altered. Certain music may inspire you, while other sounds may depress or frighten you. In sensing the world, we interact with it, and in the process we are changed.

This mysterious truth is used by the Oriental practitioner as a means of healing. The senses are tools to the inner you. Therefore, what you sense can be used to strengthen your health, or weaken it. As we will see, Oriental and alternative healers have developed elaborate systems for healing based upon the senses alone.

We want this book to be an attempt at bridge-building, or unifying two worldviews. We wish to understand and recognize the contributions of both East and West. But in reality, these contrasting ways of looking at life represent different aspects of human experience. Each of us experiences both the objective and subjective forms of reality. When it comes to contrasting East and West, we are really talking about how cultures emphasize one way of looking at life over another. But both are already present inside each of us.

Let's look closer at the human senses, and examine the evidence supporting each of these contrasting worldviews that already exists inside ourselves.

CHAPTER 18

SMELL

SMELL IS THE MOST sensitive of our senses, and perhaps the most primitive. We can distinguish literally thousands of odors and fragrances, and somehow remember them for the rest of our lives. Studies have shown that infants can identify their mothers on the basis of smell, and that mothers also can pick out their babies on smell alone. It requires only four scent-bearing molecules for us to recognize a particular smell, yet scientists still do not know exactly how odors are discerned or remembered.

Much, if not all, of our experience is associated with smell, even when we are unconscious of those smells in our environment. Consequently, memories and their related emotions can be called forth instantly by the right odor or fragrance. We can be consumed by our immediate problems while walking to work one day when suddenly, after passing a bakery or a candy store, we are enveloped in childhood memories by the smell of bread baking in the oven, or that of candy wafting innocently before our noses.

The reason that smell evokes such powerful memories and emotions is that our olfactory sense is linked directly with the brain's limbic system, one of the most primitive parts of the

In a general way I should like to raise the question whether the inevitable stunting of the sense of smell as a result of man's turning away from the earth, and the organic repression of the smell-pleasure produced by it, does not largely share in his predisposition to nervous diseases.

SIGMUND FREUD

central nervous system. The limbic system plays a central role in our ability to experience emotion and retain those experiences. It is literally a storehouse of memories, emotions, and their related odors, any set of which can be released by the right fragrance.

Smell also can arouse us sexually. Indeed, smell is among the most powerful of aphrodisiacs. After a long campaign on the battlefield, Napoleon wrote back to Josephine: "Home in three days. Don't wash."

One of the reasons that smell affects us sexually is that scent-bearing molecules also can carry hormones, called pheromones, which are received through the olfactory nerves. Research has shown that pheromones affect the behavior of sex organs. A 1971 study of Harvard women showed that, after spending sufficient time together, close friends and roommates all experienced their menstrual cycles at the same time of the month. It has long been known that animals communicate on the basis of smell, but this was the first evidence that humans were affecting one another on the basis of odors.

Later research, conducted at the Monel Chemical Senses Center in Philadelphia, showed that men help to regulate the fertility of their sex partners through their release of pheromones from their armpits. (We can only wonder if the deodorant industry isn't secretly contributing to our growing rates of infertility.) The Monel Center is now studying the efficacy of using human smells as a kind of "fingerprint" system in law enforcement and security.

Clearly, personal odor is one of the aspects of our humanness with which we are least comfortable, at least in the West. Perfume is a $4 billion industry alone. We are a people who like to be neutral-smelling, or emit mass-produced fragrances. To be identified with some unique odor is, as the TV commercial says, "uncivilized."

Recently, Madison Avenue has decided that we are olfactorily deprived and has begun scenting everything from shopping malls to magazines. You cannot pick up a copy of *Cosmopolitan* or *Esquire* without being slapped in the nose by fragrance (some would say odor).

Our capacity to identify a substance before we put it in our mouths has spared humanity much suffering and death. Eighty percent of what we perceive as taste is actually smell, though our

Nothing is more indisputable than the existence of our senses.

JEAN LE ROND
D'ALEMBERT

olfactory nerves get little of the credit. Much of what we crave from food is actually smell. According to Duke University researcher Dr. Susan Schiffman, each of us must be olfactorily sated before we actually feel satisfied by a meal. Many people are "seeking the pleasure of the odor of the food," says Schiffman. "The food doesn't tell a person to stop eating; even when they've met their caloric needs, they will go on eating until they have satisfied their hunger for smell, taste, and texture of the food."

Schiffman has been applying this principle to help obese people lose weight. She uses sprays to strengthen the fragrance of food, which in turn creates greater flavor and satiety from less volume of food. She treated a man who weighed 400 pounds who had previously said that he would rather die than give up pizza. She had a food spray created that would give the taste of pizza without the calories and fat. The man eventually lost 180 pounds with the help of the taste sprays. When food chemists and flavorists examine the world's cuisines, they point out that the typical American diet carries its flavors and fragrances in fat molecules, while the Oriental diet bears its fragrances in water.

Dr. Charles Weiner, a food chemist at International Flavors and Fragrances, and one of twenty-five senior flavorists in the U.S., says that the Oriental diet succeeds in satisfying taste without the harmful side effects. "The Oriental diet is delightfully aromatic, but there's less guilt associated with it because it's low in fat and cholesterol." Weiner says that such diets are the future. "The bland foods of twenty years ago—the meat and potatoes— are gone," says Weiner. "The demand is going up dramatically for aromatic foods and for highly seasoned foods. Twenty years ago, we didn't have so many Thai, Mexican, and Oriental restaurants. The baby-boomers want natural and healthful foods. The demand is going up for less synthetic additives and less fat, but more taste." Which really means, more smell.

The efficiency of absorption of therapeutic substances into the bloodstream by the nasal route has probably not received sufficient attention. Plant estrogens are known to exert a powerful influence upon animal behavior; the estrus of many species is triggered by the presence of plant estrogens in pasture in springtime, probably not by ingestion but by inhalation.

GERMAINE GREER

IN SEARCH OF SCENTS

Just as the ear traps sound, the nose draws odors and fragrances to itself by inhalation. At the roof of the nose, just below the eyes, lies a closely bunched set of specialized nerve endings called smell receptors. These olfactory nerves protrude downward into the

The Sense of Smell

Inhaling air through the nose allows specialized olfactory nerves called smell receptors to begin a process that ultimately can distinguish an amazing array of odors and fragrances. As yet scientists are unable to determine any microscopic difference in the smell receptors, and thus are stymied at how smells can be differentiated.

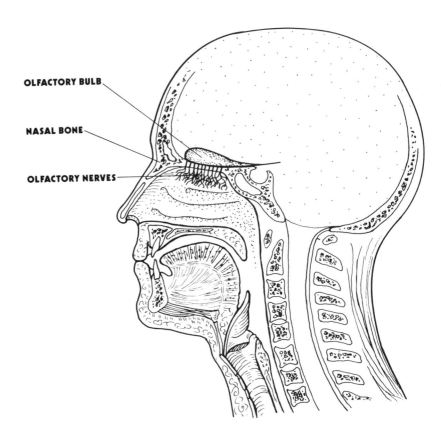

OLFACTORY BULB

NASAL BONE

OLFACTORY NERVES

nose canal. The tips of these nerves are swollen and have tiny hairs, called cilia, extending from them. A mucous membrane covers the surface of the nerves and serves to dissolve molecules that carry scent, thus making the odor accessible to the nerves.

The scent-bearing molecules stimulate the cilia, which pass sensory information onto the nerves. The nerves pass information upward to the olfactory bulbs, which are larger smell receptors that transmit the sensory information onto the olfactory nerve, which leads to the brain. The smell centers in the brain are located in the limbic system, just above the brain stem, and the frontal lobe. So far, scientists have not been able to determine any microscopic distinctions in the smell receptors. So, no one knows how smells can be differentiated.

The ability to smell varies widely among people. Some have a talent for smells, while the capacity to smell in others is relatively dull. Neither end of the spectrum is regarded as a disorder, but rather a genetic trait. However, loss of smell can occur temporarily or permanently; in both cases, our ability to taste is greatly diminished. The causes of temporary or permanent loss of smell vary widely. Swelling of the mucous membranes in the nasal passage and the development of scar tissue or lesions in the pathways or olfactory receptors can dull or even eliminate our ability to smell. Finally, disorders of the rhinecephalon or the limbic system can either diminish our ability to smell, or make it even more sensitive than normal.

SENSITIVITY AND THE SPLEEN

According to Chinese medicine, our ability to smell is governed largely by the spleen and lungs. As the Yellow Emperor says, the spleen opens in the nose, the lungs in the mouth. Since the lungs are responsible for taking in the breath through the nose, they play a major role in our ability to smell. But it is the spleen that is seen as most often responding to smells, largely because of its incredible sensitivity and its relationship to appetite and digestion. Some smells alone stimulate our hunger; others can give us indigestion. To the Chinese, this indicates the relationship between smell and the Earth Element (spleen and stomach).

When smell is weak, therefore, the Chinese recommend treating both the Metal (lungs and large intestine) and Earth Elements. (See chapters on the lungs and spleen.) In general, however, the loss of smell is regarded as a general loss of sensitivity and therefore suggests lack of circulation, fat and cholesterol plaques accumulating in the nasal passages, and a generalized weakened condition.

The Chinese also use body odor as one of the principle methods of diagnosis. Each smell corresponds to a particular element within the Five Element System, and reveals specific imbalances. According to Kiiko Matsumoto and Stephen Birch, authors of *Five Elements and Ten Stems,* the five smells and their corresponding organs are as follows: A greasy, oily odor, "like rotting flesh," indicates a liver imbalance (the Wood Element). A scorched or burnt odor indicates heart (Fire). Sweet odor points to spleen (Earth). An odor like raw fish or fat, which "clings to the nose," indicates lungs (Metal). Rancid or rotting odor "like decayed meat" is kidney (Water).

"A patient's odor is one of the things that is relevant if it is particularly noticeable," say Matsumoto and Birch. "Since these features become apparent very quickly, it will not be necessary to spend a great deal of time scrutinizing them."

FRAGRANCES THAT HEAL

Just as the word implies, aromatherapy uses fragrance to heal. The fragrances are drawn from plants in the form of essential oils. Each of these oils has its own distinct odor, which stimulates an array of emotional, psychological, and physical responses. Some arouse, excite, create alertness, or heighten sensuality; others relax, cool, and soothe. Aromatherapists say that the emotional and psychological states that these fragrances give rise to create physical responses—changes in pulse rate, respiration, perspiration, and immune response—which in turn can heal the body.

The use of fragrant oils to heal goes back 4,000 years to the Egyptians, and was later used by both the Greeks and the Romans. But it has recently begun to catch on again. Elizabeth Taylor and Princess Diana are only two of its more glamorous proponents.

The secret of aromatherapy lies in human experience—that is, how we relate fragrance to specific experiences. The odors present in a forest, a meadow, a room, or anywhere else are recorded, often unconsciously, and thus related to experience itself. To encounter that odor again will recall the emotions associated with the specific experience, even if we cannot recall the details of that experience. Aromatherapists maintain that within the fragrance lies the conditions under which the plant grew, as well. Each plant grows in specific geographical locations; it has specific characteristics; it responds to the sun, the moon, the earth, and the rain in different ways. These characteristics are also implicit in the essential oil and fragrance, say proponents of aromatherapy.

The rosemary flower, for example, is nestled deeply among its branches, close to the earth, and sends out a strong and stimulating fragrance to the entire plant. The flower has a kind of charisma all its own. It draws the sun toward itself, like a magnet, and then radiates its odors outward. Thus, rosemary offers the same characteristics to those who use it as an essential oil: it is said to stimulate, invigorate, and awaken the entire organism. It also imparts an earthly allure, drawing life toward you. For these reasons, rosemary is often found in morning lotions, day creams, or skin cleansers. Traditionally, it has been used as a purifying, warming, and decongesting herb, as well.

Lavender is just the opposite. Its flower lifts away from the plant—"almost like a cloud or a dream," says Weleda President Christine Murphy, whose company has been producing natural cosmetics and aromas for healing since her grandfather started the company with philosopher Rudolf Steiner more than sixty years ago. "Lavender leaves you feeling relaxed and light. It's wonderful after a stressful day."

Aromatherapists examine how each plant behaves in nature to discover the effects of its essential oils. Below is a short list of popular and evocative essential oils commonly used in a wide variety of natural body care products:

- *Pine:* The tree remains unaltered by the most severe winters or harshest summers, and therefore provides one of nature's greatest examples of constancy, stability, and duration in the face of life's vicissitudes. Pine is used to stimulate these same qualities, to balance the breathing, and refresh and stimulate the entire organism. As an herb, pine is used to decongest the lungs and arouse sensuality.
- *Olive:* The tree grows and produces fruit under the intense Mediterranean sun. Olive warms and soothes, creates circulation, and contains a certain fiery quality.
- *Arnica:* The plant grows high in the mountains, where the sun is pure and the air clean. It has been used traditionally as an herb for bruises and other injuries; it promotes healing, creates warmth, stimulates circulation, and moistens the skin. It arouses the senses, restores vitality, and awakens the mind and spirit.
- *Geranium:* Refreshes and arouses sensually and sexually. It lifts the mood and invigorates the senses.

When from a long distant past nothing subsists, after the people are dead, after the things are broken and scattered, still, alone, more fragile, but with more vitality, more unsubstantial, more persistent, more faithful, the smell and taste of things remain poised a long time, like souls, ready to remind us, waiting and hoping for their moment, amid the ruins of all the rest; and bear unfaltering, in the tiny and almost impalpable drop of their essence, the vast structure of recollection.

MARCEL PROUST

- *Cassia:* The tree grows in India and Southeast Asia. Its oils and fragrance are exotic, seductive, warming, and relaxing.
- *Eucalyptus:* One of the oldest traditional herbs, eucalyptus has been used to purify and decongest the lungs, as well as cool the overall condition. The essential oil has the same effects on the skin—it cleanses, purifies, and soothes and heals blemishes. It has a dispersing effect; it also enhances breathing.
- *Coriander:* Warms, relaxes, deodorizes, and soothes.
- *Chamomile:* One of the most widely used herbs and essential oils, chamomile soothes, relaxes, refreshes, and calms the overall condition.

Other evocative and popular essential oils are comfrey root, horse chestnut, lettuce, nettle, elm, tangerine, strawberry, magnolia, and sage. All of these essential oils have been used traditionally as healing herbs. Consequently, they influence the body directly, as medicinal compounds, as well as create their own atmospheres.

Essential oils are worth studying and experimenting with, especially on occasions when you want to change the mood, or heighten the senses.

CHAPTER 19

TASTE

ASTE IS PERHAPS the most immediately gratifying sense, and the one that gets us into the most trouble. The paradox of taste is that it also can be a powerful healing tool.

By itself, taste is the least refined of our senses. It relies heavily upon its sibling, smell, to compensate for its undeveloped nature. In fact, flavorists and food chemists point out that about 80 percent of what we perceive as taste is actually smell. Taste gets the credit for your gratified palate, but smell delivers most of the experience.

Humans perceive a multitude of tastes—everything from Cajun cookin' and Indian curry, to Japanese sushi and southern fried chicken seems to have its own unique spectrum of flavors. But the tongue allows us to experience only four distinct tastes: sweet, salty, sour, and bitter. All others flavors are provided to us by smell. We often hear people complain that they lose their sense of taste when they suffer from a cold or flu, but what they've really lost is their sense of smell, which dramatically reduces the ability to appreciate food.

Other factors that have little to do directly with taste play a role in our ability to taste food. These include the food's tempera-

The palate, like the eye, the ear, or touch, acquires with practice various degrees of sensitiveness that would be incredible were it not a well ascertained fact.

T. G. SHAW

ture (whether it is hot, cold, or warm), its texture (crunchy, soft, creamy), and our saliva, which helps to dissolve food and make the taste more accessible.

Taste has saved us much suffering and dying, too. Evolution has trained us to avoid certain tastes, especially bitter flavor, because it is the most common flavor carried by poisons. Conversely, we prefer sweet foods, which long experience has taught us are nutritious and especially rich in carbohydrates or energy. We also prefer salty flavor because of the presence of sodium, which is essential for proper pH balance. Children have been known to chew leather when necessary to obtain sufficient quantities of sodium.

Sometimes, we find ourselves craving certain tastes or foods, which may reflect nutritional needs. In a two-part article for the *New England Journal of Medicine* (May 26 and June 2, 1983; vol. 308, nos. 21 and 22), Duke University researcher Dr. Susan Schiffman pointed out that even infants will respond to certain foods on the basis of their perceived nutritional content. "It is clear that the ability to identify sodium chloride properly by taste in order to correct salt deficiency is innate," wrote Dr. Schiffman. "However, preferences for specific foods containing other basic nutrients, including other minerals, appear to be learned through the associations of taste with the state of need. In addition to sodium chloride, specific appetites have been reported for thiamine, calcium, potassium, and sugar in response to nutritional and metabolic imbalances."

Taste, therefore, is more than mere caprice. Indeed, at the Massachusetts Institute of Technology, researchers have identified the changes in brain chemistry that take place after a single meal consisting of protein or carbohydrates. The scientists point out that people often crave foods on the basis of their effects on brain chemistry, and the resulting mood changes that are evoked.

The next time we crave a particular food, we might ask ourselves what specifically we are looking for. Are we looking for a certain taste—sweet or salty; a certain texture—crunchy or luscious? The range of sweet foods runs from squash and fruit to apple pie and banana splits. Protein foods can be beans, fish, or beef. Calcium- and mineral-rich foods can be leafy greens (collard, kale, or mustard greens, for example), roots, or milk products. What we begin to recognize is that we have choices. Some are healthful, others not.

Beyond meeting certain biological needs, taste is a learned response to food. Parents can predispose their children to obesity, say scientists, by feeding them too many sweet-tasting foods, especially if such foods come as reward for behavior, or when a child is feeling depressed. Children also mimic their parents' food choices, even when those choices are repulsive to children. For example, Mexican parents often enjoy hot peppers that contain an irritant called capsaicin. Mexican children will eat those peppers in great quantities and suffer accordingly, because they associate the peppers with family. Eventually, the children acquire a taste for the hot peppers and even adapt to the capsaicin, but not before the peppers cause considerable pain and indigestion.

Herein lies a health secret: foods that promote health and well-being can be just as enjoyable and satisfying as unhealthful foods, if we are willing to retrain our palate. If a child can be taught to enjoy a food that burns his mouth, adults can learn to enjoy foods that are initially foreign and exotic, especially if the rewards are increased vitality, better health, and longer life.

THE FOUR TASTES OF THE WEST

Ten thousand specialized receptors, called tastebuds, give us the ability to perceive the four basic flavors: sweet, salty, bitter, and sour. These tastebuds are located mostly in the tongue, but also in the soft palate and throat. The lifespan of a tastebud is ten to twelve days.

The surface of the tongue, when magnified by a microscope, looks like a densely populated forest that's been cut down to stumps. Thousands of shoots, all closely crowded together, form what looks to the naked eye like a flat, slightly irregular surface. These tastebuds do not rest on the surface of the tongue, as many of us believe, but between crevices or pores created by these stumps, which are called papillae. Some papillae are wide (fungiform papillae), while others are narrow (filiform papillae). There are 200 to 300 tastebuds surrounding each of the papillae.

The tastebuds themselves are barrel-shaped. At one end of this taste receptor is a small opening, called a taste pore. Here, a tiny hair emerges, called a taste hair. At the other end of the tastebud is a nerve. When we chew food, saliva mixes with the food particles and dissolves them, making them accessible to the taste-buds. Molecules of food, latent with their own characteristic taste, stimulate the taste hair, which in turn triggers a nerve impulse that travels to the taste center in the brain, located in the parietal lobe.

The four tastes are located in specific parts of the tongue: the front of the tongue provides the sweet taste; the sides, near the front, respond to sour taste; further down along the sides of the tongue are located the salty taste receptors; and in the back of the tongue, near its root, are the receptors for bitter taste. Though there are regions for each taste, the tastebuds themselves are nonspecific, according to Dr. Lloyd Beidler, a taste researcher at Florida State University. No one knows exactly how food triggers flavors, or how these tastebuds identify the four basic tastes.

Specific parts of the tongue are mostly responsible for certain tastes, with the front of the tongue providing the sweet taste, the sides near the front sour, the sides near the back salty, and the very back of the tongue the bitter taste. Though there are regions for each taste, the tastebuds themselves are nonspecific, and scientists don't know exactly how these tastebuds identify the four basic tastes. Researchers are not even sure exactly how food triggers flavors at all.

The Tongue

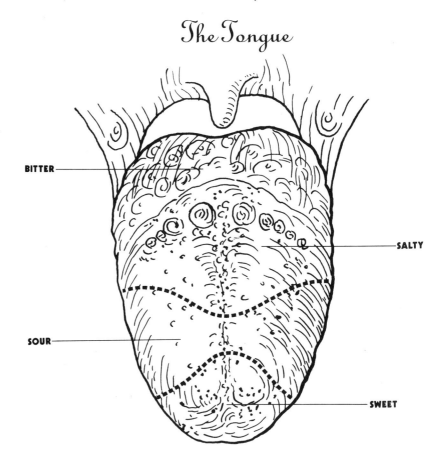

BITTER

SALTY

SOUR

SWEET

What scientists do know is that taste receptors adapt quickly to flavor, so that they need to be restimulated—either by moving the food around in our mouths or by taking another mouthful—in order for the enjoyment of food to endure.

THE FIVE TASTES OF CHINA

In Chinese medicine, taste is used medicinally to heal specific organs and restore balance to the overall system. Taste is understood within the context of the Five Element system. The five tastes, according to the Chinese Five Element system, are sour, bitter, sweet, pungent (or spicy), and salty. In moderation, each will enhance and assist the function and healing of specific organs. If all tastes are consumed in moderation, they will create balance and health. Excesses of individual tastes will excite certain organs, while controlling and diminishing others. Let's take a closer look at the effects of each of these tastes. (See chapters on specific organs for more information on the foods related to each organ and taste; see the chapter on Chinese medicine for more information on the Five Elements.)

Sour: In moderation, sour taste will help to heal the liver and gall bladder (the Wood Element) by stimulating circulation in the liver. It eliminates stagnation and thus enhances liver activity. Sour stimulates blood cleansing, and thus helps to eliminate toxins in the blood. By moving blood and qi through the liver, it balances and reduces anger. In excess, sour will cause constriction of the liver and prevent it from eliminating waste. The liver's blood-cleansing function can become stagnant. Such stagnation can cause explosions of emotion, especially anger.

Since the Wood Element controls the spleen and stomach (Earth), it will diminish the stomach and digestive functions, causing the spleen to become deficient. This will lead to lung problems and constipation. A mildly sour taste has a slight sweetness to it. Excesses cause astringency.

Bitter: Moderate amounts of bitter taste strengthen the heart and small intestine (Fire Element). Bitter tastes will improve circulation, nutrient assimilation, and digestion. Bitter taste is cleansing and stimulating. By enhancing the Fire Element, it will increase our sense of joy and wonder about life. Since the Fire Element nourishes the Earth Element (spleen and stomach), mild bitter taste enhances digestion and assists the lymph system (spleen).

Excessive bitter taste will overstimulate the heart and small intestine, causing palpitations, racing heart, or erratic small intestine function. As the Fire Element becomes excessive, the Metal Element (lungs and large intestine) will be overly controlled, causing a deficient Metal Element function. Shallow breathing, shortness of breath, and constipation can occur. Imbalances in the heart and small intestine can predispose people to hysteria.

Sweet: Balanced sweet taste strengthens the spleen and stomach (the Earth Element). It enhances digestion—hence its appeal after a meal—and improves mood (it gives people a sense of calm and stability, like the earth). Well-chewed carbohydrates provide the ideal sweetness for the spleen and stomach because the food is well-mixed with saliva, which also enhances spleen function. The spleen mediates many immune cells. It functions best when our food is well chewed, infused with saliva, and consequently slightly alkaline. Excess sweetness and acidic foods cause excessive acidity in the stomach and unbalance the spleen. The result is heartburn, gas, and stomach disorders.

Since the spleen nourishes the large intestine and lungs, spleen imbalances lead to a variety of bowel disorders. Those who eat a lot of sweets usually suffer from chronic constipation or diarrhea.

The emotion associated with the Earth Element is sympathy or understanding. Excess sweet taste causes an excess of sympathy, to the point of being maudlin. Excess sweet taste overly stimulates the Earth Element and constricts the Water Element (kidneys and bladder). This results in excessive urination, urinary tract infections, and excessive fear and anxiety.

Pungent (or spicy): Moderate amounts of pungent taste, such as that from ginger or mild spices, enhance the function of the lungs and large intestine. It cleanses the system, stimulates healthy bowel function and circulation in the lungs. Small amounts of ginger or mild spices also can help to eliminate accumulated waste in the large intestine. It promotes the elimination of grief and sadness (the emotions related to the Metal Element) and the letting go of the past.

Excesses of pungent taste overly stimulate the bowels and lungs, causing diarrhea, and rapid and shallow breathing. Since the Metal Element controls the Wood (liver and gall bladder), excesses of pungent flavor will cause the constriction of the liver function, resulting in liver stagnation and a tendency toward anger.

Salty: Moderate amounts of salt strengthen the kidneys and bladder. Salt stimulates the kidney function. It supports the kidneys in their effort to eliminate waste from the blood and maintain a balanced pH in the body. Sea salt, which contains sodium and trace minerals, also supports the immune function and alkalizes the spleen and digestive tract. By assisting these blood-cleansing and elimination organs, salt makes the kidneys' job easier. Enhanced kidney function provides a person with courage and a strong will.

Conversely, excessive amounts of salt cause the constriction of the kidneys. Tight, contracted kidneys prevent optimal circulation within the organs, which can dramatically raise blood pressure and lead to hypertension. People with kidney imbalances suffer higher-than-normal amounts of stress and fear. They also lack a strong will.

THE SIX TASTES OF INDIA

One of the great healing tools within the Ayurvedic system is the use of taste to balance and enhance each of the three doshas—vata, pitta, and kapha.

Metabolic processes release all three dosha forces, causing them to become more active and dominant. A balance of all six tastes can moderate and balance the doshas, restoring harmony and peace to the body. Imbalances of certain tastes over others, however, can increase one or two doshas, while decreasing one or two. If such imbalances are sustained, sickness can arise.

It's important to keep in mind that all of these flavors should be eaten in moderation. Mild taste is healing; extremes are weakening and unhealthful. The six tastes are as follows:

Sweet: Increases kapha, and decreases pitta and vata. It cools, relaxes, and comforts. By increasing kapha, sweet encourages the desire to be mothered and passive. In extremes, it can be counterproductive to getting anything done.

Sour: Increases kapha and pitta, and decreases vata. Sour encourages elimination, and enhances appetite and digestion.

Once I had recognized the taste of the crumb of madeleine soaked in her decoction of lime flowers which my aunt used to give me . . . immediately the old gray house upon the street, where her room was, rose up like the scenery of a theater.

MARCEL PROUST

Excesses can contribute to stagnation and the inability to get things done and can inspire jealousy of others. Excesses of sour can inspire anger because of its tendency to increase expectations (kapha and pitta) without encouraging sufficient movement and action (vata) to fulfill those expectations. A person can "sour" on life.

Salty: Increases kapha and pitta, and decreases vata. Salty increases elimination, encourages cleansing, especially of lymph, kidney, and bowels, and stimulates appetite.

Excesses can encourage rigidity of thinking, loss of creativity, fear of change, and overindulgence in food and drink.

Pungent (such as ginger, peppers, and spicy foods): Increases pitta and vata, and decreases kapha. Pungent is highly activating; it is a stimulant. Hence, it eliminates waste and burns fat (which, as potential energy, is kapha). Excesses can keep the system from relaxing, inspire greed, anger, and anxiety or nervous tension.

Bitter: Increases vata, and decreases pitta and kapha. Bitter is cooling and drying. It causes contraction. It purifies the blood, balances the system, and cleans the palate. It also increases appetite. Excesses can inspire unrealistic expectations, workaholism, and aggression. Unfilled expectation can lead to "bitterness" and grief. (There is very little balance or perspective emanating from excess bitter flavor.)

Astringent: Increases vata and decreases pitta and kapha. Astringent contracts organs, reduces all secretions (such as saliva and bile acids), and reduces the activity of the liver. Excesses can dry a person up, turn off the "juices," make one introverted and fearful.

Taste is an exotic realm, and like all exotic worlds it can lead us to self-destruction or liberation.

HEARING

$\mathcal{T}$ HE MOST WIDELY understood and appreciated connection between human beings is sound. We speak, and our words are
heard. But hearing is more than words. It is the rapturous sound
of music; the chirping of birds; the hurry of the wind; a slap-
happy river; the crash of the ocean. Hearing is an early warning
system that alerts us to the needs of a baby, and the danger of an
oncoming car. It is discerning the layers of information within
the same sound; the emotion in another person's voice; the happiness of bells; and the cry of an alarm. Hearing awakens us to
worlds where eyes cannot venture, worlds of power and soul, to
the farthest reaches of spirit, to the intimacy of the breath.

    Sound itself is composed of waves of energy moving through
a medium, such as air, water, or solid matter. These waves move
molecules very short distances—just far enough to transfer the
energy to the neighboring molecule. The process is not unlike a
line of billiard balls all slightly touching one another. When the
first ball is struck by a cue ball, all the balls move just enough to
transfer the energy down the line, yet no ball will move very far,
except the last one. This movement of energy through a medium
is understood as "vibration."

*The eye takes a person into
the world. The ear brings the
world into a human being.*

LORENZ OKEN

Sound travels at different speeds, depending on the medium. It moves through air at about 1,125 feet per second; through water at 4,856 feet per second; and through iron at 10,627 feet per second.

Technically, sound is understood as wave cycles per second, meaning the number of complete waves (from peak to peak) that occur in a single second. One cycle—a single wave—per second is called a Hertz.

Humans can hear sounds that range from 16 cycles per second, or 16 Hertz (Hz), to about 20,000 Hz. A 16 Hz sound is very low and barely audible. A person feels the vibration more than he or she actually hears it. At the other end of the spectrum is a high-pitched whistle or a shriek. A dog's hearing ranges from about 12 Hz to better than 40,000 Hz. A bat hears from 1,000 Hz to greater than 200,000 Hz; a whale, from about 120 Hz to greater than 250,000 Hz. Bats and whales navigate by sound. They send out a signal that bounces off of objects ahead and then returns to them, giving the bat or whale information about what lies up ahead and how far off that object might be.

Humans determine distances by the relative loudness of sound. Loudness is measured in decibels, or tenths of a Bel, a unit named after Alexander Graham Bell, who improved the telephone. A soft whisper can register about 30 decibels; a normal conversation usually takes place at about 60 decibels, unless you offend your friend, in which case the shouting can reach about 90 decibels. A busy street can reach 80 decibels, and an orchestra can reach 90. We start to feel discomfort and even pain at about 110 decibels, and at 120 we can suffer damage to the inner ear. Upon take-off, a Boeing 707 has a decibel level of 130, or about ten trillion times greater than the lowest whisper you can hear. A loud rock group can play between 120 and 140 decibels, which explains why some people lose hearing after a rock concert. The Saturn booster rocket can reach 180 decibels. At these ranges, hearing is not only painful, but probably shortlived.

The sounds that we listen to change our inner world. We need only contrast the inner effects of a jackhammer going full throttle with the peaceful sounds of a forest or an inspirational melody to have all the proof we need. Sound enters our inner world and changes it, leading some therapists to use sound as a tool to heal.

For the past thirty years, Dr. John Diamond, a psychiatrist in

A slight sound at evening lifts me up by the ears, and makes life seem inexpressibly serene and grand. It may be in Uranus, or it may be in the shutter.

HENRY DAVID
THOREAU

Valley Cottage, New York, has been using classical music to heal all manner of psychological and physical distress. Diamond maintains that sickness stems from an inner conflict that prevents life energy from flowing smoothly and efficiently through the body. Without life energy, cells degenerate and ultimately die. "Life energy is what makes a wound heal, what makes a flower grow," says Diamond. "I don't see how anyone can doubt that there is this quality of vitality in an individual."

Music, especially the work of the great composers, frees the body of inner conflict and thus allows life energy to flow freely again, according to Diamond. The emotional response that music evokes is a symptom of the physical changes that have occurred. Diamond, a musicologist, has studied between 30,000 and 40,000 musical recordings, as well as the lives of their composers and the background of their works.

"A composer composes to externalize his problems," says Diamond. "The composer in essence says to the audience, 'I have a problem I want to solve, and I want to tell you about it because I know that as I work my way through the ramifications of the problem, if I tell them to you step by step, I will be unstressed and energized by the process, and I will probably solve the problem, and you will also benefit.'"

Diamond maintains that all great musical compositions present both conflict and resolution. Listeners also experience the stress of these inner conflicts and also the resolution of the conflict, and are thereby healed in the process. This is the basis for the inspiration that music gives us, Diamond says.

He urges people to listen to the works of Mozart, Beethoven, Bach, and other great composers, especially when confronted with psychological or physical illness. Life's struggles and triumphs are all described in the music of these and other composers, says Diamond. Their triumph over difficulties of all kinds is found in the compositions they have left behind.

Vibration and Electricity

Hearing is made possible by the ear, which also serves to maintain physical balance. The ear is composed of three parts: the outer ear, the middle ear, and the inner ear. The outer and middle ears trap sound and channel it into the inner ear, where the sound is transformed from vibration to electrical nerve impulses.

The horn we typically think of as the ear is called the pinna, or auricle. It is composed of cartilage and folds of skin arranged in a kind of spiral that leads to an opening. That opening is the entrance to the ear's canal, also known as the meatus. The skin that lines the outer reaches of the canal is able to secrete wax, which is used to trap dust, small particles, and even bugs that fly into the ear. The canal is about one inch long in adults and leads to a thin, fibrous wall called the tympanic membrane, or the eardrum. The eardrum marks the separation between the outer ear and the middle ear.

When sound travels along the ear's canal, it changes the pressure at the surface of the eardrum. This causes the eardrum to vibrate, which conducts the sound into the middle ear.

The middle ear is composed of three tiny bones that are linked, but still able to move. These three bones, collectively referred to as ossicles, transmit sound from the eardrum, across the middle ear, to the inner ear where the sound is converted to nerve impulses that travel to the brain.

The first of these ossicles is the hammer (also called the malleus), which connects the eardrum to a second bone, called the anvil (or incus). The anvil is connected to a third tiny bone, called the stirrup (or stapes). The stirrup, so named because it is shaped like a saddle stirrup, is attached to an oval opening, or window, in the bulb of the inner ear.

These three tiny bones vibrate with every sound wave and thereby transmit sound from the eardrum to the inner ear. By the time the sound has traveled from the outer ear to the inner ear, the sound has been amplified about ninety times.

Inside the middle ear is also found the eustachian tube, which connects the ear to the throat. The eustachian tube is normally closed, but opens when swallowing or yawning. You become aware of your eustachian tubes when taking off or landing in an airplane. Pressure increases in the tube until it is released by swallowing or maneuvering the muscles in the throat so that the passageway opens and the pressure is released through the nasal cavity or mouth.

The inner ear is a bulblike structure embedded inside the

The Ear

| OUTER EAR | MIDDLE EAR | INNER EAR |

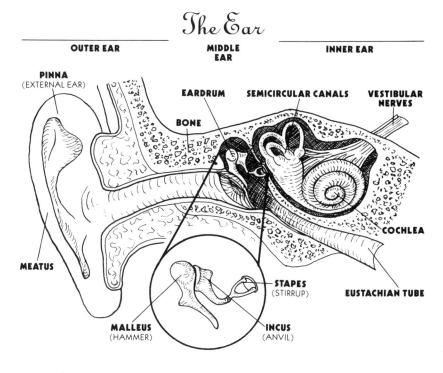

PINNA (EXTERNAL EAR)

EARDRUM

SEMICIRCULAR CANALS

VESTIBULAR NERVES

BONE

MEATUS

COCHLEA

STAPES (STIRRUP)

EUSTACHIAN TUBE

MALLEUS (HAMMER)

INCUS (ANVIL)

The ear not only allows you to hear but orients your sense of balance and position in space. The outer and middle ears trap sound and channel it into the inner ear, where the sound is transformed from vibration to electrical nerve impulses. The semicircular tubes of the cochlea in the inner ear contain fluid and tiny hairlike nerve fibers that are sensitive to gravity, speed, posture, and the positions of the head. These nerve fibers serve as a kind of gyroscope, conveying information to the brain and allowing you to make appropriate physical adjustments to maintain balance and direction.

skull. Within this bulb is a maze of winding passages, known as the labyrinth. The front part of the bulb resembles a snail's shell, within which a tube winds in a circular motion. This part of the inner ear is called the cochlea and is involved in hearing. Inside the cochlea are nerve fibers that resemble tiny hairs. At the front of the cochlea, the nerves respond to high-frequency sound waves; at the rear, or deeper into the spiral, the nerves respond to lower-frequency sounds.

The cochlea nerves pass impulses along the auditory nerve to the temporal gyrus, the auditory part of the brain. (See chapter on the brain.) In back of the cochlea are three semicircular tubes, or canals, that rise out of the bulblike structure of the inner ear. They are set at right angles to each other. Inside these canals are fluid and tiny hairlike nerve fibers that are sensitive to gravity, speed, posture, and the positions of the head. These nerve fibers serve as a kind of gyroscope, conveying information to the brain about the body's current state of balance. The brain then orders appropriate physical adjustments to maintain balance and direction.

WHAT'S THAT YOU SAY?

He who has ears to hear sees!

JAKOB BÖHME

Hearing gradually deteriorates with age in the U.S. and much of the Western world. Studies have shown, however, that comparable hearing loss does not occur in traditional societies, or among industrialized people living on a low-fat diet. A high-fat diet causes atherosclerosis in the tiny vessels and arteries of the hearing mechanism, causing the inner ear to become dulled and hardened.

One study compared the hearing of citizens living in Wisconsin with that of the African tribespeople called the Mabaans. Researchers found that not one Mabaan—even at the age of seventy—suffered the hearing loss that the average Wisconsinite had suffered by the age of thirty-five. Other research compared the hearing of Finnish people with that of Yugoslavians and found that Finnish children begin to suffer hearing loss at age ten. By the age of nineteen, they have distinct hearing impairment, especially at the higher ranges of 16,000 to 18,000 cycles per second. No such hearing loss was found among Yugoslavians. The Finns have the highest per capita blood cholesterol level (290 mg/dl) of anyone in the world, and consequently the highest rates of heart disease in the world. The average cholesterol level among Yugoslavians is 180 mg/dl.

Ear infections are among the most common and painful ailments that afflict children. They occur most often in the ear canal or eustachian tubes, where the infection causes inflammation and pus to build. The result is stabbing pain and, in extreme cases, a punctured eardrum. Antibiotics are usually prescribed to kill a bacterial infection. Excess wax and pus are aspirated from the ear, as well. Ear infections can suggest a low immune function. (See the section on naturopathic remedies below.)

Tinnitus is the perception of hearing sounds, especially ringing or buzzing, when there is no sound emanating from the environment. It can be caused by excessive wax buildup, infection, osteosclerosis (the excessive buildup of bone that immobilizes the stirrup bone, the stapes), or poor blood circulation within the inner ear. Treatment usually includes the surgical removal of the stapes, which is then replaced by an artificial stirrup bone.

THE FIVE TONES OF EASTERN MEDICINE

"The kidneys open into the ear," says the Yellow Emperor. "The kidney qi goes through the ear; if the kidney is harmonized the ear can hear the five tones." Because the kidneys provide life force or qi to the organs of the ear, hearing is dependent upon the healthy functioning of the kidneys. Diminished kidney qi will result in decreased life force to the ears, which will result in stagnation. The organs of the ear will begin to accumulate waste and toxins, such as plaque, and degeneration will proceed toward deafness. Diminished qi to the ears also can give rise to chronic ear infections.

When kidneys are deficient in qi, a person will suffer from poor circulation within the ear and possible ringing of the ears. He will suffer from poor sex drive, frequent urination, loss of hearing, and chronic earaches or infections. Conversely, excessive kidney energy can cause excessive qi to the ears, resulting in high blood pressure, excess wax in the ears, and highly sensitive hearing. Loud noises will be particularly painful.

To improve hearing, the Chinese maintain that the kidneys must become balanced and healed. Using the Five Element schematic, the kidneys and bladder are considered the Water Element. They are strengthened by mild salty flavor, beans, barley, and sea vegetables. Fat and cholesterol-rich foods clog the tiny kidney tubules and prevent blood from flowing smoothly through the kidneys, causing stagnation and degeneration. Excess sodium, which can injure the kidneys, also must be avoided.

The kidneys are controlled by the stomach and spleen (Earth Element) and nourished by the lungs and large intestine (Metal Element). Too many sweets and acidic foods cause the spleen to become excessive, which will control and limit kidney qi. For this reason, sugar and other sweet foods are often seen as the cause of ear infections and earache. They stimulate the spleen excessively, which dominates kidney qi and limits its flow to the ears and sex organs. (See chapter on the kidneys.) Consequently, all sweets should be avoided when ear infections or earache manifest.

At the same time, the lungs and large intestine should be strengthened. These Metal Element organs nourish the kidneys with life force. (See chapters on the lungs and large intestine.)

Finally, fear injures the kidneys and therefore plays a role in the flow of qi to the ears. For hearing to be healed, stress and fear must be effectively dealt with.

The five tones that the Yellow Emperor referred to above relate to the sounds associated with each organ system within the Five Elements. By listening closely to the voice, Chinese healers can recognize imbalances within specific organ systems. The greater the imbalance, the more pronounced these sounds are in a person's voice. Using the Five Element system, the five tones and their related organs are as follows:

Shouting: Associated with the liver and gall bladder (Wood Element). A person who shouts even when he or she is speaking normally, as on the telephone or when conducting routine business affairs, suffers from a liver imbalance. Chronically shouting in anger further indicates a liver imbalance.

Laughter or hysteria: Associated with the heart and small intestine (Fire Element). The tone in the voices of some people can be characterized as laughing. There is a certain playfulness, a lightness, and even lack of seriousness in the voices of many people, no matter what they are talking about. When the heart and small intestine are extremely imbalanced, hysteria is implicit in the voice and requires very little to be evoked. Both conditions indicate a heart and small intestine imbalance.

Singing: Associated with the spleen and stomach (the Earth Element). Singing strengthens the Earth organs. A singing voice indicates excessive qi in the stomach and spleen that is being discharged by a singing tone in the voice. Weak or deficient qi in the spleen and stomach also can manifest in the voice as excessive sympathy, whining, and discernible weakness.

Weeping: Associated with the lungs and large intestine (Metal Element). The Metal Element organs are associated with the emotions of grief or sadness, which manifests in the voice as a weeping quality, as if tears are implicit in the voice.

Fear: Associated with the kidneys and bladder (Water Element). Weak kidneys and bladder will stimulate a greater sense of fear and timidity. The voice will be tentative and cautious, with a palpable sense of fear in it.

THE DIETARY FACTOR

According to naturopathic medicine, the sources of most ear infections, especially among children, are dairy foods and sweets.

Mucus-producing foods, such as milk, cheese, and yogurt, refined white flour products, sugar, and fatty foods block circulation in the ear, and cause accumulation of waste products, making the environment perfect for viral or bacterial growth. Excess sugar, fruit, and fruit sugars (from fruit juice) also depress immune function. Allergies to certain foods, such as dairy or wheat, also may play a role in the onset of ear infections and other ear-related disorders, including ringing in the ears. Finally, chronic ear infections suggest a depressed immune system.

People with ear infections or earaches are urged to avoid those foods, while increasing the following foods, herbs, and supplements:

- *Foods rich in vitamin A* (beta carotene): collard greens, broccoli, brussels sprouts, squash, and carrots.
- *Foods rich in vitamin C:* broccoli (one of the richest sources of C); tangerines; leafy greens. Supplements may also be necessary for short periods.
- *Foods rich in zinc:* whole grains, shrimp, and pumpkin seeds. Short periods of supplementation may be necessary.
- *Garlic:* It is antifungal and antibacterial.
- *Mullein:* antibacterial; four drops in each ear, four times per day.
- *Chamomile:* Especially for children, as a tea. Will promote perspiration, and elimination of accumulated toxins. Take two to three times per day.

Homeopaths note that earaches and ear infections may arise as part of a generalized flu, virus, or upper respiratory infection. The eustachian tubes are connected to the throat, allowing viruses to migrate to the ears and cause infection. For earaches accompanied by colds and coughs, use the following homeopathic remedies:

Aconite: especially for earaches after a chill and exposure to cold.

Belladonna: especially for those with fever, sensitivity to light, and sore throat.

Pulsatilla: for those with yellow or thick mucus, stuffed nose, fever, chapped lips.

Hear, and your soul shall live.

Isaiah

SIGHT

$\mathcal{T}$HE EYES REVEAL the world to us and, for the keen observer, reveal each of us to the world. No other sense is so heavily relied upon to tell us what is happening outside of us. Conversely, no other organ is scrutinized more closely to reveal the inner workings of our soul.

The eyes catch light. They drink it in great drafts and send it hurtling to the nervous system and then to the brain, where the images are interpreted and, to greater and lesser degrees, understood. Their capacity to perform this task far exceeds our ability to actually grasp their magic: The eyes can perceive 10 billion gradations of light and 7 million shades of color. They give us the ability to focus on an image close at hand, dissolve it, and then refocus on another image at considerable distance within a tenth of a second. We can witness in fine detail the myriad colors of an autumnal forest and, in the proverbial blink of an eye, suddenly shift our gaze to the coarse gray hairs of a squirrel's tail.

In simple terms, sight is the happy marriage between light and the brain. To most of us, light is the neutral brightness that occurs when the sun comes up or when we throw a switch. We are lulled into thinking that light merely illuminates colors that were already in existence before the lights went on. But that's not entirely true: Light is color, or rather many colors locked together.

We are witness to these brilliant colors when light is refracted, or separated, by a prism, which then reveals the color spectrum as a beautiful rainbow. At one end of the spectrum are violet and blue, at the other end are orange and red. These colors appear when the prism divides light into its component parts: individual waves of electromagnetic energy.

Physical objects appear to us as colored because they possess pigmentation, chemical substances that absorb certain wavelengths of light, while reflecting others back at us. Pigment in skin makes it possible for an organism to hold energy from the sun's light and convert it to heat, thus sustaining body temperature. The mix of waves that is reflected back at us gives the world its color.

Sunlight is an incredible variety of electromagnetic waves that are moving, or radiating, from the sun itself. When spread out on a spectrum, some of these waves are revealed to be very short from crest to crest—as short as six quadrillionths of an inch (.000000000000006)—while other waves span eighteen miles from crest to crest.

Remarkably, we are able to perceive only a tiny fraction of all the electromagnetic energy that is around us. In fact, the extent of the spectrum that we can see is measured in billionths of a meter, distances referred to as nanometers. We are able to see exactly 300 nanometers, which, for those of us not on intimate terms with the metric system, is a microscopic fraction of an inch. The rest of the electromagnetic energy spectrum, which spans many miles, is hidden from us. Thus, we are blind to the vast majority of what is actually happening all around us.

Science has proven that many animals, such as rats and birds, see the ultraviolet rays of the spectrum, and are therefore able to "see the invisible." New theories of bird migrations maintain that birds are able to see light waves that are invisible to humans. By following these waves, birds are able to find their ways to exact locations, north and south, each year.

Despite our limited sight, our eyes nonetheless provide us with the most intense and immediate information about our world. It should come as no surprise that sight provides about 75 percent of what we perceive, unless our eyes are impaired, in which case other senses become more acute. That figure is determined in part by cultural bias, especially by our scientific orientation, which fosters the notion that "seeing is believing." Other senses could offer more information, and often do for those whose lives or professions demand that they develop greater sensitivity to touch, smell, hearing, or taste, but those senses are less obvious in comparison to the brilliance of sight.

Just as the eyes provide information, they also convey it. Intense emotions are revealed in our eyes, as well as most of our subtle feelings. The eyes laugh, cry, convey happiness and sorrow. They respond to many physical changes in the body, from the condition of the liver, heart, and kidneys, to the health of the endocrine and nervous systems. The eyes even reveal the amount of oxygen in our bloodstream (the pupils dilate when oxygen is depleted) and become irritated when the immune system is mobilized.

The eyes are "dim windows of the soul," as William Blake

The human eye is a highly complex organ. Anatomical estimates put its number of working parts at close to one billion. Its light receptors, the rods and cones on the retina, can perceive ten million gradations of light and seven million shades of color. The rods and cones themselves represent about 70 percent of the body's total sense receptors. The eye works by taking in light and transforming it into electrical impulses that are sent to the brain, where 90 percent of vision occurs.

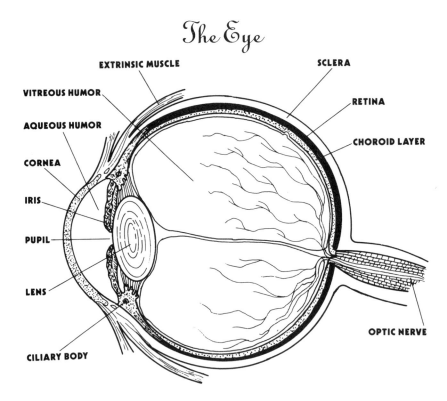

The Eye

EXTRINSIC MUSCLE

VITREOUS HUMOR

AQUEOUS HUMOR

CORNEA

IRIS

PUPIL

LENS

CILIARY BODY

SCLERA

RETINA

CHOROID LAYER

OPTIC NERVE

said. Indeed, the amount of information they convey seems limited only by our ability to decipher it.

An Inside Look at the Eye

Light enters the eye through the cornea, a clear convex window made of cells which permit light to pass without bending or scattering the electromagnetic waves. Immediately behind the cornea is the aqueous humor, a watery alkaline fluid that provides nutrition to the cornea and sustains just the right amount of pressure so that the cornea bulges slightly.

Behind the cornea is the pupil, the dark spot that expands and contracts to permit greater or lesser amounts of light to enter the eye. The pupil is controlled by the iris, the colored disc in the center of the eye. The iris is lined with muscle and autonomic nerves that control the opening or narrowing of the pupil. The parasympathetic nervous system causes the eye to contract, while the sympathetic nervous system causes it to expand.

The iris is colored by the presence of melanin, the pigment-giving substance that also colors the skin and hair. The amount of melanin determines the color of the eyes: greater quantities of melanin make the eyes brown; less makes the eye blue. Shades of green and gray are determined by greater and lesser amounts in between.

Behind the pupil is the crystalline lens, a bulblike structure that is shaped like a rounded diamond, with the wide end right behind the pupil, and the narrow near the center of the eye. The shape of the lens is continually being altered in order to focus on an object. This is called accommodation, meaning the ability of the lens to adjust to the distance from the object being focused on. Typically, the lens becomes less elastic and flexible with age, requiring eyeglasses for most older people. This loss of accommodation is more common in the West than among traditional peoples, however, a fact often referred to by many optometrists who argue that visual acuity is determined in large measure by lifestyle, attitudes, and overall health, as well as overuse of and overdependence on the eyes.

The lens changes shape, thus focusing on near and far objects, thanks to the ciliary body, a muscular ring that surrounds the

Two lights brighten our world. One is provided by the sun, but another answers to it—the light of the eye. Only through their entwining do we see; lacking either, we are blind.

Arthur Zajonc

The mechanics of eyesight are so well understood by now that they can be imitated artificially: robot eyes have been developed that can detect light and send it to be stored and decoded by a computer. The only problem with this impressive cracking of the visual code is that the experience of seeing has been entirely missed. Robot eyes are never bored by what they look at, or enthralled by beauty. They do not prefer crimson to scarlet, or vice versa. They do not relish the softness of the shadows in Titian's paintings or the stark melodrama in Caravaggio's. None of the qualities of light that really matter, in a human, personal sense, can be translated into mechanical terms.

DEEPAK CHOPRA

lens. When the eye focuses on a near object, the ciliary body contracts, causing the lens to become more convex. When the eye focuses on a distant object, the ciliary body expands, causing the lens to relax. The ciliary body is connected to fibers of the autonomic nervous system, which allow the brain to tell the ciliary ring to expand or contract, depending upon what the brain needs in order to see the image clearly. Focusing the eye is thus an involuntary action.

Since muscles within the iris and the ciliary body focus the eye, many leading eye therapists maintain that visual acuity is largely a function of eye-muscle fitness. Indeed, numerous exercise programs have been developed that can successfully restore visual acuity to those suffering from a wide variety of eye disorders.

The lens is surrounded by vitreous humor, a transparent jellylike mass that allows light to pass from the lens to the retina. The vitreous humor makes up most of the mass of the eye and maintains the shape of the eyeball.

The retina is a tiny flap of nerves, no thicker than a postage stamp, that catches the light. It sits at the very back of the eye and surrounds much of the vitreous humor. The retina is composed of photoreceptors, or light-sensitive nerve cells. These nerves are divided into two groups, rods and cones. There are an estimated 120 million rods and 7 million cones in the human eye. The rods detect low-intensity light; we rely upon them most heavily for night vision. Rods tend to perceive light in shades of black and white. Cones, so named because of their shape, respond to bright light and are capable of perceiving color.

Rods and cones react to different degrees of light because of their differing chemical natures. Rods contain the chemical rhodopsin, or visual purple. Cones contain a group of substances called opsins, which are highly sensitive to the wavelengths of the three primary colors, red, blue, and yellow.

When bright light hits the rods, rhodopsin bleaches, permitting the cones to become the dominant light-perceiving cells. When the light is dim, rhodopsin increases in volume, thus causing the rods to become the dominant photoreceptors. Whether the image we see is primarily black and white or full of color depends upon the degree of light available, and thus which nerves of the retina—rods or cones—are employed. Inside the retina, both rhodopsin and the opsins bind with vitamin A. When light hits the rods and cones, it interacts with vitamin A to create an electrical signal that flows from the retina to the vision center of the brain, thus allowing us to perceive images. It is this dependency upon vitamin A that created the folk wisdom—now known to be true—that carrots are good for the eyes.

Interestingly, the image that the retina receives is actually reversed, or upside down, due to the light being refracted or bent while it travels through the various layers of the eye. The brain corrects this error.

Your eyes are so coordinated that if you cover one eye and shine a light in the other, both pupils will contract. Motor nerves inside the brain and the eye manipulate six small muscles that surround each eye to coordinate their movements.

Because vision is so accurate at discerning the physical world, we tend to believe that the eyes serve as mere windows. On the contrary, the brain works more like a computer, putting together an incredible array of complex information to form its own picture, which corresponds with the outside world. This information is coordinated by the left and right hemispheres of the brain. For example, when you look at a baseball at rest, your right eye will perceive both the left and right sides of the ball; the left eye does the same. Hence, each eye will have left and right fields of vision. The brain treats the left and right fields of vision of each eye differently, however. The right field of vision for both eyes will be interpreted by the left hemisphere, while the left field of vision will be deciphered by the right hemisphere. The brain puts these four separate images together to form a coherent picture.

The eye is a master, the ear a servant.

JAKOB GRIMM

WHEN VISION IS LESS THAN PERFECT

Many illnesses of the brain, nervous system, and the eye will affect vision. Below is a review of the most common disorders affecting the eyes.

Nearsightedness occurs when light rays are focused at a point before they reach the retina. So, distant objects are blurred. What is actually happening is the eyes are over-focusing. The lens is not relaxing (or expanding) sufficiently, causing the image to be focused before it reaches the retina. The condition is corrected by

Oh thou most excellent eye, elevated above all that God created! What exalted praises are capable of expressing thy nobility? What peoples, what tongues, can describe thy abilities? Through the window of the eye the soul regards the world's beauty.

LEONARDO DA VINCI

concave lenses, which expand the image and compensate for the exaggerated focusing action of the eyes.

Farsightedness occurs when the cornea and lenses are unable to focus (or contract) sufficiently, causing nearby objects to be blurred. Convex lenses are used to contract the image for the eye, thus correcting the distortion.

Glaucoma, one of the most common eye disorders, is a condition caused by excessive pressure within the eye, causing damage to the nerve fibers of the retina and the tiny blood vessels inside the choroid layer. The result is diminished vision and often total blindness. Orthodox physicians use drugs to lower the pressure, or several types of surgery to open a drainage canal so that the aqueous fluid can escape.

With cataracts, the lens loses its transparency and becomes increasingly opaque. This happens when proteins within the lens degenerate, forming white patches that move from the center of the lens to the periphery. Treatment usually involves the surgical removal of the lens and the insertion of a plastic artificial lens.

THE LIVER CONNECTION

According to Chinese medicine, the eyes are nourished by the liver, meaning that the life force, or qi, flows from the liver to the eyes. The Yellow Emperor states that the liver "opens" into the eyes. "When the liver receives the blood it strengthens the vision," says the Yellow Emperor's Classic. A healthy liver will provide optimal qi to the eyes and therefore support visual acuity. Conversely, excessively yin or yang conditions of the liver will result in various types of eye disorders.

"When the liver is deficient (empty), then the eye becomes blinded and can no longer see," says the Yellow Emperor. Deficient qi flowing to the eyes will manifest as stages of illness, proceeding from small impairments of sight toward the gradual degeneration of the eyes until blindness sets in. An expanded or swollen liver will most often result in deficient liver qi, and thus inadequate qi to the eyes. The result will be an inability of the cornea and lens to contract, or focus on nearby objects (farsightedness).

Initially, an overly contracted liver will usually cause excessive liver qi because blood flow will likely be backed up inside the organ, causing a fiery condition. The eyes will therefore receive excessive life force, causing over-focusing or nearsightedness. However, as the condition in the liver worsens, a contracted liver also will result in diminished life force to the eyes, causing a variety of eye disorders, including glaucoma and cataracts.

Dim windows of the soul.

WILLIAM BLAKE

The reason: the liver provides life force to the eyes. Therefore, all cellular maintenance and metabolism within the eye depends upon the liver, which is the eyes' source. As the liver degenerates, the condition of the eyes also will worsen. Cellular reproduction and metabolism within the eye will become deformed, causing a buildup of waste within the eye (glaucoma) and cellular degeneration (cataracts).

According to Chinese medicine, the spleen also can be involved in eye disorders. The spleen nourishes the muscles, while the liver controls them (see chapters on the liver, spleen, and Chinese medicine). Muscle weakness within the eyes—which prevents the ciliary body from contracting and thus focusing on nearby objects—can be caused by both a liver and spleen imbalance. Whatever weakens the liver will ultimately affect vision, say the Chinese.

In the Five Element schematic, the liver is nourished by the kidneys (Water Element) and controlled by the lungs and large intestine (the Metal Element). The conditions and emotional states related to these organs also can play a role in the health of the liver and thus in visual acuity. For instance, the liver is associated with anger. Too much anger will injure the liver, often causing liver qi to become initially excessive, but eventually tired and lethargic. Hence, excessive or repressed anger, especially in childhood, can result in visual impairment.

The kidneys are associated with fear and the will. Kidney imbalances and excessive fear will cause the kidneys to become weak, thus preventing them from passing sufficient life force onto the liver. Without adequate qi from the kidneys, the liver condition will degenerate, thereby ultimately impairing vision.

When the qi of the lungs and large intestine is excessive, these organs will control the liver excessively, causing it to be deficient in life force, and thus diminishing the life force to the eyes. The lungs and large intestine are associated with grief or sadness. Consequently, these emotions, too, may play a role in how well or how poorly we see. While the liver is the primary organ of concern with all eye-related problems, the health of other organs, especially the kidneys, lungs, and large intestine, also may be involved. Restoring healthy vision always begins with treating the liver, but these organs may be involved secondarily. (See chapters on the liver, spleen, kidneys, bladder, lungs, and large intestine for healing foods and herbs associated with these organs.)

Ayurvedic healers associate the eyes with the pitta dosha and the Fire Element of the Indian Five Element system. The pitta dosha serves to balance the more kinetic energies of vata, and the potential energy of kapha. Pitta is associated with both the Fire and Water Elements, creating harmony between these two opposites (and antagonists) within the body. When the pitta dosha is strong, the eyes see clearly. It is increased by sour, salty, and pungent tastes, and is decreased by sweet, bitter, and astringent flavors.

The following foods are said to promote the pitta dosha:

- *Grains:* barley, oats, rice, and wheat.
- *Vegetables:* cabbage, broccoli, brussels sprouts, asparagus, cauliflower, green beans, leafy greens, lettuce, mushrooms, okra, parsley, peas, sprouts, zucchini.
- *Beans:* All beans are considered supportive, except lentils.
- *Animal foods:* shrimp, chicken, turkey, egg whites.
- *Fruit:* apples, grapes, oranges, pears, prunes, raisins.
- *Seeds and nuts:* All nuts are considered harmful. Sunflower and pumpkin seeds are considered healthful in small amounts.

Seeing is not a separate isolated function. It's a process involving the entire human organism. The child sees with his whole being; it is profoundly integrated with the total action system of the child—his posture, his manual skills and coordination, his intelligence, and his personality.

ARNOLD GESELL

BODY-MIND RELATIONSHIPS

During the past fifty years, a new school of optometrists has emerged. These men and women, who refer to themselves as behavioral optometrists, believe that visual acuity is a learned response to the environment and that various emotional and psychological factors play a role in how well or how poorly we see. Also, physical capabilities, especially coordination, dexterity, and confidence, play fundamental roles in how well our eyes perform. Because all the physical senses, and indeed the body at large, develop together, vision is a whole-body function. Certain behavioral optometrists maintain that particular body types and personalities are associated with specific visual disorders, including nearsightedness and farsightedness. Others maintain that particular physical characteristics, especially lack of physical coordination, poor concentration, or poor self-awareness, conspire to bring about eye disorders.

Behavioral optometrists use a wide variety of exercises for the eyes and the whole body, such as relaxation techniques and mental imaging methods, to improve sight. Behavioral optometry has its roots in the work of pioneer vision therapist Dr. William Bates, who developed exercises to improve vision. The Bates Method was used successfully by many young men who wanted to be fighter pilots during World War II, but were unable to pass the eye exam at the first try. Among the most common practices: lie on a bed and trace the outline of your room where the walls meet the ceiling at a steady and rapid pace. You are rotating your eyes and thus exercising the muscles that focus the eye. Bates also encouraged reading for short periods—ten to twenty minutes—without the use of glasses. When the eyes get tired, rest them, and then read again for as long as possible until they tire again. This time stop. Bates encouraged people to do as much as possible without the use of eyeglasses, which tend to weaken the eyes by making them dependent upon the corrective lenses.

Nathan Pritikin was an expert on the eye and vision. He maintained that both high-fat and high-protein diets contribute to eye disorders by causing fat, cholesterol, and protein by-products (such as uric acid crystals) to infiltrate the eye from the choroid layer. These substances can migrate into both the vitreous humor and aqueous humors of the eye. They also can block the filter meshwork and canal of Schlemm, thus preventing optimal elimination of waste products from the eye. As the filter meshwork and canal of Schlemm become less efficient, aqueous fluid is prevented from flowing out of the eye and thus causes interocular pressure to build, resulting in glaucoma.

Who would believe that so small a space could contain the images of all the universe?

LEONARDO DA VINCI

CHAPTER 22

TOUCH

The human body is the best picture of the human soul.

LUDWIG
WITTGENSTEIN

WE ALL NEED to be touched and to touch one another. There is abundant scientific evidence showing that touching the skin, especially the skin of infants, promotes the development of life-sustaining systems, such as the nervous, respiratory, lymph, and circulatory systems. Breast-fed babies seem to possess a variety of superior physical characteristics, including enhanced immune and gastrointestinal functions, which scientists point out are not entirely attributable to breast milk alone. Studies have shown that infants who are not sufficiently touched have lower immune function and suffer higher rates of infection and even mortality. Touching a child is essential for the healthy psychological status of both the infant and the mother. Even in adulthood, some people who are deprived of the touch of loved ones experience a variety of antisocial behaviors and even violence.

The same occurs with other members of the animal kingdom. Domestic animals typically lick their young. Studies have shown that this licking stimulates the development and function of the gastrointestinal and urinary tracts, as well as the sex organs. Other research has shown that when animals are deprived of this licking, they frequently die.

Touch is your most basic means of experiencing the physical world. It is your most immediate way of understanding the nature of things: their temperature, texture, weight, size, and shape. Humans touch other people to communicate affection, to satisfy the desire for sex, to show love, and to receive love in return.

Still, despite the necessity of laws and mores that regulate touching, few things are more healing and essential than the touch of love. Every culture has had its form of healing touch, whether it is the laying on of hands, massage techniques, or bodywork. Today, therapeutic touch is returning in many forms. In the past twenty years, there has been a veritable explosion of bodywork therapists in the U.S., Europe, and Japan. Many nurses and other health-care professionals are providing therapeutic touch in hospital settings.

After decades of repression in which doctors were loathe even to touch a patient, the power and importance of touch is now being reevaluated. It's a good thing, for who among us can live without the gentle awakening that comes when another human hand is received in peace?

THE SENSATIONS OF TOUCH

Your sense of touch is located in the skin, including the lips, tongue, eyes, nose, genitals, and scalp. Many thousands of specialized cells in the skin respond to external stimuli and communicate to your brain the characteristics of the things with which you come in contact. These characteristics include five specific sensations: touch, pressure, pain, heat, and cold. Secondary sensations, such as tickling and itching, are muted variations of touch and pain, and are conveyed by the same nerves that provide both of these more common experiences.

The body's parts possess varying degrees of sensitivity. Some parts of the body possess greater sensitivity to temperature than others. The feet are more sensitive to heat than the hands, for example. Other parts are more sensitive to pain. The cornea is several hundred times more sensitive to pain than the bottoms of the feet. Other parts of the body have selective sensitivity, such as fingertips, which have excellent powers of recognition but are not particularly sensitive to pain.

To a significant degree, our body, face, and voice reflect our habits, emotions, thoughts, and lifestyle. Our innermost thoughts, neuromuscular tensions, and habits form, in large part, the shape of our bodies and the topography of our faces.

DAN MILLMAN

Like other senses, touch has greater potential for sensitivity than most of us will ever experience. People who lose one of the physical senses or whose professions demand that they develop their potential for touch demonstrate far greater perception and sensitivity than most of us. The blind read Braille with their fingers, for example, while a massage therapist may develop an ability to assess another person's health with his or her hands.

The skin contains many types of touch receptors. In general, these are divided into two main categories. One type is made of a long nerve fiber that may rest near the surface of the skin or attach itself to a hair follicle and respond when the hair is moved. The other possesses a specialized nerve ending, called an end organ, that is capable of reacting to a specific stimulus, such as pressure or pain. These are more common in nonhairy parts of the skin, such as the lips and fingertips.

Touch receptors pass electrical nerve impulses from the point of origin (the fingertips, for example) to sensory nerves that flow to the spinal cord. The spinal cord then passes the information on to the thalamus in the brain, and from there to the sensory cortex, where it is interpreted and often made conscious. We are not aware of much of the physical stimuli that our nervous systems process. For example, you are probably unconscious of the interaction between your buttocks and your chair, or the feeling of this book in your hands, or even of the smell in the room. We remain unconscious of much of the information available to us.

The specialized touch receptors that are embedded at various depths within the skin provide information about specific sensations. Each group of receptors has its own responsibility and nature. Also, several types of touch receptors may be involved in the same chore. For example, touch and light pressure are conveyed to us by several types of specialized nerves, including Meissner's corpuscles, long tentaclelike nerves with round, flat nerve endings that look like tennis rackets; Merkel's discs, which are multiple branches of nerves that spring from a single stem; free nerve endings, which look like trees with many long limbs; and hair-root plexuses, which collect around hair follicles and respond when hairs are stimulated. Most of these nerves are right below the surface of the skin and respond to slight touch.

Deep pressure is conveyed by a type of nerve fiber called Pacinian corpuscles, which look like elongated donuts with a long string attached to them. Pacinian corpuscles are deep within the skin. You need to press on something before they are stimulated. Cold is communicated via the end bulbs of Krause, which possess a circular end organ with many thin stringlike fibers inside the circle. Heat is communicated by the end organs of Ruffini, which look like inverted umbrellas on long handles. Pain is conveyed by free nerve endings, which are very fine branches with knobs at their ends. Free nerve endings are distributed throughout most tissues, but especially just below the surface of the skin.

There are two types of pain. Somatic pain involves the external parts of the body, while visceral pain occurs in internal organs. Somatic pain can occur superficially, at the surface of the skin, or deep within the tissues, such as at the bone, tendons, muscles, and ligaments. Generally, pain is described as pricking, burning, or aching. Pricking occurs at the surface of the skin from a pin prick, a cut, or a pinch; burning pain is experienced from excessive heat or scraping the skin; aching or throbbing is a deep and persistent pain, often of low intensity.

Pain usually arises from disease, disorder, or injury. It is among the most important and primitive sensations of the human body. It alerts the conscious mind of danger. It informs you that remedial action or change is necessary and must be made immediately. The kinds of actions to be taken depend upon the source of the pain. It may require nothing more than moving your hand away from a flame, or more long-term actions, such as altering habits and lifestyle. Unlike other senses, such as taste or smell, adaptation to pain does not occur easily. Pain persists and will be perceived consciously until appropriate action is taken.

Pain is a symptom, a means of communication, caused by some underlying disorder. It is essentially a teaching mechanism. It is the body's way of telling you about its immediate condition, and instructing you on the effects of your behavior. It is this latter function that guides you in your understanding of which behaviors support health and life, and which are destructive. In this sense, pain is essential for continuation of life.

Pain is often seen as an inconvenience in modern society, hence the success of the analgesic industry. Painkillers cover up pain by eliminating your ability to feel it. They do nothing for the underlying cause of the pain, however. Consequently, the underlying problem may grow worse until a crisis manifests and you are forced to undergo more radical action.

FROM SHIATSU TO ACUPRESSURE

In the Orient the value of touch has been explored and elevated to highly evolved healing and spiritual disciplines. Touch is among the most important methods of healing in the East. It an important means of transmitting the life force from one person to another.

The healthful and efficient functioning of the human form depends upon the presence of optimal amounts of qi or prana. Traditional health care in the East is essentially the promotion and maintenance of the life force within the body. For the Oriental, we are literally standing in the midst of infinite energy. Our health and fulfillment depend upon our being receptive to this universal energy.

The oldest tradition that combines this understanding with the body is Indian yoga. Yogic tradition sees the body as the physical manifestation of the mind and spirit. All three are interrelated as one unit. Consequently, your consciousness, the way you feel about yourself, about others, and your world, is manifest in your physical body in a variety of ways. Those aspects of you that are developed, evolved, and at peace will be reflected as flexibility, strength, and vitality in your body. Those aspects that are in conflict will be reflected in your body as places of tension, rigidity, and structural abnormalities. Thus, to heal the body is also to heal the mind and spirit. Yoga employs postures and exercises to free the body of unnatural or abnormal restrictions that arise from past trauma and delusions.

Healing is the act of balancing the life force within the body to restore the overt biological functions to normalcy. The human body receives life force from the environment at large. It utilizes this life force to maintain its own health; at the same time, the body—if strong enough—can also transmit qi to others. Healing touch is the healer's act of transferring universal energy from the environment at large to the patient, by using his own body as a conductor.

Healing touch, such as the laying on of hands and various kinds of massage therapy, especially acupressure and shiatsu, are methods of transferring healing energy to another human being. The laying on of hands is a less specific way of transferring qi to another person. The premise is to enrich another person's overall life force, which, it is hoped, will help him or her to overcome illness.

Acupressure and shiatsu, just two of many Oriental disciplines, are massage techniques for transferring qi to specific acupuncture points and meridians. Rather than use needles, which work as antennae to draw qi into the body at specific points and along certain meridian lines, healing touch is used to stimulate qi and unblock meridians. This results in the reestablishment of the life force and the restoration of health.

Reflexology is also based upon the concept of meridians and life energy. Foot reflexology is the therapeutic massaging of the feet at energy points that are said to correspond to specific organs and systems.

The Bible is full of references to healing through touch. So, too, are the Dead Sea Scrolls. Indeed, the laying on of hands has been one of the oldest and primary means of restoring health in the Western world.

During much of this century, these traditions were practiced only among a few esoteric therapists. But since the 1960s, healing touch emerged as if from below ground in the form of a variety of bodywork therapies. These practices concentrate on places of tension and restriction in the body, and also on movement and posture. Among the most widely practiced bodywork therapies today are the Hellerwork, Rolfing, Feldenkrais, and Alexander techniques. While the techniques differ somewhat, the basic principles are essentially the same: the body, mind, and spirit are a unified entity, and by healing the body, one frees the mind and spirit of conflicts, distress, and illness.

Among the pioneering practitioners of bodywork in the West is Dr. Alexander Lowen, who has been exploring for decades how emotional conflicts in childhood keep people from experiencing their feelings. The failure to feel deeply is transferred to the body, which also becomes numb. The result is a parallel degeneration among the body, mind, and spirit.

"You grow up as a child with so many traumas," says Lowen,

"so much unfulfillment, so much pain and despair, that you can't stand it and the only way to stand it is to numb yourself. So you have to numb your body, because that's where feeling is. Then you can't function in a healthy way anymore because there's numbness. You're not sensitive to other people, you're not sensitive to your own needs."

The results, says Lowen, are a wide variety of physical distortions, changes in breathing, and ultimately disease. Lowen, who is the author of several important books on the relationship between the mind and body, including *Language of the Body* and *Love, Sex and Your Heart,* says that by working on the body, by "softening it" and removing its "armor," health can be restored.

He describes the process of going from sickness to health this way: "Health is aliveness, spontaneity, gracefulness, and, especially rhythm. We describe the process of getting well in three stages. First, the person has to become self-aware. You've got to feel yourself, know yourself, before you can work through. The second step, after you learn to know yourself, is to learn how to express yourself. You've got to be able to cry, to get angry, to feel sad or frightened. To be free to express feelings. The third step is self-possession, which means you have to have all your feelings available to know exactly how to use them." Lowen, who terms his work *Bioenergetics,* says that by working with the body, all three of these steps can be accomplished.

PART FOUR

The Systems

THERE ARE NO Oriental approaches to the body's systems, per se. An understanding of the nervous and endocrine systems, for example, is possible only with the help of the modern sciences, such as biochemistry and electricity. The fact that we know such systems exist at all is due exclusively to the work of Western medicine.

Yet, the Oriental systems, particularly the Chinese, do have their own classification of illnesses that are diagnosed today as diseases of the nervous or endocrine systems. What is recognized today as Parkinson's disease, an illness affecting the nervous system, was once diagnosed as an imbalance of the triple heater, for example. Swollen glands, a disorder of the lymph system, was seen in Chinese medicine as related to a spleen imbalance.

While you are reading these chapters, keep in mind the basic yin-yang dialectic used by the Chinese. Though the Chinese knew nothing of these systems, their most essential tool for understanding the human body—the premise that the body functions by virtue of a polarity between pairs of opposites—is consistently in evidence in the physiology of the systems.

We provide some of these crossover relationships, but also offer a variety of other alternative approaches to common illnesses that afflict these systems. In many cases, the alternatives are grounded in traditional understandings of health care. For example, we offer some of the cutting-edge insights into such illnesses as multiple sclerosis, diabetes, and osteoporosis. The approaches we describe often are grounded in the existing scientific evidence, as well as the ancient healing traditions of the East and West.

CHAPTER 23

THE CIRCULATORY SYSTEM

*T*HE CIRCULATORY SYSTEM is well-known today because, in most industrialized nations, it is the part of the body most likely to fail in a way that causes death. In fact, there have been few epidemics in world history as deadly as cardiovascular disease. Today, sixty-six million Americans suffer from illnesses that afflict the heart and arteries, including coronary heart disease, high blood pressure, and stroke. Some 800,000 Americans die annually from these diseases, accounting for half of all deaths in the U.S.

The cost, not only in lives but in dollars, is staggering. Americans spend nearly $100 billion a year on medical care and lost wages from cardiovascular disease. Much of the medical bill goes to surgery, such as coronary bypass operations. Some 350,000 coronary artery bypass surgeries are performed annually, about 70 percent of them on men, at an average cost of about $20,000 apiece.

Ironically, cardiovascular disease is almost unheard of in the Third World and among Orientals living on traditional diets. The reason is simple: the diets of traditional peoples tend to be low in fat and cholesterol, and rich in whole grains, vegetables, and fish. That diet protects them from many illnesses, but especially from heart disease.

The rule of the artery is supreme.

ANDREW STILL

251

Drugs and surgery are all too often given as substitutes for understanding and changing what I believe are the primary underlying causes of coronary heart disease: harmful responses to emotional stresses, a high-fat, high-cholesterol diet primarily based on animal products, and cigarette smoking.

DEAN ORNISH

New research has shown, however, that such traditional diets not only prevent cardiovascular disease, but also cure it. In November 1989, Dr. Dean Ornish, director of the Preventive Medicine Research Institute in Sausalito, California, reported a study showing reversal of the cholesterol plaque (known as atherosclerosis) that clogs the arteries to the heart and is the underlying cause of cardiovascular disease. He cured the illness by having patients follow a program that included meditation and a diet low in fat and cholesterol. Ornish's research is the first to show that diet and lifestyle alone can reverse atherosclerosis in the coronary arteries in humans. Unlike other studies that demonstrated reversal, Ornish's study used no cholesterol-lowering drugs.

What is unfortunate is that the circulatory system is known for what goes wrong with it, rather than what it actually does. Your circulation provides every cell in your body with what it needs to stay alive right this instant: oxygen, nutrition, immune protection, and the elimination of waste.

A TALE OF TWO CIRCUITS

Human circulation is essentially a two-circuit system. Systemic circulation brings oxygen-rich blood to cells throughout your body, while pulmonary circulation returns carbon dioxide–rich blood to the lungs. Let's take a closer look at each, beginning with the first circuit.

After your blood receives oxygen in the lungs, it flows to the upper chamber, called the left atrium, of the heart, and then down into the left ventricle, the lower chamber. There, a powerful contraction of the heart muscle forces the blood out of the heart and into the main artery, the aorta, which runs down the center of the body and branches off into smaller arteries, called arterioles. These arterioles flow to organs and muscle tissue.

Inside the organ or muscle, the arterioles branch into a network of capillaries. Capillaries are made of semipermeable membranes that allow oxygen and nutrients in the blood to pass through the capillary wall to the cells that surround the tiny vessel. At the same time, carbon dioxide and other forms of waste can pass from the cells through the capillary wall and into the blood. While this exchange is taking place, the blood turns from

The Circulatory System

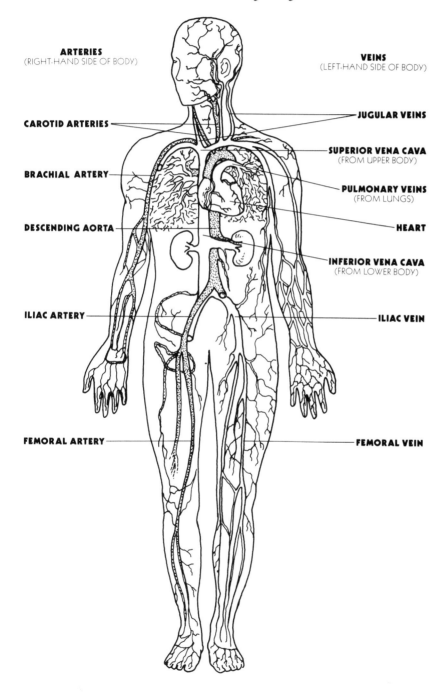

ARTERIES
(RIGHT-HAND SIDE OF BODY)

VEINS
(LEFT-HAND SIDE OF BODY)

CAROTID ARTERIES

BRACHIAL ARTERY

DESCENDING AORTA

ILIAC ARTERY

FEMORAL ARTERY

JUGULAR VEINS

SUPERIOR VENA CAVA
(FROM UPPER BODY)

PULMONARY VEINS
(FROM LUNGS)

HEART

INFERIOR VENA CAVA
(FROM LOWER BODY)

ILIAC VEIN

FEMORAL VEIN

The human body's dual circulation system brings oxygen-rich blood to cells through the arteries and returns carbon dioxide–rich blood to the heart and lungs through the veins. A series of interlinked loops ensures that all parts of the body are infused with nutrients and essential constituents, and that blood is constantly cleansed by the liver and kidneys.

253

its bright red, oxygen-carrying color, to a reddish purple, its color while carrying carbon dioxide (CO_2).

After the blood has received the CO_2, it flows from the capillaries to small veins, called venules. These small veins flow to larger veins that eventually join with one of two venae cavae that flow into the heart. The superior venae cavae flows into the right atrium of the heart from above; the inferior venae cavae flows into the same atrium from below.

The heart pumps blood into the lungs via the pulmonary artery. In the lungs, the blood flows into another network of tiny capillaries that join with millions of tiny sacs, called alveoli. Here, the blood gives up its carbon dioxide load and receives oxygen. Once again, the blood flows to the left atrium, then to the left ventricle, and then to the aorta.

The heart pumps blood with considerable pressure, but that pressure is diminished on its way back to the heart, especially in the legs and arms. Circulation is assisted by a valve system within the veins which prevents blood from flowing backward.

The circulatory system is actually a series of loops within the body that ensures the blood will pass through specific parts of the body such as the neck and head and then back to the heart. Once blood returns to the heart, it goes to the lungs again for oxygen, and then back to the heart, and then onto another loop.

For the blood to nourish cells, it must receive adequate supplies of nutrition. It does this by passing from the aorta to the stomach, intestines, spleen, and pancreas. These organs provide the blood with vitamins and minerals, blood sugar (glucose), immune cells, and various other blood constituents. From there, it passes to the liver.

The liver receives blood from two sources. The hepatic artery carries oxygenated blood to the liver, while the portal vein carries nutrient-rich blood from the digestive organs and spleen. The liver cleanses the blood of impurities, infuses it with thousands of enzymes and immune cells, and obtains the nutrients essential for its health. From the liver, the blood goes back to the heart, where it receives a new supply of oxygen and then flows to the next loop, the kidneys, where it will be cleansed and nutrients will be balanced. From the kidneys, the blood returns to the heart, and then onto another circuit, the lower extremities. Because all the loops within the system are linked, the blood is always being infused

With advances in modern medicine, and especially transfusion technology, blood is losing much of its sacred and symbolic meaning, and instead is often being seen and treated as little more than an increasingly valuable commodity in the medical marketplace. Currently, blood is the most commonly sold human body "product."

ANDREW KIMBRELL

with nutrients and essential blood constituents, and being cleansed by the liver and kidneys. Thus, no part of the body is deprived.

High blood pressure, or hypertension as it is also called, is the most common cardiovascular illness in the U.S. It can lead to heart attack, kidney damage, pancreatic disease, and disorders of the eye. High blood pressure often results in aneurysms, "blowouts" of arteries leading to the brain that result in a stroke. Blood pressure is considered high when it exceeds 140/90. Many insurers will not carry a policy on someone when the lower number of the blood pressure scale exceeds 85.

Blood pressure is caused by the expansion and contraction of the heart. The diastolic phase occurs when the heart relaxes and opens, allowing blood to flow into the chambers. The systolic phase occurs when the heart contracts, causing blood to be pumped into the arterial system and throughout the body.

Contrary to what many people believe, elevated blood pressure is not an inevitable consequence of aging. Blood pressure increases with age in the U.S. and much of the Western world, but in populations that still follow traditional diets, blood pressure tends to remain within the healthy range throughout life.

The three principal causes of high blood pressure are atherosclerosis, excessive salt intake, and kidney disease. Atherosclerosis raises blood pressure by narrowing the passageways within arteries. This causes pressure to build behind the blood that is backed up. The effect is analogous to pinching a hose to increase the pressure of the water that flows out.

Excessive salt intake causes edema, which increases the plasma or liquid portion of the blood. Greater quantities of plasma mean increased blood flow within arteries and veins that have distinct limits. Salt also causes the tiny renal arteries in the kidneys to contract, which causes blood to back up behind the kidneys and thus increases pressure.

Sweating therapy can be used to restore circulation. It will raise body heat and metabolism, burn off toxins, and relieve congestion.

You can lower blood pressure simply by reducing the amount of fat in your diet. In most cases, blood pressure will be reduced even if salt is kept at a constant.

Ornish's study proved conclusively that by lowering fat and

Blood will tell, but often it tells too much.

Don Marquis

Americans and Europeans are literally eating themselves to death, gorging on marbled beef and other grain-fed animal products, taking into their bodies massive amounts of saturated fats and cholesterol. The fatty substances are building up in the blood-stream, clogging arteries, lining cell walls, blocking passages, triggering metabolic and hormonal changes, stimulating cell growth, and rupturing organs. The "good life" promised by the beef culture has metamorphosed into a cruel joke as Americans, overweight and plagued by the diseases of affluence, suffer from their own excesses.

Jeremy Rifkin

cholesterol, even advanced atherosclerosis can be cured. Ornish enlisted the cooperation of forty-eight men and women, all of whom had coronary artery disease and were scheduled for angio-grams, a test used to determine the amount of atherosclerosis clogging the coronary arteries. All forty-eight people showed significant closure of the coronary arteries after their angiograms.

The test subjects were divided into two groups of twenty-four. The control group was given the standard medical advice for heart disease: they were encouraged to adopt a 30 percent fat diet, stop smoking, and do aerobic exercise three times per week.

The experimental group was placed on a vegetarian diet that derived only 8 percent of its calories from fat. The foods that the experimental group ate were primarily whole grains and vegeta-bles. They also received instruction in stress management, yoga, and aerobic exercise. All of the members of the experimental group stopped smoking, as well.

The two groups were followed for one year. Before they began receiving their treatment, the average blood cholesterol level in the experimental group was 213 mg/dl. At the end of the year, their cholesterol levels fell to an average of 154 mg/dl. The control group started out with an average cholesterol level of 251 mg/dl, and managed to bring that down to 230 on the 30 percent fat diet.

Doctors also performed angiograms once again on the remaining participants of both groups. (Seven had dropped out of the study, two from the experimental group and five from the control group. Interestingly, compliance was better among the experimental group than the controls, who received the less demanding program.) Of the twenty-two remaining participants in the experimental group, eighteen members showed reversal of atherosclerosis in the coronary arteries. That is, the atherosclerotic plaque in the arteries leading to the heart got smaller, making the passageway within the artery larger. In the control group, ten of the remaining nineteen members showed a worsening of the atherosclerotic plaque. Three members remained the same, and six got slightly better.

After reviewing the study, Dr. Claude L'Enfant, director of the National Heart, Lung and Blood Institute, stated, "This is a tremendously important study in the control of coronary artery disease without pharmaceutical intervention."

Ornish's work and other recent studies suggest that heart disease is much more than a pump in need of repair. In addition to being fed a healthful diet, your heart requires emotional and spiritual sustenance. According to Ornish, "Many people are in pain, spiritually and emotionally. Without addressing that pain, it's hard to get any further. But when it is addressed and when you show people ways of dealing with that, the transformations can in many cases be dramatic."

Ornish points to the case of a volunteer in his study who had reduced his cholesterol level from 271 to 192, an admirable reduction but not yet sufficient, Ornish thought, to cause reversal of arterial blockage. An angiogram revealed, however, that the man's arteries had indeed opened. Ornish attributed the surprising success to the man's eagerness to open himself to a higher power, to explore his feelings of isolation and loneliness and do something about them, and to avoid the factors Ornish says are "most toxic to the heart": excessive self-involvement, hostility, and cynicism.

Much more than a pump, the heart is a symbol of love, compassion, affection, and spirit, as has been recognized by various societies throughout the world. By keeping it healthy, you can keep the rest of your body well, and also contribute to the overall health of friends, partners, family members—indeed, all those with whom you come in daily contact.

For the blood is the life.

DEUTERONOMY

THE MUSCULAR SYSTEM

*Exercise is more than burning
up calories. Movement is more
than stretching. The presence
of a mind in our person, and
all that this means, from
sensation to higher forms of
reasoning, is paradoxically
most obvious in the way
our bodies move.*

TED KAPTCHUK

USCLES ARE MOVEMENT. Muscles are Michael Jordan soaring across a basketball court and descending on a rim. They are José Canseco driving a baseball out of a stadium with an awesome swing of the bat. They are the physical comedy of Steve Martin, the sensuality of Madonna. Muscles provide much of the power and beauty of the human body.

Though the word *muscle* shares a Latin derivation (*mus*) with the word *mouse* (from the perceived resemblance between the movements of a mouse and a muscle), muscle also has come to mean sheer power and brute force. To "muscle in" is to be able to make one's way or take control by strength or force. Was it an accident that the 1980s, a decade that admired corporate "strong-arming" and business bullies, was the decade of pumping iron, Arnold Schwarzenegger, and the bodybuilding craze? What is it about muscles and the body's muscular system that inspires such varied views?

There are some 656 muscles in the body. Each works by pulling, thus drawing bones closer to one another. For this to happen, muscles must be coordinated; as one set pulls, another relaxes and stretches. Thus, when you lift something heavy with your arms, your bicep muscles contract while the tricep muscles (located in the back of the arm) relax and stretch. Conversely, when you want to extend your arms, your tricep muscles contract while the biceps relax. In this way, all movement occurs: your leg is straightened or bent, your head is turned, your eyes are opened. Healthy, well-toned muscles provide strength and endurance.

But their utility is only half the picture. Muscles are the foundation of human beauty. They are expressions of poised power. In their motion lies our capacity for physical grace, agility, speed, force, and flight. In the sculpture of ancient Greece and the painting of Renaissance Italy can be found perhaps the fullest expressions of the muscular system's archetypal beauty. Among God's most wondrous creations is the muscular body, said the Italian sculptor and painter Michelangelo.

AN INSIDE LOOK AT MUSCLES

Muscles and bone are joined by tendons, and are so closely wedded that many consider them one musculoskeletal system. Indeed, if we fail to use one, both will atrophy into nonexistence. A third dimension is often considered, as well. Muscles are coupled to nerves in a neuromuscular system. Bones, muscle, and nerves form the trinity of movement within the body, each one dependent upon the other, none fully understood without the other two.

There are three types of muscle: smooth, cardiac, and skeletal. Smooth muscles, which are located in the digestive tract and the walls of organs and blood vessels, are controlled by the autonomic nervous system and are largely involuntary. They serve four functions: to propel materials, such as food and waste, along the digestive tract; expel body fluids from organs, such as bile from the gall bladder and urine from the bladder; regulate the size of openings, such as the sphincter muscle of the anus or the pupil of the eye; and close blood vessels and other passages, such as bronchial tubes.

Cardiac muscles are found in the wall of the heart. Fibrous and striated, and arranged in parallel bundles, these muscles are made of cells that rhythmically expand and contract. The cells and bundles of muscle tissue function as one, partly by virtue of the coordinated electrical impulses fired by specific nodes within the heart.

Screw up the vise as tightly as possible—you have rheumatism; give it another turn, and that is gout.

ANONYMOUS

The skeletal muscles are what we typically think of when we picture muscles. They control posture, locomotion, and the movement of the head, neck, torso, back, limbs, and fingers. The skeletal muscles are long, cylindrically shaped, and composed of many striated fibers that lie parallel to one another. These fibers are grouped in bundles, called fasciculi, and enclosed in membranes called perimysium. The entire muscle is enclosed in a sheath called the epimysium. Sheets of connective tissue, called fascia, separate individual muscles.

Skeletal muscles are capable of both expansion and contraction. They work by stretching and shortening. The elasticity gives them the ability to regain their original form once their work is done and they relax. Muscles move thanks to nerve impulses which are triggered by a variety of stimuli, among which are changes in temperature and pressure. A weak stimulus causes a less intense response of shorter duration; a strong stimulus results in a more intense response that usually lasts longer. Continual stimulus results in sustained contraction, called tetanus.

When muscles are exercised they require more fuel in the form of oxygen and glucose. Thus, circulation is increased dramatically to muscle tissues. As tissue is changed into energy and waste products, new cells form, making the muscles stronger, bigger, and more efficient. Meanwhile, waste products that have been stored in the muscles are released into the blood stream and eliminated from the body. Fat, surrounding muscle tissue, is burned as fuel, causing muscle tone to be enhanced. As skeletal muscles become stronger and more fit, they act as auxiliary hearts, pumping blood more efficiently throughout the body and taking stress off the heart.

All muscles except the heart are susceptible to cramping, or sustained contraction, which can be painful. Inefficient and out-of-shape muscles are far more susceptible to cramping than well-toned muscles. Overall, muscle efficiency is dependent upon the frequency of exercise.

MUSCLES IN CHINA AND INDIA

In Chinese medicine, the spleen and liver control muscle condition and development. The Yellow Emperor says that the liver

The Skeletal Muscles

The long, cylindrically shaped skeletal muscles control posture, locomotion, and movement by expanding and contracting, stretching and shortening. This elasticity gives them the ability to regain their original form once their work is done and they relax.

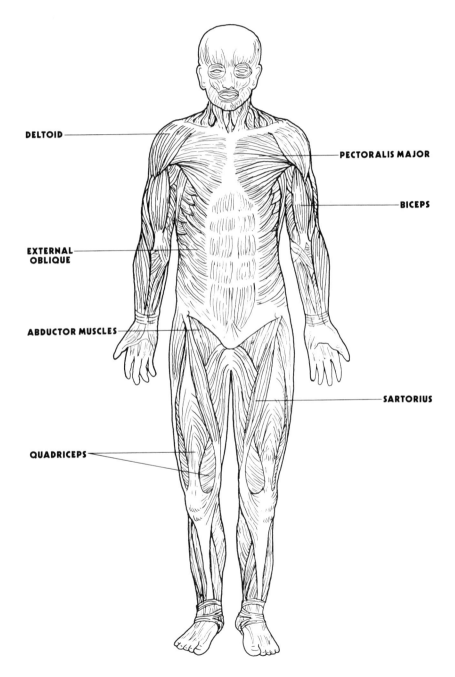

DELTOID

PECTORALIS MAJOR

BICEPS

EXTERNAL OBLIQUE

ABDUCTOR MUSCLES

SARTORIUS

QUADRICEPS

controls the muscles and muscle activity. But it is the spleen that sends qi to the muscles and is responsible for muscle tone. (See chapters on liver and spleen for information concerning these organs and the foods and herbs that will strengthen muscle development and tone.)

From the point of view of Ayurvedic healers, all three doshas come into play in the utilization and maintenance of muscles. Vata controls all body movements, and therefore plays a central role in muscle activity. It is responsible for making glucose and other nutrients available to muscles, and for moving waste from muscle tissue. Kapha ensures that muscles have potential energy, sustains their essential form, and lubricates and cleanses the muscles with lymph. Pitta provides the fire that burns the glucose as energy.

Each of the three archetypal constitutions is revealed through a specific body type. Kapha has excellent muscle development, tone, and coordination. The kapha type is the most likely to be athletic, yet is prone to being overweight. The pitta constitution will have moderate muscle development, good athletic abilities, and will likely remain thin or moderately built. The vata type has the least muscle development, has little interest in athletics, and may appear to be wasting away.

Kapha types need vigorous exercise of any type and regular activity because their muscle development is potentially the greatest of the three constitutional types, and therefore the one most in need of continual attention to maintain balance. Pitta types are attracted to competitive sports and can sustain long periods of exercise. A vata person needs light exercises, such as yoga and tai chi, because he or she easily becomes exhausted.

CHAPTER 25

THE SKELETAL SYSTEM

HUMANS WOULD BE a race of odd-shaped worms if not for the skeleton. You owe your ability to stand upright to your bones, which also, along with the muscles, allow you to walk, run, and dance. In addition bones protect and support the organs within the body, especially the brain, encased in the skull; the spinal cord, encased in the vertebrae of the spine; and the heart, lungs and other thoracic organs within the rib cage. Some 99 percent of the body's calcium is stored in the skeleton. Bones are the stones of the human body, the mineral world within.

Bones are composed of several layers, the first of which is a thin membrane, the periosteum, which contains blood vessels and nerves. Beneath this outer layer is the hard dense shell that we typically think of as bone. Below that is the spongy marrow, which contains tissues that produce red and white blood cells. Calcium and phosphorus act as mortar to make bones hard, while collagen, a protein, forms a latticelike connective tissue upon which calcium and phosphorus accumulate.

As we have seen in virtually every other part of the human body, the bones remain healthy by virtue of opposing functions within them. In this case, these opposing functions arise from

The human body is an instrument for the production of art in the life of the human soul.

ALFRED NORTH
WHITEHEAD

263

two types of bone cells. Osteoblasts build bone tissue by causing calcium to be added to the collagen foundation, while osteoclasts break down bone by causing calcium to be removed from the bone and added to the blood.

New bone tissue is continually being formed within the bone, while old bone is being broken down in the paradoxical functions of metabolism and catabolism. Endocrine glands determine which of these functions is more active. Growth hormone from the pituitary, estrogen or testosterone from the sex organs, and calcitonin from the thyroid stimulate osteoblasts to form more bone, while parathyroid hormone encourages osteoclasts to remove calcium from bone tissue and increase blood levels of calcium.

The Skull

The skull is made up of twenty-nine mostly hollow bones, thus keeping the head light and maneuverable. The various cavities and holes in the skull allow it to hold such vital organs as the brain, mouth, eyes, and nose, and allow the entrance and exit of nerves, blood vessels, and the brain stem.

PARIETAL

TEMPORAL

FRONTAL

NASAL

OCCIPITAL

MASTOID PROCESS

MANDIBLE

A Jigsaw Puzzle of Bones

Most people possess 206 bones, though some have an extra vertebrae while others are missing a digit in a finger or toe. The skeleton also consists of ligaments, which are fibrous tissues that hold bones together at the joints and also connect organs to one another, and cartilage, which covers the ends of bones at the joints and serves as the foundation for some of the body's structures, such as the ears and nose.

The bones of most people do not reach their maximum density until around the age of thirty-five. After that, all of us experience some degree of bone loss, usually about 1 percent per year on the average.

There are four types of bones: long, found in the limbs; flat, in the skull, ribs, and sternum; short, in the wrist and ankle; and irregular, found in the spine and skull. The skeleton can be divided into general categories: the axial and the appendicular. The axial consists of eighty bones that make up the skull, spine, ribs and sternum (or breastbone).

The skull is made up of twenty-nine bones, all of them flat or irregular. Many of them are hollow and thus lighter, making it easier for you to move your head. Small bones within the skull include the hyoid, located in the back of the tongue, and three tiny bones in each middle ear. There are also various cavities and holes in the skull. The cavities hold the brain and form the mouth, eyes, and the nasal hole. The holes allow nerves and blood vessels to enter and exit, and allow the brain stem to enter from below.

The skull rests on the top vertebra of the spine, called the atlas, that allows extensive though limited movement of the head. The spine contains twenty-six bones, all of them small vertebrae. They are the seven cervical bones (or the upper section of vertebrae); the twelve thoracic (middle section); five lumbar (found in the small of the back); the sacrum (lower end of the spine); and the coccyx or tailbone.

There are 126 appendicular bones, including sixty-four bones in the shoulders and upper limbs. Your body has two collarbones (clavicles), two shoulder blades (the scapulas) capping each upper arm (the humerus), forearm bones (the radius and ulna), eight short bones in the wrist (carpals), five shorter bones in each hand (metacarpals), and fourteen bones in the digits of each hand (the phalanges, two in each thumb and three in each finger).

The lower extremities are composed of sixty-two bones, including the hip or pelvis, one bone in each thigh (the femur), a kneecap (the patella), the inner side shin (tibia), the outer side shin (fibula), seven short bones in each ankel (tarsals), five short bones in each foot (metatarsals), and fourteen bones in the digits in each foot (two in each big toe and three in each of the other toes).

WHEN BONES BECOME BRITTLE

Osteoporosis, a disease in which bone tissue becomes more porous and thus prone to fracture, afflicts approximately 25 million Americans. Fractures occur most commonly in the forearm, various spinal vertebrae, the hip, the pelvis, and the femur. Osteoporosis afflicts more women than men, and more Caucasians and Orientals living in the U.S. than African-Americans, who tend to have greater bone mass. It is more prevalent in the Western, industrialized world than in poorer Third World nations, a fact that many scientists point to when making the argument that lifestyle plays a significant role in the onset of the illness.

Osteoporosis is a controversial illness, with leading scientists and physicians disagreeing about the best methods for preventing and treating it. Some doctors maintain that diet and lifestyle should be given greater emphasis in both the prevention and the treatment of the illness, while others say that the singular treatment for osteoporosis is hormone replacement therapy. Much is still unknown about the illness. Though it has been diagnosed for centuries, it was only in 1984 that the National Institutes of Health termed the disease a major threat to public health. Regardless of whatever disagreements exist, both sides agree that all women should know the risk factors for contracting the illness.

In addition to gender and race, the other important risk factors for osteoporosis are:

- *Diet:* The scientific evidence demonstrates that the availability of certain nutrients increase bone mass, while too much of others contribute to bone loss.

The more I have studied the medical literature, the harder it has gotten for me to listen to the dairy industry's promotion of "milk for strong bones." *In spite of its high calcium content, milk, because of its high protein content, appears actually to contribute to the accelerating development of osteoporosis. The occurrence of this condition has reached truly epidemic proportions in the United States, and the promotion of dairy products as an* "answer" *to the suffering of millions seems to me to be not only self-serving, but even criminal.*

JOHN ROBBINS

- *Exercise:* Like muscle tissue, bones grow stronger with physical exercise, and atrophy from inactivity.
- *Smoking:* Nicotine and tars in cigarettes prevent calcium assimilation and bone development, and smoking has been shown to lower estrogen levels in women.
- *Alcohol:* The leading cause of osteoporosis among men, alcohol causes male sex organs to produce lower levels of testosterone.
- *Certain pharmaceutical drugs:* Prednisone, commonly prescribed for asthma and inflammation, is among the most destructive medications to skeletal health available on the market today.
- *A family history of osteoporosis.*
- *Blood levels of vitamin D.*

Once a woman reaches menopause, her rate of bone loss increases dramatically because she loses most, though not all, of her ability to produce estrogen. After menopause, the ovaries stop producing eggs and secrete far less estrogen. The adrenal glands compensate somewhat by producing additional hormone, but the total quantity of estrogen in a woman's body decreases sharply after menopause.

Estrogen in women and testosterone in men are essential for producing and maintaining bone tissue, though scientists still do not understand exactly how these hormones perform such tasks. Since men do not undergo menopause, their rate of osteoporosis is far lower than that of women. However, men can reduce the amount of testosterone their bodies produce by consuming too much alcohol, which will substantially decrease the male hormone and consequently diminish bone mass.

Women experience the sharpest decline in bone mass during the first five years after menopause, when they can lose anywhere from 2 to 6 percent of bone mass per year. Subsequently, bone loss tends to level off to an average of 1 percent per year. How that loss affects the overall health of the skeleton depends a great deal on how much bone reserve the woman has accumulated during her first thirty-five years. According to Jeffrey S. Bland, publisher of *Complementary Medicine,* a journal for health professionals, "All women after menopause lose bone, but they will not necessarily develop demineralization diseases of bone such as osteoporosis. If bone density is high before menopause and the rate of loss after menopause is slowed, the onset of bone demineralization disease may not clinically appear until the individual is 150 years old."

Once a woman reaches menopause, many doctors prescribe estrogen replacement therapy to prevent osteoporosis, even to women whose bodies are still producing some estrogen, because the hormone slows the rate of bone loss and encourages replacement of bone tissue. The effectiveness of hormone therapy has made it the principal line of defense against osteoporosis for many physicians, despite studies showing an increased risk of cancer.

Robert Lang, who taught medicine at Yale University Medical School for a decade and is an expert in osteoporosis, is a prominent proponent of diet and lifestyle as a means for both preventing and treating the disease. Lang argues that estrogen therapy, though essential for many patients, is not necessary for all women suffering from osteoporosis. "Medication, when it is needed, must be more individualized to the person's risk factors," says Lang. "Some people can do well without estrogens." He says that physicians should be more cautious in prescribing estrogens. Lang encourages women to follow a healthful diet to prevent and treat osteoporosis. He recommends:

- Between 40 and 50 percent of the total diet should be made up of whole grains such as brown rice, whole wheat, bulgur, corn, millet, barley, and oats.
- Women should eat large quantities of leafy greens, preferably twice a day, and a variety of other vegetables. Leafy greens are rich in calcium and other minerals essential for healthy bones. Among the most nutritious greens are collard, kale, mustard greens, and cabbage. Also include broccoli, squash, carrots, turnips, and other vegetables. In addition to vegetables, various seaweeds such as arame, hijiki, and nori and sardines with the bones still intact are excellent sources of calcium.
- Avoid or limit foods rich in fat and cholesterol, and if you crave dairy products, eat those low in fat, such as skim milk. In place of fatty animal foods, eat low-fat fish such as had-

Even your body is not really your own. It belongs to life, and it is your responsibility to take care of it. You cannot afford to do anything that injures your body, because the body is the instrument you need for selfless action.

EKNATH EASWARAN

dock, cod, flounder, scrod, and sole, and, if you crave it, small amounts of chicken.
• Avoid sugar, caffeinated beverages, and salt.

Contrary to popular opinion, the high rate of osteoporosis in the U.S. is not due exclusively to insufficient calcium consumption. In perhaps the most comprehensive study of diet and disease patterns ever undertaken, in 1990 Cornell University and Chinese researchers reported that rates of osteoporosis, cancer, and heart disease are low in China, even though the population consumes a diet that is far lower in calcium than the average American's. After examining the nutrient intake of 6,500 people living in China, the researchers found that the Chinese consume an average of 544 mg of calcium per day, as opposed to an American average of 1,143 mg per day. The U.S. recommended daily allowance (RDA) ranges between 1,000 mg to 1,500 mg, with older adults being urged to consume the higher amount.

Research on other cultures, such as the Bantus of Africa, has shown that native populations often consume small amounts of calcium yet have little evidence of osteoporosis. Why the discrepancy? Scientists have known for years that an excess of certain nutrients, especially protein, promotes bone loss. The reason, say researchers, is that protein metabolism increases the acid levels in the bloodstream. This causes the body to secrete more calcium, an alkalizing substance, to neutralize or buffer it, a task that takes place in the kidneys.

"The component in protein which is affecting the calcium loss is the sulfur-containing amino acids," says Robert Heaney, a specialist in osteoporosis at Creighton University in Omaha, Nebraska. Those amino acids "are converted to sulfate in the body and then excreted in the kidney," says Heaney. "The sulfate load tends to wash some calcium out with it. In a sense, it is kind of the endogenous equivalent of the acid rain problem."

There is also considerable evidence that animal proteins have a more harmful effect overall on the body than vegetable proteins, though scientists are still uncertain if animal proteins interfere with calcium metabolism more than vegetable proteins do.

Not only do the Chinese consume far less protein than Americans (an average of 64 grams per day compared to 91 grams for the Americans), but the vast majority of the Chinese protein comes from vegetable sources (60 grams, as compared to 27 for the Americans). Heaney notes, "Vegetarians get less protein than carnivores, and more calcium."

Dairy products contain relatively large amounts of protein and therefore are not ideal sources of calcium. On the other hand, leafy green vegetables are rich in calcium but low in protein. Protein, however, is not the only problem with dairy foods. Milk, eggs, and meat contain phosphates, which research suggests may inhibit the body's absorption of calcium.

Not all leafy greens are good sources of calcium, however. Popeye's panacea, spinach, contains calcium but also has oxalic acid, which binds with calcium and prevents its absorption by the body. Beet greens, rhubarb, sorrel, and Swiss chard also contain oxalates, which makes these vegetables less desirable for people concerned about osteoporosis.

Like protein, sodium promotes calcium loss through the kidneys. It also increases parathyroid hormone and thus contributes to bone loss.

Finally, vitamin D is essential to healthy bone metabolism. While only twenty minutes of sunlight twice a week will provide adequate vitamin D to maintain healthy bone, deficiencies of D often occur among the elderly who are shut-ins, undergo lengthy indoor convalescence, or are hospitalized. Physicians recommend that even if people are unable to walk, they should sit outdoors and get some sun periodically.

While Lang emphasizes the importance of a healthful diet, he encourages those who need calcium supplements to take one that combines calcium and magnesium. Researchers have established that magnesium promotes the body's ability to utilize calcium. "Ten years ago, health food stores were promoting supplements that combined calcium and magnesium, but doctors didn't think much of the research supporting that recommendation," comments Lang. "Now, there's good evidence to show that magnesium does promote better calcium utilization."

Finally, certain drugs can interfere with calcium metabolism and bone health. Of primary concern are the corticosteroid group, the most common of which is prednisone, prescribed for inflammation and asthma. For many, it wreaks havoc on bone tissue.

In light of the evidence showing how humans age, and how bone mass accumulates during the first half of life, exercise has become an increasingly important part of the formula for healthy bones. Two types of exercise are essential. Weight-bearing exercises, such as walking, stimulate the bone-forming osteoblast cells to create new bone. Consequently, people who exercise have denser bone at all ages, from the very young to the very old. Also, weight-bearing exercise speeds the rate of bone turnover. Old bone is broken down and eliminated and new, healthier bone replaces it.

"All of us experience micro-fractures," says Lang. "However, when bone turnover is low, these micro-fractures accumulate and become major breaks." Exercise makes muscles stronger and better able to carry body weight, thus taking the stress off bone tissue.

Stretching exercises are also important because they reduce cramping and muscle spasm. Lack of activity makes muscles contract and become shorter, causing them to apply more tension to the bone. Such contractions can cause fractures by themselves.

Every part of a bone she [nature] makes bone, every part of the flesh she makes flesh, and so with fat and all the rest; there is no part she has not touched, elaborated, and embellished.

GALEN

JOINT PROBLEMS

There are several kinds of arthritis, the most common of which are osteoarthritis, rheumatoid arthritis, and gout. All of them are characterized by swelling, pain, stiffness, and redness in the joints. The illness may involve many joints, or be concentrated in just a few, such as the hands.

Osteoarthritis, the most common form of the illness, usually afflicts older people. It is a degenerative condition in which the cartilage in the joints becomes deformed and enlarged. These bony outgrowths, called osteophyte, cause pain and prevent normal movement in the joint. Three times as many women as men contract osteoarthritis. The illness is treated with painkillers, anti-inflammatory drugs, physical therapy, and sometimes corticosteroid drugs (which also treat inflammation). Surgery also may be used to replace joints or immobilize them. The cause is unknown.

Rheumatoid arthritis is an autoimmune disorder in which the body's immune system attacks the tissue lining the joints, especially in the hands, feet, and arms. Like osteoarthritis, it affects two to three times as many women as men. Treatment includes painkillers, anti-inflammatory drugs, immunosuppressant drugs, and antirheumatic drugs, including gold and penicillamine, which may slow the growth of the disease. The underlying cause is unknown.

Gout occurs when uric acid accumulates in the body and migrates to the joints, where it forms crystals that cause inflammation and pain. The illness is associated with kidney stones and, when sufficiently advanced, kidney failure. It is extremely painful. Gout is treated with anti-inflammatory drugs, pain relievers, and changes in diet to reduce the level of protein, which causes higher levels of uric acid.

Traditional people the world over who live on diets low in fat and protein show few signs of any type of arthritis. Conversely, arthritis is epidemic among people living in affluent industrialized countries living on high-protein, high-fat diets. Gout, for example, was especially prevalent among the aristocracy of seventeenth-century England, who ate a diet rich in meat.

Nathan Pritikin, the pioneer nutritionist, theorized that arthritis is caused by an increase in uric acid and purines. The uric acid crystals and the purines stimulate an immune response, which views the uric acid crystals and purines as foreign substances. White blood cells attempt to consume uric acid crystals in the cell's acid-rich stomach. But the crystal cannot be digested by the white cell and, instead, may puncture a hole in the cell, causing the acid to spill out onto the joints and sensitive joint tissues. This gives rise to the associated pain, swelling, and stiffness of arthritis. Pritikin contended that by eliminating high-protein foods, especially animal foods, gout can be eliminated.

Other forms of arthritis are often relieved in the same way. Animal proteins, of course, come with fat, which reduces circulation and oxygen levels in joints. Blood and oxygen are essential for tissues to function properly. As fat and cholesterol increase in the blood, red blood cells become sticky and begin to adhere to one another, a condition called "rouleaux formation." These cells clump together and thus are unable to pass through smaller capillaries. This prevents blood and oxygen from getting to cells, thus causing cells to suffocate and die. Another effect is edema, or swelling within the joints, caused by rouleaux formation within the bloodstream.

CHAPTER 26

THE NERVOUS SYSTEM

$\mathcal{T}$HE HUMAN NERVOUS SYSTEM is the most advanced communications network on earth. At every instant it receives untold bits of information, prioritizes them, and offers a range of appropriate responses—everything from forming words, to changes in internal chemistry, to beautifully coordinated movements. It governs a universe of cells, glands, and organs within us. At the same time, it allows us to experience life in orderly patterns and gives us the ability to respond to those patterns so that we can meet our needs and those of others around us.

At this very moment, every color, shape, and smell within your environment, every physical thing that touches your body, the very taste in your mouth, are all vying for your attention. The book you are holding, the words on this page, the sounds in the background, the faint smells in the air, the clothes you wear, and the chair on which you sit are all sending signals to your brain. You could be overwhelmed, but your nervous system's ability to organize this profusion of stimuli, and prioritize it according to your needs, makes the environment seem both calm and innocuous, at least most of the time.

Suddenly, a bee nears. Before you see the bee, you hear it

The environment is considered a candidate for healing along with the individual person.

DAVID J. HUFFORD

The nervous system has a fundamental characteristic: We cannot carry out an action and its opposite at the same time. At any single moment the whole system achieves a kind of general integration that the body will express at that moment. Position, sensing, feeling, thought, as well as chemical and hormonal processes, combine to form a whole that cannot be separated out into its various parts. This whole may be highly complex and complicated, but is the integrated whole of the system at that given moment.

MOSHE FELDENKRAIS

buzzing. The sound is recognized and given priority over all other forms of information. Your eyes search for the bee. You notice that it is coming at you! In the blink of an eye, your heart and respiration rates quicken. Your bloodstream is filled with adrenaline, giving you lightning-quick reflexes. You drop the book and swat at the bee. Though you miss it, your flailing motion is enough to dissuade the bee's curiosity. It's gone.

Now your priorities change. The words on the page draw your attention once again and sounds exist in the background of consciousness. Without your awareness, your nervous system is working furiously to slow your heart and breathing, lower your blood pressure, relax your muscles, and change the hormonal composition of your blood. It performs these tasks while it observes the words on the page, translates the symbols into meaning, remembers important facts, and relates the information sequentially so that each paragraph makes sense in light of its predecessor. In short, it is miraculous.

The nervous system is a symphony of billions of instruments that, in health, never miss a beat. It rules an infinite series of events so complex and so varied that no computer—no matter how big—could duplicate its abilities.

AN ELECTRICAL AND CHEMICAL MARVEL

Both the nervous and endocrine systems coordinate, integrate, and control all bodily functions. The nervous system operates largely through electrical and chemical mechanisms, while the endocrine system functions through chemical (hormonal) means. They are so interdependent that they are sometimes referred to as the neurohumoral system.

The nervous system, of course, is the seat of consciousness, intelligence, and memory. It is the physical tool for all higher mental activities, such as reasoning, thinking, judgment, and emotion. Much is known about how the nervous system works, yet much remains a mystery. Scientists do not fully understand how nonphysical events such as thoughts and emotions trigger physical changes in nervous function. Nor do they understand where memory is stored and how such information is called forth when needed.

Interestingly, many of your thoughts have specific effects on nervous and endocrine function. This is the basis for the relatively new science of psychoneuroimmunology, the study of how thoughts and emotions change the kinds of messages and chemical responses experienced by the nervous and endocrine systems.

There are two main physiologic divisions of the nervous system: the central nervous system, consisting of the brain and spinal cord, and the peripheral nervous system, which is made up of the nerve fibers that infuse the sense organs, skin, muscles, internal organs, and glands. The peripheral nervous system is connected to the central by twelve pairs of cranial nerves at the brain, and thirty-one pairs of spinal nerves at the spinal cord.

Sense organs send information from outside the body to the central nervous system. At the same time, receptor nerves within the peripheral nervous system monitor internal organs such as the heart, lungs, and bladder, and relay that information to the central nervous system. The central nervous system then decides what kind of response is necessary and orders a range of reactions that usually involve muscles, internal organs, and glands. Such reactions translate into human behavior, everything from external speech and physical movement to internal hormonal and biochemical changes.

There is also a functional division within the nervous system, known as the autonomic and the somatic (or voluntary) nervous systems. The autonomic nervous system works automatically or unconsciously. It regulates internal organs and performs reflex responses. All smooth muscle functions, which include digestion, respiration, and circulation, are controlled by the autonomic nervous system. When your body changes the size of your pupils, constricts and dilates blood vessels in the scalp, secretes hormones, or creates goose pimples on the skin, it is due to responses controlled by the autonomic nervous system.

The somatic or voluntary nervous system is under your conscious control. It performs the tasks that you consciously order at a particular moment: eating, drinking, scratching your head. The somatic or voluntary nervous system works by translating thoughts into physical responses. It does this by controlling skeletal muscles, such as those in the arms and legs, neck and feet, and face and mouth. Inside the brain and spinal cord are programs that coordinate specific muscular and skeletal activities so that orderly

The Nervous System

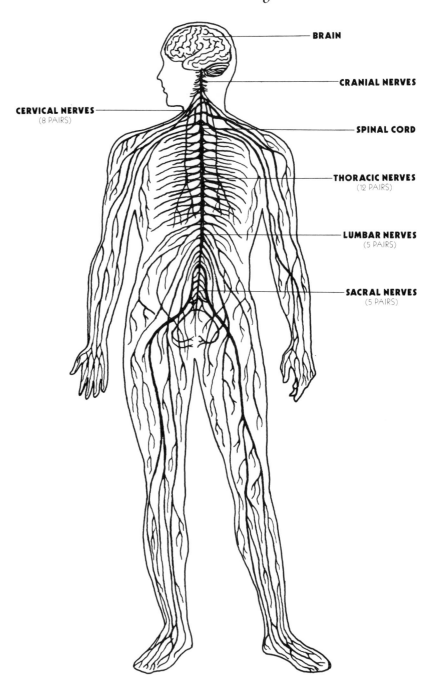

The body's many nerves are part of either the central nervous system, consisting of the brain and spinal cord, or the peripheral nervous system, made up of the nerve fibers that infuse the sense organs, skin, muscles, internal organs, and glands. The peripheral nervous system is connected to the central by twelve pairs of cranial nerves at the brain, and thirty-one pairs of spinal nerves at the spinal cord.

BRAIN

CRANIAL NERVES

CERVICAL NERVES
(8 PAIRS)

SPINAL CORD

THORACIC NERVES
(12 PAIRS)

LUMBAR NERVES
(5 PAIRS)

SACRAL NERVES
(5 PAIRS)

movement occurs. Consequently, when you want to, say, lift a piece of bread from a plate and bring it to your mouth, you experience the act as a fluid motion and not as a series of commands. Your nervous system is, however, in fact directing a series of individual commands, which were learned and perfected in childhood. Each of these commands must be performed at precise moments so that you can reach out, grasp the bread with your fingers, bring it to your face, bite off a small piece, and, while chewing the bread, return it to the plate. This simple act can involve as many as fifty muscles and thirty bones, all acting as one unit.

Such actions are made possible by billions of individual units within the nervous system called neurons. While individual neurons vary somewhat in shape, they are usually star-shaped with several short "arms" or projections emanating from the cell body, and a single long projection. The short arms are called dendrites; the long radiant is called an axon.

A nerve impulse occurs when an electrical signal is fired from the cell body and down along the axon. The impulse causes the tip of the axon to release a chemical called a neurotransmitter. This chemical neurotransmitter passes over a space called a synapse between the axon and the neighboring neuron. One of the dendrites on the neighboring neuron, or the cell body itself, will catch the neurotransmitter, which in turn will stimulate another electrical impulse within that cell body. The newly triggered electrical charge will trigger an electrical charge to flow along that cell's axon and cause the release of another neurotransmitter at the axon's tip. That chemical will breach the synapse and trigger another electrical impulse in an adjacent cell. In this way, nerve impulses are transmitted through the nervous system. And it all happens in the blink of an eye.

Each resting neuron is a polarized cell, meaning that the outside of the cell is surrounded by positively charged particles (or ions), which come from sodium. Inside the cell are negatively charged particles, which come from potassium. When the neuron is stimulated, such as the moment you touch something, the positively charged particles enter the cell and combine with the negative particles to release a flow of electrons which streak down the axon to stimulate the production of a neurotransmitter.

The chemical neurotransmitter then stimulates another electrical impulse in a neighboring neuron, but causes a specific re-

A state of "dis-ease" in the body is always a reflection of conflict, tension, anxiety, or disharmony on other levels of being as well.

SHAKTI GAWAIN

sponse within the tissues of that part of the body. For example, some neurotransmitters cause muscles to contract. Others cause muscles to relax, while still others cause hormones to be released from glands.

Neurons cannot be replaced after the nervous system has been fully developed in fetal life because individual neurons lose their ability to reproduce. Radiation, infection, aging, lack of oxygen, and poisoning, such as from drugs or alcohol, cause neurons to die. Depriving the body of oxygen for more than about four minutes can cause irreparable damage to the central nervous system.

Nerve cells are covered with an insulating tissue called a myelin sheath, which is composed of proteins and lipids (fats) that keep the nerve impulse conducted along its proper path and prevent it from stimulating adjacent fibers. The speed with which the nerve impulse fires through the body is awesome. Depending upon the size and thickness of the nerve cell, and whether it is covered with the insulating myelin sheath, the speed can vary from about three feet to 400 feet per second.

Like the brain, the central nervous system is composed of both gray matter and white matter. In the brain, the cerebral cortex is composed of gray matter, which makes possible all the higher functions: thinking, reasoning, perception, judgment, and emotional experience. Within the central nervous system, gray matter is found deep within the spinal cord. Nerve impulses are received by the gray matter. The information is analyzed and organized, and a response is initiated. White matter is found beneath the cerebral cortex, in the peripheral nervous system, and in the outer or surrounding portions of the spinal cord. Its primary role is to conduct nerve impulses.

THE YIN AND YANG OF THE NERVOUS SYSTEM

Though the Chinese do not have a concept for the nervous system, as such, it is revealing to consider it in terms of polarity and opposition: the autonomic versus the voluntary, the parasympathetic and the sympathetic systems. For instance, the parasympathetic can be seen as restrictive, contracting, and yin. The sympathetic system works on the overall system to excite, quicken, expand vessels, and create a fiery or yang effect. Also,

How the Nerves Work

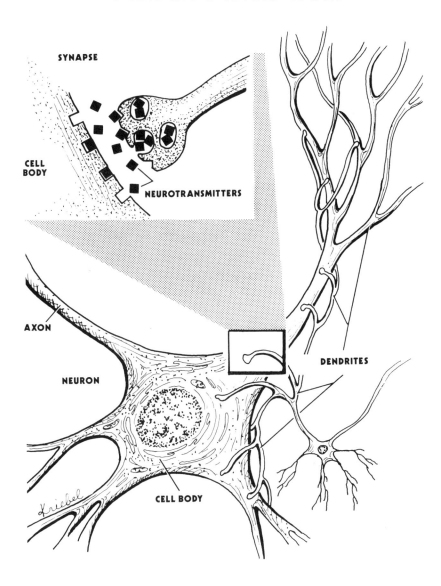

SYNAPSE

CELL
BODY

NEUROTRANSMITTERS

AXON

NEURON

DENDRITES

CELL BODY

Nerves send their messages to the brain with the help of billions of neurons. These tiny, star-shaped units have short arms called dendrites, and usually a single longer one known as an axon. A nerve impulse occurs when an electrical signal is fired from the cell body and down along the axon. The impulse causes the tip of the axon to release a chemical called a neurotransmitter. This chemical neurotransmitter passes over a space called a synapse between the axon and the neighboring neuron. One of the dendrites on the neighboring neuron, or the cell body itself, will catch the neurotransmitter, which in turn will stimulate another electrical impulse within that cell body, triggering another electrical charge and release of neurotransmitters. In this way, nerve impulses are transmitted through the nervous system.

the function of individual neurons is made possible by the presence of positively (yang) and negatively (yin) charged particles. These particles create polarity, which make an electrical charge possible. Thus, the nervous system, too, can be seen in the larger dialectical terms of the East.

279

ATTACK OF THE IMMUNE SYSTEM

Multiple sclerosis is a progressive disease of the central nervous system in which the immune system attacks sections of the myelin sheath, the insulating cover of the nerve fibers. The immune system actually recognizes parts of the myelin sheath as foreign substances. Patches of scar tissue form, thus preventing nerve impulses from flowing along the nerve tissue. Often, the degeneration goes beyond the myelin sheath to the white matter below. Symptoms include numbness in the tips of the fingers and limbs, weakness in the limbs, spastic and uncoordinated movements, stiffness, slurred speech, unsteady gate, incontinence, vertigo, pain in the face, and double vision. The cause of the illness is unknown.

Scientists point out that both environmental and genetic factors seem to play a role in the onset of multiple sclerosis. The disease is more prevalent in temperate climates than in tropical or desert zones. At the same time, those with a family member afflicted by the disease are eight times more likely to contract the illness. The ratio of women to men affected by the disease is three to two. The illness usually attacks young adults between ages of twenty and forty. Treatment generally includes corticosteroid drugs to suppress immune function.

According to Roy Swank, at the University of Oregon Medical School, a low-fat and low-cholesterol diet could be effective in the treatment of multiple sclerosis. His studies in the 1960s and 1970s led him to believe that fat and cholesterol adversely affect the myelin sheath that covers nerve fibers.

After reviewing the scientific literature, Nathan Pritikin concurred, but offered a diet even lower in fat and cholesterol than Swank's. Like Swank, Pritikin maintained that exercise was vital to the improvement of the nervous system. Pritikin urged those with multiple sclerosis to walk daily. The person afflicted with MS should walk as far as he or she could, said Pritikin, rest for as long as necessary, and then walk home.

People with MS who have followed Pritikin's suggestions have improved somewhat. Laura Ornstein of New York City was counseled by Pritikin for several years. She reported that after following the program for several months, she was able to improve her walking distance from a hundred feet to a half-mile without assistance. Her right eye had begun to drift prior to adopting the Pritikin program, but after following Pritikin's recommendations she experienced an improvement in her vision and the correction of her right eye.

Naturopath Ross Trattler has suggested that in addition to improvement in exercise and dramatically lowering fat and cholesterol, the person with MS must abstain from all animal foods, artificial ingredients, and pesticides. He cites studies showing a link between MS and exposure to heavy metals, such as lead. Trattler's recommendations include taking supplementary vitamin A, B complex, C, D, E, and the minerals calcium, magnesium, manganese, selenium, and zinc.

CHAPTER 27

THE ENDOCRINE SYSTEM

Nature is liberal to provide for the necessities of the poor and has sent forth many matters of medicaments, that they may be found everywhere and with little art may be prepared.

NICHOLAS CULPEPER

HORMONES SUCH AS TESTOSTERONE, estrogen, and thyroxine are ghostly substances that we often associate with moods and behavior—or, rather, misbehavior. These strange chemicals move in the blood and lymph and affect people in powerful but sometimes bizarre ways. Often, when a coworker or family member experiences a sudden mood change, someone will say derisively, "It must be hormones." The word itself has become synonymous with unpredictable change. Yet, contrary to popular perception, hormones are among the most consistent performers in human biology. So important are they in health and development that if they were not so dependable, there would be scarcely any consistency in human anatomy and physiology.

The word *hormone,* from the Greek for "to stimulate" or "excite," was not used in connection to the body until 1905, when these strange and powerful chemical substances were discovered. Scientists soon learned that only some of these endocrine chemicals excite, while others inhibit physical reactions. Consequently, the word *chalone,* from the Greek "to slacken," was originally used to designate those inhibiting substances within body tissue. In time, the word *hormone* came to be applied to both the exciters and the inhibitors, and *chalone* is no longer used. Since 1920, knowledge of the endocrine system has steadily accumulated, but endocrinology is still considered a young science and much about the hormonal system is still unknown.

Hormones are produced by endocrine organs, called glands, and transported through the blood and lymph. Every organ that produces hormones can be considered an endocrine gland. These include the pituitary, thyroid, parathyroid, adrenals, pancreas, testes, ovaries, thymus, pineal, skin, kidneys, and intestines. Hormones can be targeted to specific organs or tissues, or have a general effect on the overall body.

The chemical composition of hormones varies. Some are made up of amino acids (the building blocks of proteins). Others are composed of whole proteins. Some are steroids, a classification of chemicals produced by the adrenal glands and sex organs, or fatty acids. Still others are peptides (fragments of proteins, made of two or more amino acids).

Whatever their composition, hormones are uniformly powerful. Tiny amounts of adrenaline, also known as epinephrine, will trigger rapid increases in respiration, heart rate, and energy consumption, for example. Once a hormone reaches its target, it effects some type of change in the organ, tissue, or blood. When the job is done, excesses of the hormone are broken down by the liver and turned into bile, or excreted by the kidneys.

Hormones control virtually every fundamental human function, including growth and development, maturation, reproduction, and most of human behavior. "Much of a person's behavior and most of the traits that collectively constitute personality depend on the normal functioning of the endocrine glands," write Steen and Montague in *Anatomy and Physiology.*

Endocrine glands work in harmony with one another, and with the constituents that make up the blood, which determines how much of a particular hormone is released by a gland. For example, the amount of blood sugar present determines how much insulin is released by the pancreas. Or the quantities of calcium in the blood determine how much parathyroid hormone is released by the parathyroid gland. In other words, endocrine glands are continually responding to the current conditions within the bloodstream, and to what the other glands are doing, as well. As we will see below, dietary factors greatly influence how particular

Burgeoning research on relations between the nervous, endocrine, and immune systems has revealed the body's great redundancy of healing (or homeostatis-maintaining) process. Because of this redundancy, particular kinds of physiological repair or mood alteration can be mediated in more than one way.

MICHAEL MURPHY

glands work, and how effective certain hormones—especially insulin—are.

Other important endocrine glands include the testes, ovaries, and mammary glands, all of which are dealt with in the chapter on the reproductive system. Let's have a look at the primary endocrine glands and their functions.

THE MASTER GLAND

Located in the base of the brain, within the brain stem, the pituitary is a pea-sized gland sometimes referred to as the "master gland" because it regulates the activities of other endocrine glands. The pituitary is itself controlled by the hypothalamus, which influences the pituitary function through its own hormones and a series of nerve fibers. (See hypothalamus in the chapter on the brain).

The pituitary gland, also called the hypophysis, is made up of three lobes, each of which has its own distinct functions. Like the hypothalamus, the pituitary gland seems to have a finger in virtually every important aspect of human physiology. Indeed, the hormones produced by the pituitary regulate the following functions of human behavior:

- Physical growth and development, made possible by growth hormone.
- Milk production in lactating women, made possible by the hormone prolactin.
- Regulation of the adrenal glands, which, among other things, accelerate reflexes in emergency situations (such adrenal responses are made possible by the pituitary's production of adrenocorticotripic hormone [ACTH]).
- Maintenance of metabolism through the production of thyroid-stimulating hormone (TSH).
- Healthful function of male and female sex organs, through the production of luteinizing hormone (LH) and follicle-stimulating hormones (FSH).
- Skin color, made possible by the production of melanocyte-stimulating hormone, which causes skin pigmentation.
- Proper water balance in the bloodstream, through the production of antidiuretic hormone (ADH), which signals the

The Endocrine System

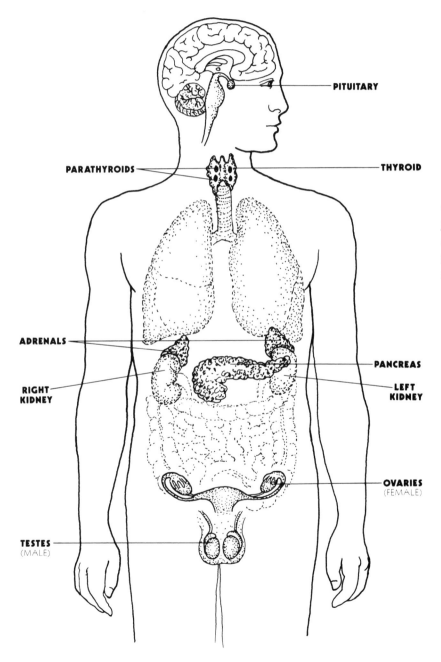

PITUITARY

PARATHYROIDS

THYROID

ADRENALS

PANCREAS

RIGHT
KIDNEY

LEFT
KIDNEY

OVARIES
(FEMALE)

TESTES
(MALE)

The endocrine system regulates the body's production and
use of hormones, ghostly substances that intimately affect
your moods and behavior.
While much about the hor-
monal system is still
unknown, scientists have
identified a number of endocrine organs, including the
pituitary, thyroid, para-
thyroid, adrenals, pancreas,
testes, ovaries, skin, and
kidneys.

kidneys to retain more water and decrease urination, and thus increases the water content of the blood.

- The ability of a woman's uterus to contract during childbirth and expel milk from her breasts, through the production of oxytocin.

That this little gland is involved in so many fundamental and vital functions boggles the mind. But perhaps the pituitary demonstrates best how powerful and important hormones really are. Tiny quantities of these chemicals enact life-altering changes in the body's biochemistry.

YOUR BODY'S METABOLISM COP

The thyroid gland is found at the base of the neck, toward the front. It is composed of two lobes, one on each side of the windpipe or trachea. The thyroid is responsible for regulating metabolism, the term used to describe the many processes that take place in the body. Metabolism is divided into two categories: catabolism, which is the breaking down of substances into still smaller parts; and anabolism, in which the body uses smaller substances to build larger structures, such as using minerals to produce bone tissue, or amino acids to create proteins. Catabolic processes release energy, while anabolic actions consume it. The rate of such metabolic processes depends to a great extent on the activities of the thyroid gland.

The thyroid produces two primary hormones, thyroxine and calcitonin. For the most part, thyroxine promotes catabolism. It regulates respiration and oxygen consumption by cells, as well as the body's utilization of carbohydrates and fat for energy. It's also essential in the promotion of protein synthesis. That is, it helps join amino acids so that the body can form proteins and thus build and replace tissue. In this way, the thyroid assists in normal growth and development. In addition the thyroid helps maintain the central nervous system.

Calcitonin, on the other hand, promotes anabolism, using calcium to form bone tissue. When blood levels of calcium are high, calcitonin is secreted by the thyroid to promote absorption of calcium and the formation of bone matter. It does this by promoting the activities of osteoblasts, the cells that produce bone, and depressing the activities of osteoclasts, the cells that break down bone tissue. Calcitonin performs the opposite task of parathyroid hormone, which is secreted by the parathyroid to increase calcium levels in the bloodstream.

The thyroid is dependent upon iodine, which is derived from foods such as iodized salt, fresh saltwater shellfish, seaweeds, and foods grown in iodine-rich soil. Deficiencies of iodine result in a range of disorders, including insufficient production of thyroxine and the creation of a goiter, which is the swelling of the thyroid gland.

Illnesses associated with the thyroid generally fall within two categories: hypothyroidism, the underproduction of thyroid hormones, and hyperthyroidism, the excess production of thyroid hormones. Tumors can form in the thyroid and lead to malignant cancers. Exposure to radiation is among the most common causes of thyroid cancer.

Traditional Chinese healers consider the thyroid gland part of the Fire Element within the Five Element system, and clearly thyroxine possesses all the characteristics of the Fire Element: catabolic, scattering, and heat-producing. Fire Element foods are used to enhance the thyroid function, especially when it is deficient, though such foods should not be considered a substitute for thyroxine for people with diagnosed hypothyroidism.

Naturopaths and other alternative healers often recommend various foods, vitamins, and minerals to help alleviate disorders of the thyroid, including vegetables such as radishes, mushrooms, watercress, collard and other leafy greens, squash, carrots, and broccoli; grains such as corn, wheat, and millet; garlic; shiitake mushrooms; vitamins A, B6, and E; and the minerals zinc and copper.

DISTINGUISHING SELF FROM NOT-SELF

Western medical scientists have only recently begun to appreciate the thymus. Only a few decades ago, doctors believed it was a useless organ, especially in adulthood, because it usually begins to shrink after puberty. Today, scientists know that the thymus gland is essential to a healthy immune system.

A doctor is a person who still has his adenoids, tonsils, and appendix.

LAURENCE J. PETER

Located in the upper part of the chest just below the breast bone, the thymus is slightly smaller than a fist, with two lobes that are packed with tiny immune cells called lymphocytes. The function of the thymus gland is to produce lymphocytes and to train them to distinguish self from not-self, or one's own cells from disease cells. The thymus also trains the cells to act appropriately in the face of disease by either tagging diseased cells with an antigen, or by attacking the cell and destroying it. Once trained, these lymphocytes are called thymus cells, T-cells for short.

The thymus is essential to healthy immune function. Children whose thymus glands are impaired suffer higher rates of infection and severely impaired immune function. The thymus gland also influences the behavior of the immune system once the lymphocytes leave the thymus.

Studies have shown that the thymus gland shrinks and its functions are impaired as a consequence of chronic stress. Exposure to radiation and chemical pollutants also cause the thymus to shrink. In addition, the absence of various minerals in the diet, especially zinc, has a detrimental effect on both the thymus and the overall immune system. On the other hand, there's evidence that positive emotions and a more optimistic attitude toward life cause thymus function to be enhanced.

Like the thyroid gland, the thymus is considered part of the Fire Element in traditional Chinese medicine and is therefore supported by Fire Element foods, herbs, and medicinal preparations. Not surprisingly, the Fire Element is associated with joy and is suppressed or controlled by the Water Element, whose associated emotion is fear. Increased joy and a diminution of fear enhance thymus function, from the Chinese point of view. A diet rich in minerals, and Fire, Wood, and Earth Element foods and herbs, is essential to the healthy functioning of the thymus gland.

KEEPING BLOOD SUGAR IN BALANCE

The pancreas is a narrow organ, shaped like a horn of plenty, located in the center of the abdomen directly behind the stomach. The wide end of the pancreas is at the right and narrow end near the spleen, on the left. The pancreas serves two essential functions. It secretes digestive juices into the duodenum, thus assisting digestion, and it produces hormones (most notably, insulin) that make possible the utilization of blood sugar as fuel.

Most of the organ is composed of tissues that produce and secrete alkaline digestive juices (see chapters on the stomach, small intestine, and gall bladder). These enzymes are secreted directly into the small intestine where they help break down food particles.

Nestled among these tissues, however, are the endocrine cells that produce hormones. These cells, called the islets of Langerhans, are of two types: alpha and beta cells. The beta cells produce insulin, a hormone that promotes the uptake and utilization of blood sugar by the cells, especially those of muscle and liver cells. In the liver, blood sugar (also known as glucose) is changed to glycogen, the stored form of energy. In the muscles, the blood sugar is burned as fuel.

How insulin promotes the utilization of glucose is not completely known. It is believed that insulin coats the cell membrane, causing it to become more permeable. This greater permeability allows sugar to enter the cell and thus be burned as fuel.

To illustrate, picture the cell as a room in which there are many doors. These doors or insulin receptor sites are the places that allow blood sugar to enter, but only with the assistance of insulin, which somehow makes the doors open. When you eat a food that contains carbohydrates, your blood sugar levels increase, and your pancreas secretes insulin so that blood sugar can be used by the cells.

The pancreas's alpha cells provide the opposite effect on blood sugar. They produce glucagon, which increases blood sugar by promoting the conversion of glycogen (sugar stored in the liver) into glucose, or blood sugar. When you are in need of more fuel in your bloodstream but are unable to eat, the pancreas will secrete glucagon, which will raise your blood sugar level.

Glucose levels in the blood increase when we eat foods rich in carbohydrates. The rate of increase, however, is dramatically different among complex carbohydrates, such as those found in whole grains, beans, vegetables, and many fruits, and simple carbohydrates, such as those in white sugar and refined sweets. This is because refined sugars are small molecules that are able to enter the bloodstream immediately upon touching the tongue and other tissues in the digestive tract. This causes a quick and dramatic increase in blood sugar levels. The pancreas responds to this rapid rise in blood sugar by secreting quantities of insulin, which makes the glucose available to cells as fuel. This interaction of insulin and blood sugar gives you an immediate rush of energy. That fuel is quickly spent, however, leaving you with depressed energy levels. You may also experience a depression in mood, a rise in anxiety and nervous tension, and a hunger for more sweets to bring sugar levels back up. Such a low blood sugar state is called hypoglycemia.

On the other hand, the complex carbohydrates found in whole grains and vegetables are long chains of atoms that must be broken down slowly by enzymes in the mouth and small intestine. The body responds to these long chains by metabolizing them slowly as energy is demanded by the body, causing the person to experience long and enduring flows of energy. Complex carbohydrates thus provide ongoing supplies of energy and endurance, without the depression and anxiety normally experienced by people with hypoglycemia.

Doctors distinguish between two types of diabetes. Type I, or juvenile diabetes, is a genetic disorder in which the pancreas fails to produce insulin, thus preventing the body from metabolizing blood sugar. Juvenile diabetics usually experience rapid weight loss and require insulin in order to survive. Type II, or adult-onset diabetes, is a condition in which the pancreas produces adequate amounts of insulin—in some cases, even more insulin than is necessary—but cells are still unable to absorb glucose. It usually occurs later in life, and it is the much more common type of diabetes, counting among its victims 11 million of the 12 million Americans with diabetes. Both types of diabetes are associated with a number of other serious illnesses, including cardiovascular disease, blindness, gangrene, progressive loss of hearing, impotence, and palsy.

Adult-onset diabetes is among the most serious and misunderstood illnesses today. For decades, doctors believed that adult-onset diabetics were unable to produce sufficient quantities of insulin to sustain health. Consequently, doctors gave these patients insulin injections or oral medication. In addition, patients with adult-onset diabetes were told to avoid all carbohydrates, even complex carbohydrates from whole grains, vegetables, and fruits. These foods were believed to be harmful to diabetics because carbohydrates are sugars, which the diabetic cannot metabolize. Instead, doctors recommended that diabetics consume a high-protein, high-fat diet, consisting mainly of red meats, dairy products, and eggs.

And then, in 1970, new information began to surface. Or, to put it more accurately, old information surfaced again. That year, scientists recognized that adult-onset diabetics were in fact producing insulin—sometimes even more insulin than non-diabetics. But the insulin could not make glucose available to cells. Something was preventing the insulin from working. As researchers looked more carefully at the existing scientific evidence, they unearthed a cache of studies demonstrating that the problem for adult-onset diabetics was not the insulin but a high-fat diet that was preventing the insulin from working.

As far back as 1935, Dr. H. P. Himsworth had discovered that a healthy person could be made to test diabetic by placing him or her on a high-fat diet for as short a time as one week. Remarkably, Himsworth also found that he could reverse the process and restore health by placing the same person on a low-fat diet. Other researchers corroborated Himsworth's discovery, but it failed to gain the recognition it deserved until almost four decades later.

One of the first people to recognize Himsworth's work in the modern era was Pritikin, who theorized that dietary fat covers the cells and prevents insulin from attaching to the insulin receptor sites, preventing glucose from entering the cell and thus giving rise to diabetes. Consequently, the cells cannot obtain fuel and die. (Scientists have demonstrated that dietary fat and cholesterol coat immune cells, as well.) Pritikin demonstrated that most adult-onset diabetics could be cured with the use of a low-fat, low-cholesterol diet made up primarily of whole grains and vegetables.

Recent research done during the 1970s and 1980s by James Anderson at the University of Kentucky Medical School proved Pritikin's hypothesis. Anderson demonstrated that a high-fat diet does indeed give rise to a diabetic state, and that a low-fat, high-fiber diet can reverse adult-onset diabetes and restore blood sugar levels to normal. Anderson showed that soluble fiber, such as that found in brown rice, barley, and oats, binds with the fat and cholesterol and eliminates it from the body.

Other researchers confirmed Anderson's findings, which

caused the American Diabetics Association to reverse the standard dietary advice for diabetics. The ADA now urges diabetics to eat a diet low in fat and cholesterol and rich in whole grains, vegetables, and fiber. Doctors still prescribe insulin and oral medication for adult-onset diabetics, though for many patients dietary and lifestyle changes offer the hope of eventually discontinuing insulin intake. The diet also helps to prevent such diabetes-related illnesses as atherosclerosis, blindness, and gangrene.

Meanwhile, the Pritikin Longevity Center's success in treating adult-onset diabetes is well-documented. Loma Linda University researchers who conducted a study reviewing the effects of the Pritikin Program found that of those attending the Center who were taking insulin, half left the Center after a thirty-day program off insulin and free of all diabetic symptoms. Of those who arrived on oral medication for adult-onset diabetes, 80 percent left the Center symptom-free and off all medication.

In Chinese Medicine, the pancreas is considered part of the Earth Element and, therefore, supported by Earth and Fire foods, herbs, and activities (see chapters on the spleen and stomach). It is balanced by moderately sweet foods, round vegetables (especially squash), millet and sweet corn, and certain herbs, such as liquorice. On the other hand, it is injured by excessively sweet foods. (People with pancreatic problems, including diabetes, should follow the dietary recommendations outlined in the chapter on the spleen.)

THE STRESS GLANDS

There are two adrenal glands, each one triangular-shaped and sitting on top of a kidney. Each adrenal gland can be thought of as having two functional units. The cortex, or outer region, secretes groups of hormones, some generally referred to as corticosteroids and others as mineralocorticoids. These play a vital role in protein metabolism, mineral balance, immune response, and the health of bones. The cortex also secretes sex hormones. The interior region of the adrenals, called the medulla, secretes another set of hormones, most notably adrenaline.

The corticosteroids include hydrocortisone and cortisone, both of which assist in protein formation and metabolism. These hormones also have anti-inflammatory properties and, when released in excess, depress the immune system. The mineralocorticoids include aldosterone, which regulates the body's water balance and maintains sodium and potassium balance. Other hormones released by the cortex cause inflammation of tissues, especially when the body is experiencing an allergic reaction.

Adrenaline increases heart rate, respiration, and blood pressure. It also causes smooth muscles to relax and bronchial passages to contract, thus explaining how adrenaline can play a role in the onset of allergies or an asthma attack. The medulla also secretes dopamine, a neurotransmitter that triggers heightened alertness and aggression. Together, these hormones and neurotransmitters cause virtually instant release of energy. They also stimulate the sympathetic nervous system to provide quick reflex muscle reaction, the so-called "flight or fight" reaction.

The adrenals are highly susceptible to stress. During stressful situations, the pituitary gland secretes ACTH, which signals the adrenal glands to secrete hydrocortisone and adrenaline, which in turn can suppress immune function, create inflammation, and increase susceptibility to illness.

Traditional Chinese healers consider the adrenals part of the Water Element. The glands are, therefore, supported and enhanced by foods, herbs, and therapies grouped under the Water and Metal Elements (see chapters on the kidneys, bladder, lungs, and large intestine). Like the kidneys and bladder, the adrenals are highly vulnerable to fear and stress.

THE THIRD EYE GLAND

The pineal gland is a tiny cone-shaped organ in the brain stem. It grows only from gestation to puberty, but continues to function for the rest of your life. According to the *Atlas of Human Anatomy,* by Samuel Smith and Edwin B. Steen, "Some evidence suggests that it is a vestigial organ, the remnant of a third eye." For centuries, the pineal was regarded strictly in spiritual or religious terms. The seventeenth-century French philosopher René Descartes maintained that it was the seat of the soul. Until recently, scientists believed that the pineal gland had no function because, in adults, it became infiltrated with calcium deposits or "brain sand." New research, however, is showing that the pineal gland has a range of vital functions, including the maintenance of biorhythms, brain chemistry, and mood.

The pineal produces the hormone melatonin and the neurotransmitter serotonin. Increased blood levels of melatonin are associated with depression, irritability, lethargy, and the need for more sleep. The pineal produces more melatonin at night and in darkened environments, but stops producing melatonin when the eyes are exposed to sunlight. The sun stimulates nerve fibers in the eyes that send impulses to the pineal, via the optic nerve, to cease production of melatonin.

This research has explained the medical basis for the depression and lethargy suffered by millions of people living in northern climes during the fall and winter months. Scientists now refer to this condition as SAD, or seasonal affective disorder. People with SAD feel depressed and withdrawn when there is less sunlight, and they also overeat and crave foods rich in carbohydrates.

According to research conducted at the Massachusetts Institute of Technology, carbohydrates stimulate production of serotonin, a neurotransmitter that promotes deep and restful sleep, feelings of well-being, and the ability to focus the mind on a desired subject. Thus, melatonin and serotonin appear to have opposite effects on brain chemistry and mood. Also, carbohydrate cravings may be the body's way of counteracting melatonin production. Research suggests that melatonin can be created from serotonin, and that as melatonin levels increase, serotonin levels decrease.

Curing SAD is simple enough: expose the eyes to full-spectrum bright light, either from the sun or from special, high-intensity full-spectrum fluorescent lights, for up to thirty minutes per day. Studies have shown that 60 to 80 percent of people with SAD lose their symptoms when they are exposed to that much full-spectrum light per day.

"People who talked of hating winter all of a sudden become big fans of winter," notes Dr. Martin Teicher, chief of the chronobiology laboratory at McLean Hospital in Belmont, Massachusetts. "They take up skiing. They love Christmas. The holidays are no longer a matter of conflicted memories."

More than two dozen studies have demonstrated that light has antidepressant qualities. Light also has been shown to reduce the

rates of violence among prisoners who had previously been confined to cells that allowed little or no natural light to enter. Interestingly, studies also have shown that blood-cleansing organs,
especially the liver, function better when the body is exposed to
more sunlight than when it is kept in darkened quarters.

The scientific finding that the pineal is sensitive to light adds
to—and indirectly supports—the widespread traditional view

The Chakras

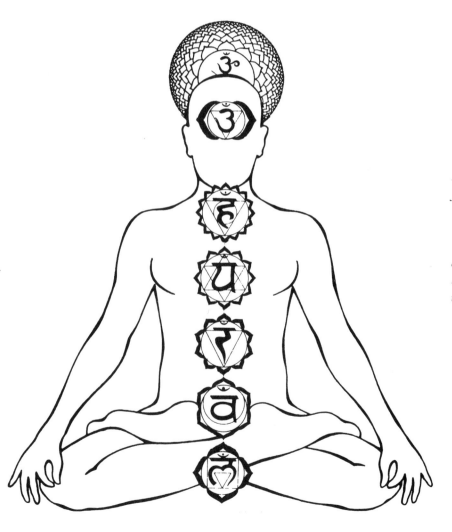

*According to a number of spir-
itual traditions, the body contains a chain of seven spheres
or "chakras" of energy aligned
down the middle of the body.
Each energy center corre-
sponds with particular bodily
functions and characteristics.
The pineal corresponds to
the third eye chakra located
in the middle of forehead, seen
as the source of intuition and
the ability to perceive
universal truth.*

that the pineal bears some relevance to human spirituality. Light has traditionally been seen as the medium of the soul and the higher spiritual realms. Ancient spiritual traditions, especially the Hindu, have conceived of the body as being a chain of seven spheres of energy. These spheres, called chakras, are aligned down the middle of the body at specific points: the top of the head, midbrain (or third eye), throat, heart, solar plexus, sacral (known in Japan as the hara), and sex organs. Each energy center corresponds with particular human characteristics. The pineal corresponds to the third eye chakra, the source of intuition and the ability to perceive universal truth.

CHAPTER 28

THE REPRODUCTIVE SYSTEM

*I*N ANCIENT TIMES, and especially in the East, sex was seen in an altogether different context than it is today. Rather than being the great temptation, the surest road to hell, it was considered a path of spiritual development, and thus a way toward greater intimacy with the divine.

That divinity is seen as a state of wholeness and completeness that is implicit in all of us. In the traditions of the East (especially in Taoism of China and Tantra of Tibet), man and woman represent opposite halves of that universal whole. Each is an earthly manifestation of the two cosmic creative forces, whose intermingling bring forth all phenomena. When man and woman unite in sex, heaven and earth are joined. The sexual experience offers a glimpse of that wholeness within. It is thus one of the great gifts of humanity, offering a relatively accessible experience of peace and harmony, and thus serving as a metaphor for the larger purpose of life. That purpose, said the sages, is to achieve peace and harmony through unification of opposites. Look around you, Lao Tzu might say, and recognize man and woman as yet another expression of the same cosmic duality that creates day and night, winter and summer, positive and negative, north and south, heaven and earth. Bring together these opposites and the world collapses in spiritual ecstasy, say the Taoist teachers.

We tend in this "scientific" age to explain human sexuality only in terms of anatomy and physiology. That might cover the matter well enough for rabbits, but human beings are vastly different.

BENJAMIN SPOCK

"In man and woman are found all the materials and experiences of the world," writes Ehud C. Sperling in his publisher's preface to *Sexual Secrets,* by Nik Douglas and Penny Slinger. "When they unite, these experiences and materials can be distilled into a vision of and a harmonization with the dynamic unity underlying all of reality. For centuries this vision of unity has been obscured by individuals and institutions that have promoted a schism between body and mind, between religious feelings and sexuality."

As Douglas and Slinger point out, sex is a powerful form of human energy that can be channeled and utilized for many purposes. "Tantra is a philosophy, a science, an art and a way of life whereby sexual energy is consciously and creatively utilized," write Douglas and Slinger. "The mystical treatises known as the Tantras contain a broad spectrum of practical techniques for enhancing sexual awareness and achieving transcendence. The hidden potency of the sexual act is the seed of all creativity. Through an understanding of the practical teaching of Tantra, a whole new experience of life opens up."

This same teaching is implicit in the mystical writings of the Egyptian, Hebrew, Greek, and Arab cultures. Each tradition understood sex as a gateway toward greater self-knowledge, personal health, power, and the experience of the divine.

Through most of its history, the West has focused primarily on the dark side of sex. Today, we are suffering the terrible consequences of our attitudes. At the same time, we stand at a crossroads in our maturity, in which it is possible to explore our sexual dimension in new and exciting ways.

Just as our disease patterns have forced us to change our dietary habits, and our environmental crisis causes us to alter our relationship with the earth, AIDS is forcing us to reexamine sex. AIDS challenges us to better understand ourselves, our potential, and our natural limits. Hence, another paradox: there may be a gift in our collective nightmare, yet.

THE ORGANS OF SEX

The male sexual anatomy is made up of two testes; a penis; the prostate gland; and a duct system that connects the testes, prostate, and penis, thus allowing sperm and seminal fluid to pass out of the penis during ejaculation.

The Male Reproductive System

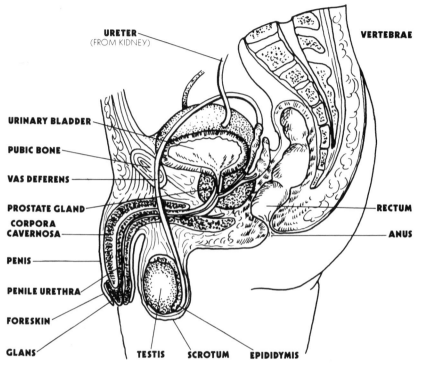

URETER (FROM KIDNEY)

VERTEBRAE

URINARY BLADDER

PUBIC BONE

VAS DEFERENS

PROSTATE GLAND

CORPORA CAVERNOSA

PENIS

PENILE URETHRA

FORESKIN

GLANS

TESTIS   SCROTUM   EPIDIDYMIS

RECTUM

ANUS

A man's two testes produce sperm, the male sex cells. During ejaculation, the sperm make their way upward to the penis by first passing into a canal called the epididymis and then into the vas deferens, tubes that run from the testes to the prostate gland at the root of the penis. Ducts within the prostate allow sperm to mix with seminal fluid and then to pass into the urethra and down through the erect penis.

The testes produce spermatozoa, the male sex cells, and sex hormones, called androgens, which convert to testosterone. The testes are suspended in a sac, called the scrotum. This sac is capable of expansion or contraction, allowing the testes to rise or fall, and thus draw closer or farther away from the body. This maintains and regulates the temperature of the testes to ensure a harmonious environment for sperm production.

The inner body of the testes is divided into lobules, or chambers, which contain tiny tubules, called seminiferous tubules. It is here, in these tiny tubules, where sperm is produced. The sperm makes its way upward to the penis by first passing into a canal called the epididymis, and then into one of two primary tubes that run from the root of the penis to the testes, called the vas deferens. The vas deferens run to the prostate gland. During ejaculation, sperm travels up from the testes and is mixed with prostate fluid. This seminal fluid is slightly alkaline, and made of zinc, magnesium, acid phosphatase, and numerous enzymes.

Ejaculation occurs at the height of sexual excitement, causing rapid contractions which pump sperm from the testes to the prostate, where it is joined with seminal fluid. From there, the sperm and seminal fluid passes down through the urethra and out the tip of the penis. An average ejaculation produces between 200 million and 400 million sperm. Each sperm has a long tail that it uses in a whipping motion to swim. Sperm can remain active for several days, but can fertilize an ovum for only twenty-four hours.

The female sexual anatomy consists of two ovaries, two Fallopian or uterine tubes, a uterus, vagina, and external genitalia. Breasts, or mammary glands, are considered accessory sex organs.

The ovaries produce reproductive cells, called ova, and the female hormones, estrogen, progesterone, and relaxin. They also create specialized cells called follicles, or groups of cells, that surround the ovum and assist in its development. About 200,000 follicles are present at birth and gradually decrease in number until no more remain at menopause. In a mature, premenopausal woman, an ovum and follicle develop together until they emerge from the ovary, at which time the ovum is released—a process called ovulation. Ovulation is assisted by various hormones that are under the direction of the pituitary gland. In health, ovulation takes place every twenty-eight days. Only one ovum is produced every twenty-eight days.

Once the ovum leaves the ovary, it enters the uterine tube. If there are no sperm present, it will gradually degenerate and leave the body during menstruation. Menstruation is the process in which the uterine wall becomes engorged with blood, caused by the cyclical death of tissues and blood vessels within the uterine wall. This part of the uterus, the outer layer, is called the endometrium, and is shed every twenty-eight days. An unfertilized ovum is released with the flow of blood, which usually lasts four to six days.

If sperm are present in the tube and the ovum is fertilized, the fertilized ovum, or zygote, will move from the uterine tube to the uterus, where it will attach itself and begin to develop. This movement requires four to five days and is assisted by cilia (tiny hairs inside the uterine tube) and muscles within the walls of the tube. The fertilized ovum draws nourishment from the endometrium, which would otherwise have been shed had not fertilization occurred.

The Female Reproductive System

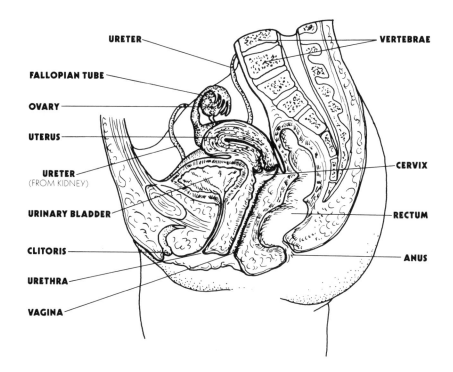

URETER

FALLOPIAN TUBE

OVARY

UTERUS

URETER
(FROM KIDNEY)

URINARY BLADDER

CLITORIS

URETHRA

VAGINA

VERTEBRAE

CERVIX

RECTUM

ANUS

A woman's ovaries produce a reproductive cell, or ovum, every twenty-eight days or so. With the help of various hormones, at ovulation the ovum leaves the ovary and enters the uterine or Fallopian tube. If there are no sperm present, it will gradually degenerate and leave the body during menstruation. If sperm are present in the tube and the ovum is fertilized, the fertilized ovum, or zygote, will move from the uterine tube to the uterus, where it will attach itself and begin to develop. This movement requires four or five days and is assisted by tiny hairs inside the uterine tube and muscles within the walls of the tube.

Just outside the vagina, toward the front of the pubis, is the clitoris, which is a small erectile structure containing many highly sensitive nerve endings. The clitoris is the homologue of a man's glans penis. Stimulation of the clitoris and vagina results in female orgasm. Unlike the vast majority of men, women can have multiple orgasms in close succession.

The Tao of Love and Sex

The most advanced Eastern approaches to sex are those of China (Taoism), Tibet (Tantra), and India (yoga). The Tantric practices of Tibet are based on both Taoism and yoga. All highly developed Oriental philosophies, including those of Japan, are based upon these three essentially similar philosophies.

In the traditions of both Taoism and Tantra, sex is considered the aspect of humanness from which all creativity flows. All our desires and abilities to create flow from our sexual nature, whether it be art, music, literature, or fashion. It is our sexual energy that makes creativity possible, according to Taoist and Tantric traditions. Procreation is but one aspect of that creativity.

The words sex and creativity might be interchangeable in this context; however, by saying sex we better identify a source of those creative energies within us.

For a full presentation of Taoist and Tantric practices, you will have to turn to other books devoted entirely to the subject of sex. Among the best of these are *Sexual Secrets,* mentioned earlier, *The Art of Sexual Ecstasy* by Margo Anand, and *The Tao of Love and Sex* by Jolan Chang. However, all Taoist and Tantric sexual practices begin from certain common and fundamental tenets. The first is that the body is the temple of the divine, and therefore must be treated with absolute care and respect. To abuse the body with unhealthful foods, drink, thoughts, or behavior is to destroy the very home of the universal spirit. Conversely, to respect and understand the body is to understand the universe itself, for the body is the microcosm of all that exists.

Second, the mind, body, and spirit are a single whole that is unified by a larger body of energy that permeates our physical form. This larger body of energy is itself arranged in a highly complex pattern. Among the most important parts of this energy pattern is a channel of energy that flows along the spine, beginning at the sex organs and running to the top of the head. Along this channel, or spiritual axis as it is sometimes called, are six energetic chakras, representing levels of consciousness, or aspects of our mind.

At the sexual center is located a pool of powerful energy, conceived of as a coiled snake, or a female deity, called kundalini. During sex, this powerful energy can be coaxed out of its potential state and made to move upward along the spiritual axis, causing each state of consciousness, represented by the specific chakras, to be transformed and illuminated. Ultimately, the kundalini reaches the head, in a place between the eyebrows, called the third eye, known in esoteric traditions of both East and West as the place of cosmic consciousness. When the kundalini energy unifies all the chakras and unites with the Third Eye, you experience "the joyous ecstasy of oneness with the universe, outside the limitations of time," write Douglas and Slinger in *Sexual Secrets.*

A great yogi, called Anandagiri, described the rise of kundalini this way: "The inner woman, entering the 'royal road,' takes rest at intervals in the secret centers. Finally She embraces the Supreme Lord in the lotus of the head. From that union flows an exquisite nectar that floods and permeates the body; then the Ineffable Bliss is experienced."

The way to stimulate the rise of the kundalini is through visualization during meditation and sex, and by controlling your breath. Breath is the single greatest tool in learning to prolong sex, control your inner energy, and, in the case of the man, forestall orgasm. Tantric and Taoist practices teach that breathing should be deep and abdominal. The stomach should move outward, and take the shape of a pot. Also, the breath should be held, anywhere from one to four counts, and then exhaled fully. As we describe in the chapter on the lungs, we take in life energy in the form of our breath. Every breath can revitalize us. The retention of the breath allows the qi to permeate the body and enrich health and inner power. On the inhalation, you can visualize the movements of the qi to specific organs. Retain this breath and see the qi revitalize your organs, and restore health and vitality. Breath retention is one of the keys to greater personal power, vitality, and wisdom. By controlling the breath, you control the mind, say yogis.

With the exhalation, you free yourself from all negative thoughts and feelings. Make the exhalation long. See the dark clouds of negative thoughts and emotions, of illness and dark attachments, leave the body and rejoin the earth, where they are purified.

By learning to control the breath, we learn to control our more subtle energetic, nervous, and muscle systems. This gives us greater body control, and thus allows us more fulfilling lovemaking. Tantric and Taoist practitioners also suggest that lovers learn to breathe together and to share their breath, in order to experience sex at a deeper and more intimate level.

In the Taoist, Tantric, and yogic traditions, sex is a means of self-development. Tantra says that such self-development cannot take place without love, trust, and commitment to one's partner. All the higher human values must be joined with sex in order to make it elevating and spiritually uplifting. In such a context, sex is a way to the ultimate center within.

CHAPTER 29

THE IMMUNE SYSTEM

States of health or disease are, at heart, the organism's success or failure at adapting to environmental challenges.

RENÉ DUBOS

*I*N 1981, a mysterious and chilling disease surfaced in the United States that rendered the human immune system powerless to fight against an array of deadly diseases. Initially, the illness appeared to be confined to homosexual men, a fact that prompted medical doctors to begin calling it "gay-related immune deficiency," or GRID.

A year later, the number of cases had increased significantly and the old acronym was changed to AIDS: acquired immune deficiency syndrome. At the time, the cause of the illness was still unknown. But in 1983 French scientists at the Pasteur Institute in Paris isolated the virus that was causing AIDS. The French called the organism human immunodeficiency virus, or HIV.

In 1984, U.S. scientists officially recognized HIV as the cause of AIDS. Scientists learned quickly that the illness was spread through the exchange of body fluids, primarily through sexual relations, intravenous drug use, or blood transfusions. It was also learned that a latency period existed between the moment HIV invaded the body, and the point at which it became sufficiently virulent to manifest as AIDS. One could carry HIV for as long as a decade before it became AIDS.

Despite the obvious dangers the disease posed, there was little if any public education concerning AIDS in the early 1980s. As Randy Shilts points out in his book *As the Band Played On: People, Politics and the AIDS Epidemic,* researchers were initially dissuaded from even investigating the AIDS virus because it was thought to be confined to homosexuals, and therefore did not warrant the serious attention of the scientific community. It was not until the French made important discoveries in AIDS research that American scientists began to investigate the illness with greater urgency.

The belief that AIDS was confined to the homosexual population also provided the American public with a false sense of security. That feeling of safety quickly evaporated in 1985 when Rock Hudson, a symbol of American manhood, contracted the disease. Hudson's subsequent decline and death provided a very public education, as much of the world looked on in horror. One of the most handsome faces in the world soon became a skull covered with paperlike flesh. By the time Rock Hudson died, everyone knew what AIDS did to people. But it was just the beginning.

Following Hudson's death, several people contracted AIDS from blood transfusions given at hospitals. Suddenly, the true nature of the illness was clear: This was not simply a "gay disease," but an illness that afflicted people regardless of their sexual preference.

The media turned their full attention to what was being called the "AIDS epidemic." By 1986, the word most often used to describe the public attitude towards AIDS was "hysteria." Education campaigns shifted into full throttle, warning everyone from the third grade onward of the dangers of "unsafe sex" and random use of intravenous drug needles.

By 1991, more than 160,000 men and women had contracted AIDS in the U.S., and more than 100,000 had died. That year Centers for Disease Control (CDC) officials estimated that more than 1.5 million Americans were infected with HIV, and that by 1994, more than 215,000 will have died of AIDS. The Hudson Institute, one of the world's leading think tanks, stated in 1989 that by the year 2002, 14.5 million Americans would be infected with HIV, and the vast majority of them would develop AIDS unless a cure was found.

Most of those who are afflicted with AIDS in the U.S. are young (between the ages of twenty-five and forty-four) homo-

Health is not equivalent to happiness, surfeit, or success. It is foremost a matter of being wholly one with whatever circumstances we find ourselves in. Even our death is a healthy event if we fully embrace the fact of our dying.

MWALIMU IMARA

sexual men or intravenous drug users. However, a growing proportion of those with AIDS are young women, who now represent nearly 10 percent of AIDS sufferers.

The U.S., of course, makes up only a fraction of the picture. AIDS is spreading most rapidly among black Africans. According to the World Health Organization, the more than 2 million African people with AIDS represents only the tip of the iceberg. In Uganda alone there are 800,000 cases of HIV infection, which represents 20 percent of the population and 88 percent of the prostitutes, who are among the principal sources of the illness within the population. Ugandan health officials estimate that by the year 2000, one out of every two Ugandans will be infected with HIV.

AIDS research is now one of the world's top medical and scientific priorities, but scientists maintain that a vaccine will not be ready in this century, and that a cure is even further off. The principal means of protection is prevention, specifically safe sex and, for drug users, sterilized needles.

The scourge of AIDS has awakened us in many ways, especially to the miracle of the body's defense system. We live in a world alive with microorganisms, chemical pollutants, radioactive waste, and simple dust. Many of these foreign substances are deadly. Yet despite the fact that we breathe them into our bodies in virtually every inhalation, we are able to destroy them without ever being aware that they existed in the first place. Such are the wonders of this marvelous system called immunity.

THE PHASES OF IMMUNE DEFENSE

The body's first wall of defense is the skin, which serves as a barrier against an onslaught of innumerable organisms and poisons that bombard us at every moment. Those foreign substances that penetrate the skin are dealt with initially by tears, sweat, and saliva, all of which neutralize and evacuate the foreign invader.

Nevertheless, diseases do get inside the body. When a virus enters a cell, it causes the cell to reproduce the virus many times over, making cells factories for disease. More times than not, however, the immune system destroys the virus and the virus-producing cells before we become aware that we are infected. The same is true of a cancer cell. From time to time, the DNA or genetic code of a cell becomes deformed and causes the cell to replicate uncontrollably. Nevertheless, the cancerous cells are usually destroyed by the immune system before they gain a foothold in the body. No matter what the problem—an environmental toxin, a virus, or a cancer cell—the immune system has an answer, most of the time.

The system responds to an invader in several phases: first, it recognizes the invading enemy as "not-self"; second, it creates a specific and effective response; third, it carries on a highly coordinated battle, using multiple approaches; finally, it determines that the war has been won and calls off the immune response, lest it consume the body itself. Having called the army to a halt, the immune system resumes its everpresent vigil, continually alert. Let's look a little closer at each of these stages.

Once a virus appears in the bloodstream or tissues, it is immediately encountered by a group of large white blood cells called macrophages or phagocytes. These cells are the body's neighborhood cops. They patrol the bloodstream looking for bad guys. The macrophage cells can respond to an invading virus or groups of virally-invaded cells in several ways: they can gobble up as many invaders as they can; or consume a portion of the cell's membrane, thus destroying the cell; or mark the cells that they cannot destroy with a sign, called an antigen, that will distinguish the invader as "not self." This is important because the body must be able to tell self from not-self throughout the course of the battle to keep immune cells from destroying healthy tissue.

The presence of the antigen serves to call out other immune cells, the first group of which are the helper-Ts or T-4 cells, so named because they are schooled to react to disease by the thymus gland before they are set free to roam the body. These T-4 cells, which like other helper-Ts are part of the general category of immune cells called lymphocytes, rapidly multiply and join the fray.

T-4 cells are the battlefield generals. They do not engage the invader themselves, but organize the body's response to the invading pathogen. Once set into action, the T-4 cells lock onto the virus and signal the macrophage to secrete a chemical called Interleukin-1, or Il-1, which scientists maintain allows the immune cells to "communicate" with one another.

The Interleukin-1 stimulates the body to produce fever and deep sleep. Scientists now speculate that fever may actually be an important first step in the body's efforts to destroy an enemy

We should love our disease because it is keeping us healthy. Without the disease we have, we might have a worse illness. Disease is always a creative attempt to solve problems. When we accept this, we can move toward wellness by thanking our disease and discovering in relationship with other people—a group or our doctor—other ways to solve the problems which the disease is addressing.

LEWIS MEHL

invader, perhaps raising the body's temperature to make the inner environment hostile to the invading organism. Sleep is induced probably in an effort to allow the body to direct its energies to the task of destroying the enemy.

T-4 cells then secrete another chemical, Interleukin-2, or Il-2, which activates another type of lymphocyte called killer-T cell. Killer-T cells destroy virally-infected cells by attacking their cell membrane. This keeps the virus from replicating.

While the killer-Ts attack the invading organism, the T-4 cells call out another arm of the immune system, the B-cells. B-cells make specialized antibodies, composed of proteins, to fight the virus. In an extraordinarily complex array of maneuvers, B-cells mutate and shuffle genes to create the unique antibody that will destroy the virus. B-cells are literally on-site laboratories. They are perhaps the most prolific chemists ever created, capable of creating more than one million kinds of antibodies. They are also capable of producing immunoglobulins, proteins that also serve as antibodies against illness.

While the B-cells are creating the right chemical agent, the T-4 cells help select the perfect antidote to the invader. Once it is found, the T-4 cells stimulate the B-cells to multiply and produce more antibodies.

Macrophages, helper-Ts, killer-Ts, B-cells, and antibodies— these are the main soldiers on the body's inner battlefield.

When the appropriate antibody is found, as it is in better than 99 percent of the occasions, the immune system "records and re-members" the formula. It is now capable of warding off the patho-gen the next time it is encountered. We are said to be "immune" to the measles, mumps, or chicken pox after we've been afflicted with them once. This means that whenever that pathogen is en-countered again, the immune system instantly whips up a batch of the effective antibody and force-feeds it to the illness, thus kill-ing it before we ever feel a sniffle or any other symptom. In this way, the immune system also acts like a giant computer that keeps genetic information on hand. The body's immune record is al-ways available. The immune system is vigilant and prepared the next time you or I breathe a familiar flu or chicken pox virus.

Once the battle is won, the immune system must call off the fight, lest it ultimately destroy healthy tissue and, indeed, the body itself. To call off the attack, suppressor cells, called T-8s, are called

There is no riches above a sound body.

APOCRYPHA

308

out. These cells literally suppress the immune response by sending out a chemical that tells T- and B-cells that the fight is over and that they are to shut down their activity. This allows the immune system to return to a state of balance, or restful surveillance.

Immune cells are involved in virtually every disease and healing process, including the onset and recovery of cardiovascular disease (see chapter on circulation), cancer, and arthritis, just to name a few.

The immune system is powerful and effective, but at the same time it is highly sensitive to how we think, how we feel, and what we eat. These factors often decide whether or not we become ill, and how quickly we recover. Let's have a closer look at how the mind and nutrition affect immune function.

MIND AND IMMUNE FUNCTION

It is now well established that the mind plays a vital role—sometimes even a determining role—in the efficacy of immune function. The evidence began to pile up in the 1940s when pioneer researcher Hans Selye determined that the mind could greatly influence how the body functioned. He found that stress can have immediate and accumulated effects on the body. The body has been trained through evolution to either escape danger or confront it. However, in the modern world, we are often forced to face a dangerous situation and resist both urges. For example, when a police officer orders you to stop your car because you failed to stop at a red light, your natural impulse is to press down even harder on the gas pedal and flee, or get out of the car and tell him to get off your back. Unfortunately, you can do neither. It may be the same with your employer, or the banker, or some other member of your circle with whom you have a difficult relationship. When this natural instinct is repressed, the accumulated tension can cause a wide range of negative physical reactions, including hormonal, respiratory, cardiovascular, and nervous system disorders. These imbalances, said Selye, could cause kidney damage, cardiovascular disease, and even death.

In the 1960s, Dr. Meyer Friedman and Dr. Ray H. Rosenman articulated the so-called type A and type B personalities. Type A is goal-oriented, driven by deadlines, and heavily invested in the outcome of events; type B is more centered in the moment, more

Healing is a matter of time, but it is sometimes also a matter of opportunity.

HIPPOCRATES

309

Your immune system is your interface with the environment. If it is healthy and doing its job right, you can interact with germs and not get infections, with allergens and not have allergic reactions, and with carcinogens and not get cancer. A healthy immune system is the cornerstone of good general health.

ANDREW WEIL

relationship-oriented, and less concerned about the outcome of events. These respective personalities, Friedman and Rosenman showed, have very different impacts on cardiovascular health. Type A behavior causes elevated levels of corticosteroid hormones, adrenaline, and blood cholesterol, and runs a much higher risk of heart disease and stroke than type B. The research of both Selye and Friedman-Rosenman demonstrated that stress has potentially devastating consequences. How effectively a person deals with stress can determine both the quality and length of that person's life.

From then on, mind-body research began to explore the behavior of immune cells themselves. It has been known for years that people who suffer the recent loss of a loved one are at greater risk of succumbing to disease and death than those who have not undergone such a trauma. This is typically referred to as dying of a broken heart. Scientists at Mount Sinai Medical Center found that bereavement sometimes has a deadening effect on lymphocytes. Dr. Stephen Schliefer and his colleagues found that the lymphocytes in some bereaved men sometimes fail to respond in the presence of a virus or foreign body. If the bereaved person survives long enough after the death of the loved one—usually about six months after—the lymphocytes mysteriously resume their normal behavior and function perfectly.

At Harvard University, Dr. John B. Jemmot found that the immune systems of type A students were weaker than those of type B students. The scientists studied the quantity of immunoglobulin A, or IgA, produced by the B-cells. During the rigors of the school year, especially during exams, the Type A students lost more IgA, and took longer to restore the IgA, than did the type B students. The research confirmed that Type A people tend to be more heavily invested in the outcome of events, often viewing such events as "life and death" situations. The Type B students were far less identified with the outcome of the tests. Therefore, their immune systems were not as depressed.

While negative emotional states have a harmful effect on immune response, scientists have found that positive thoughts and images can help restore immune function. The mind can be used intentionally to reinvigorate immune cells. Such cases as Norman Cousins, who used laughter and a positive attitude to prolong his life with a terminal illness; the work of O. Carl Simonton, an oncologist who has reported that visualization can help patients extend their lives and, indeed, overcome serious illness, including cancer; and the enormous body of evidence showing that people who maintain longstanding supportive relationships live longer and enjoy more fruitful lives, all point to the dramatic influence the mind has over the body.

New studies are showing that laughter has impressive benefits on hormones, respiration, and heart function. One showed that even smiling alters both mood and brain chemistry for the better. Finally, meditation and positive imagery routines have been shown to have a strengthening effect on immune function.

All of this research points to the need to maintain balance in life. People who are singularly focused and heavily identified with one aspect of life tend to have weaker immune responses than those who live more varied and balanced lives. Something in the human condition needs variety.

Here the unity of mind and body are unequivocal: health is an outcome of a balance among work, supportive relationships, and self-esteem.

Diet and Immune Function

Numerous studies have shown that dietary factors, such as fat and cholesterol, vitamins, minerals, and fiber content play important roles in the relative strength or weakness of the immune system. These studies show that by enhancing the diet and reducing the number and severity of the toxic influences on the body, the strength of the immune system can be recovered.

In general, scientists have long recognized that inadequate nourishment causes depressed immunity and vulnerability to a host of pathogens. Malnutrition has been associated with a wide range of illnesses, from scurvy to malaria to blindness. But research has demonstrated a far more specific and powerful relationship between the body's defenses and our daily eating habits.

Saturated fat has been shown to affect a macrophage by adversely changing the cell's membrane and reducing its sensitivity. Macrophages, or scavenger cells, depend on the sensitivity of their cell membranes to identify and destroy pathogens. Failure to identify a pathogen renders this first phase of the immune response ineffective.

Once inside the system, dietary fats oxidize or become rancid. These rancid fats further break down into substances called free radicals, highly charged molecules that are extremely reactive within the system. Free radicals destroy DNA and cause cell mutations.

Scientists have discovered that foods rich in beta carotene, such as broccoli, carrots, and squash, and vitamins C and E, are "free radical scavengers," or antioxidants. These foods donate electrons to imbalanced atoms, thus restoring stability to molecules and tissues. Foods rich in beta carotene and vitamins C and E have been shown to prevent free radical formation, and to stop the chemical changes that otherwise create havoc in human tissues and immune cells.

Beta carotene has been shown to have powerful protective properties against the onset of cancer, even among cigarette smokers. The National Research Counsel of the National Academy of Sciences has encouraged Americans to increase their intake of foods rich in beta carotene to reduce their chances of contracting cancer.

Deficiencies of vitamin A have been shown to reduce the size and number of T- and B-cells. Iron deficiency has been shown to decrease the effectiveness of white blood cells.

Minerals, such as zinc, selenium, manganese, magnesium, copper, and calcium, dramatically affect immune response. In a study published in the *American Journal of Clinical Nutrition* (March 1987), scientists reported that zinc deficiencies cause atrophy of the thymus gland and reduce antibody response to antigens. The scientists compared two groups of infants, one whose diets were supplemented with zinc, while the other was given a placebo. The scientists found that the zinc-supplemented group had lower rates of infection and higher blood levels of white cells than the group given a placebo. Scientists familiar with the evidence have maintained that diet does indeed have a role to play in the treatment of AIDS and other immune-related diseases.

Writing in *Nutrition Update,* Dr. Brian Leibovitz of the University of California's Department of Food Science stated, "Two very important areas of research are being neglected: the control of viral expression and the enhancement of immune response by nutritional means. It is my firm belief that these are the two most important areas to be studied with regard to AIDS."

A variety of new and exciting studies examining the relationship between nutrition and immune function are now being done. The early research seems to convince scientists that healthful eating is essential to a strong and optimal immune response.

AIDS: A MULTIPLICITY OF CAUSES

While it is now well-established that HIV infection is the prerequisite for the contraction of AIDS, scientists have found that a long series of insults to the immune system is necessary before HIV turns into full-blown AIDS. Such information is important because it demonstrates that lifestyle factors can help prevent AIDS from manifesting, even after HIV infection has occurred.

In one of its early studies, the Centers for Disease Control (CDC) discovered that gay men with AIDS had a history of heavy drug use. The CDC reported in 1982 that of the 87 men with AIDS studied, 97 percent said they used poppers, or amyl nitrate; 93 percent said they smoked marijuana; 68 percent used amphetamines; 66 percent used cocaine; 65 percent LSD; 59 percent Quaaludes; 12 percent heroin. The CDC also found that, as a rule, the men were multiple drug users, consistently using a variety of "street drugs," not just one.

Poppers and other drugs have long been known to depress the immune function and cause anemia, intestinal disorders, and liver damage. Some studies suggest that poppers may be directly associated with the onset of Kaposi's sarcoma. Drug addiction has long been known to depress immune function; heroin, for example, has been found to deplete the number of T-cells.

The introduction of sperm into the male body, especially through anal intercourse, has been known to suppress the immune cells. The walls of the intestines are only one cell thick. Researchers describe the thin intestinal lining, or mucosa, as having the strength of wet tissue paper. The intestinal wall is easily torn, allowing sperm and infection to spread rapidly into the bloodstream. (By contrast, the vagina is lined with a thick protective layer of mucosa cells that protect against the invasion of sperm and other substances directly into the bloodstream.)

Sperm is a concentrated protein containing purines, ammonia, and other chemicals that can be toxic to the blood and tissue. The introduction of sperm into the blood causes rapid deployment of immune cells, which must be directed away from other infections.

The CDC also reported that 80 to 90 percent of the gay male population with HIV harbors intestinal parasites. Parasites are cited as a potentially important contributing factor in the onset of AIDS among heterosexuals in Africa and the U.S. Intestinal parasites have been dealt with by the gay community with the use of antibiotics. But research has shown that antibiotics have a depressing effect on the immune system. In 1982, W. E. Hauser and J. S. Remington reported in the *American Journal of Medicine* that antibiotics depress at least four immune components.

All of this is in addition to the fact that so many men with AIDS have been previously infected with a variety of sexually transmitted diseases, including syphilis, herpes, hepatitis B, gonorrhea, and amoebic dysentery. These diseases are also immunodepressant.

Meanwhile, scientists at Johns Hopkins University in Baltimore discovered that a minority of patients—about five in 2,000—test positive for HIV after exposure, but are discovered to be seronegative several months later. These people are apparently able to destroy the virus once it manifests in their bloodstreams.

AIDS and other immune deficiency illnesses, such as Epstein Barr and chronic fatigue syndrome, demonstrate both the power of the immune system, and its delicacy. Research is showing increasingly that the power of immune response is very much in our own control, but that oftentimes we unwittingly depress immune function and sometimes even destroy it.

For additional information regarding specific conditions, see the related organs, systems, and senses described throughout this book.

Foods that boost the immune system include the following:

- *Allium vegetables:* Vegetables such as onions, garlic, leeks, chives, and scallions are immune-enhancing and protect against stomach cancer. Fifty or more pounds per year of these vegetables can prevent gastric cancer, according to some studies.
- *The cabbage family:* Broccoli, cauliflower, brussels sprouts, cabbages, and kale. These vegetables protect against colorectal, stomach, and respiratory cancers. Cole slaw and sauerkraut are good substitutes and can be equally effective.

- *Fish:* Fish oils can increase the activity of white blood cells, which detect and attack foreign cells. They have been shown to prevent metastasis in early stages of cancer.
- *Miso:* Contains high levels of lecithin and linoleic acid, which break down fatty deposits. It coats the inner wall of the colon with beneficial flora of lactus bacillus; it also improves digestion and assimilation of nutrients. Miso creates an alkaline blood and intestinal environment.
- *Organic foods:* Farmers in the corn belt have the highest incidence of leukemia and prostate and pancreas cancer deaths. In 1945, chlorinated hydrocarbon pesticides became available in South Dakota, Iowa, Minnesota, New Hampshire, Arkansas, Nebraska, Kansas, Oklahoma, Oregon, and Washington, and this brought about the rise in these diseases. Wheat farmers, who use considerably less insecticide, don't show these problems. These synthetic insecticides put large numbers of farmers at risk after heavy exposure for prolonged periods and put the general public at risk also, but to a lesser extent. Some of these pesticides are passed through the water supply and the food chain. Avoiding foods that have been treated with such pesticides by eating organically-grown fruits and vegetables is a wise idea.
- *Sea vegetables:* Rich in calcium, iron, zinc, and other trace minerals. Sea vegetables gather heavy metals and strontium 90 from the body and create insoluble salts, which are flushed from the body.
- *Shiitake mushrooms:* Immune-enhancing and antitumor. The *U.S. Journal of Cancer Research* reported that six out of ten mice suffering from sarcoma (a type of virally induced cancer) and treated with shiitake extract over short periods of time had complete tumor regression. At higher concentrations all the mice showed tumor regression. Shiitake dramatically lowers blood cholesterol. Animal studies have shown a drop in blood cholesterol between 25 to 45 percent, in a few days. The impact is stronger when a whole mushroom is consumed. Five to six mushrooms a day lower cholesterol 12 percent in a week. They contain cortinelin, a broad-spectrum antibacterial agent, which kills a wide range of pathogenic bacteria. A sulfide compound purified from shiitake has been found to have an antibiotic effect

Be careful about reading health books. You may die of a misprint.

MARK TWAIN

315

upon ringworm and other skin diseases. Researchers at Japan's Yamagushi University School of Medicine have reported that shiitake extract had a "protective effect" that inhibits the cell-destroying effects of the HIV virus.

- *Whole grains:* They contain B vitamins essential for proper functioning of the immune system and fiber to enhance digestion and intestinal function. They are rich in complex carbohydrates for long-lasting energy and contain protein, a wide variety of vitamins, and minerals.
- *Zinc:* It is immune-enhancing and essential to production of thymic hormones, needed to foster maturation of immune cells. An excess of zinc also can depress immunity, so it is safer to get it in foods than to take supplements. Good sources: seafood, whole wheat, whole wheat flour, bulgur wheat, cashews, most beans, and black-eyed peas.

There are also nutrients that boost the immune system. These include:

- *Argenine:* An amino acid. Stimulates immune reponse in patients whose immune systems are undermined by drugs or surgery. In animal studies, adding this amino acid to the diet enhanced immune responses and preserved immune function in the face of malnutrition and advancing cancers. Found in fish, beans, and grains.
- *Beta carotene:* Beta carotene is immune-strengthening, acts as an antioxidant, and protects against cancer and heart disease. Sources: carrots, squash, broccoli, bean sprouts, collard greens, brussels sprouts, peaches, apricots, prunes, watermelon.
- *Calcium:* Regulates lymphocyte function and the synthesis and functioning of prostaglandins. Good sources: leafy greens, especially collard, kale, and mustard greens, and sea vegetables.
- *Chlorophyll:* Found in green vegetables, blue-green algae, and chlorophyll supplement drinks, it can help rejuvenate the immune system, rebalance the body's physiology, rejuvenate the thymus, and act as a powerful detoxifier.
- *Fiber:* Sources: Whole grains, vegetables, fruit. Protects against colon cancer and, some studies suggest, breast cancer.

Let thy food be thy medicine.

HIPPOCRATES

- *Selenium:* Essential for the formation of antibodies and enzymes that participate in immunity. It is found in seafood, whole grain cereals, and garlic.
- *Vitamin B complex:* Immune-enhancing. Deficiency reduces production and efficiency of B-cells and T-cells, and causes atrophy of lymph tissue, poor antibody production, and diminished activity of thymic hormone. B6 deficiency impairs cellular and hormone-regulated immunity. Good sources are greens, whole grains, legumes, potatoes, corn, nuts, avocados, green peppers.
- *Vitamin C:* Immune-enhancing. Vitamin C strengthens the body's general resistance to viruses and stimulates eliminative process. It has been shown to protect against cancer of the esophagus and stomach. Good sources are broccoli, cabbage, strawberries, oranges, grapefruit, cantaloupe, leafy greens, sauerkraut, squash, and red and green peppers. Rose hips and hibiscus tea are especially rich sources of C.
- *Vitamin E:* Immune-enhancing; it is a free radical scavenger, meaning it can penetrate cells, restore tissue, and stop decay resulting from oxidation; it can also protect against ozone-induced free radical damage and slow aging. Researchers estimate that dietary measures that control oxygen radical damage could add five or more years to life. Vitamin C can help to regenerate Vitamin E. Sources: whole grains, especially wheat and bulgur; seafood.

Herbs that boost the immune system including the following:

- *Echinacea:* Boil the root to use as a tea or place fifteen to thirty drops in water. It stimulates and strengthens the body's immune system, and acts as an antibiotic. Echinacea is one of the most powerful and effective herbs against all forms of infection.
- *Goldenseal:* Herbalist Michael Tierra reports in his book *Planetary Medicine* (Lotus Press, 1988) that goldenseal is "effective against flu, fevers, and infections of all kinds; and in treating hemorrhoids, vaginal yeast infection and as an eyewash for inflamed eyes." Tierra warns against long-term use of goldenseal as a preventive, however, because it can weaken the flora in the intestinal tract.

A NEW WORLDVIEW OF HEALTH AND HUMAN POTENTIAL

If any thing is sacred, the human body is sacred.

WALT WHITMAN

WHAT IS HEALTH? Simple questions, such as this one, are often the most difficult to answer. If we fully understood the meaning of health, we would better understand what it means to be human. We would see more clearly our human potential, and even get a glimpse of where we are headed in our evolution.

Perhaps because the question of health leads to such a mine-field of subject-areas, the American Medical Association doesn't even attempt to answer it. It defines health as the absence of physical and mental disease. Unfortunately, that's like defining sunlight as the absence of darkness. Such an answer doesn't tell us a thing about sunlight, or about health. We'd like to have some pictures. Or, to use the vernacular of Western medicine, we'd like to know the "symptoms" of health. Does a healthy person possess more energy than an unhealthy person, for example? How does a healthy person age? What kinds of work do healthy people do? Is a healthy person more likely to have supportive or destructive relationships? Does a healthy person better understand himself in relationship to life?

These are the kinds of questions that we want to have answered when we consider the meaning of health. They get us thinking in the right direction, because, at bottom, we are wondering if health better equips us to answer the questions that life presents. If that is true, then health has got to be more than merely the absence of disease, because life itself is a struggle against ignorance and confusion as much as against illness.

Our medical system's inability to define health is at the very core of our health care crisis. Ours is the only medical system ever to exist that offers no unified definition of health, or what causes it. Without such a broad understanding of health and illness, we have been unable to offer an integrated approach to disease prevention, or health enhancement. Medical doctors have not begun to understand how the body heals itself. No one knows what the underlying power is that motivates wounds to heal, or the body to rid itself of disease. Doctors can describe part of the process, but cannot explain what causes it. The fact that the body makes a concerted and valiant effort to achieve health itself suggests all kinds of things about the nature of life, but scientists haven't got a clue as to how the human body might be linked to the larger forces of the universe.

As medical doctor and author Andrew Weil says in his book *Health and Healing,* "Allopaths may say that health is the absence of disease, but they have no clear conception or theory of what disease is, nor any general concept of treatment . . . Lack of a coherent philosophy of the abstract notions of health as wholeness, perfection, and balance encourages allopaths to pay attention mostly to the concrete manifestations of illness."

The current Western medical system is founded exclusively upon material values. When medical doctors look for health, they examine the behavior of cells and organs. They consult machines to determine the condition of the body and the causes of disease. In other words, the current medical system focuses on the elements of the earth for the answers to questions of health and illness. Moreover, it sees health and illness as conditions that are often outside of human control. You breathe in a flu virus and, bingo, you've got a cold. You suddenly manifest a cancer cell and your life is in jeopardy.

Such thinking is the basis for genetic research because it is believed that by altering the most fundamental aspects of human biology, the genes, illnesses such as cancer, diabetes, heart disease, and other disorders might be averted. In genetic research, modern

"M.D." does not stand for "Medical Deity."

BERNIE SIEGEL

I can compress what we have learned about the causes of these modern killers in three summarizing sentences: We are killing ourselves by our own careless habits. We are killing ourselves by carelessly polluting the environment. We are killing ourselves by permitting harmful social conditions to persist— conditions like poverty, hunger, and ignorance— which destory health, especially for infants and children.

JOSEPH CALIFANO

science has taken its materialistic values to an extreme, for it discounts behavior and spirit entirely. Rather, it focuses upon genetically redesigning the body.

In traditional medicine, health was defined to embrace virtually every aspect of human experience because the sages of East and West maintained that the body, mind, and spirit are a single unified whole. All three of these human aspects are harmonized by an underlying entity that the ancients called the life force, a kind of spiritual energy that permeates the universe and manifests as individual beings—you and me. When you are fully infused with this life force, the body and mind function optimally; that is, all of your cells, organs, and systems function at their full potential. In the same way that the whole is greater than the sum of its parts, you would fully realize your potential. All your talents and abilities would be available to you to express as you desired. Such a state, said the sages, brings with it an experience of unity with the ultimate reality, a harmony with the creator of life itself. This philosophy defined the methods used to maintain health and treat disease.

Thus, the path to health was, and is, a path of spiritual development. Through self-study, we come to understand ourselves so thoroughly that we come to know what supports our physical and spiritual health, and what detracts from it. Since humankind is directly linked with the natural environment, the fruits of that environment are relied upon to treat disease and restore health.

This "holistic" understanding of health is the one that humanity has held for the longest time. It is only in modern times, specifically the last 400 years, that we have redefined health to mean something strictly limited to the body. At the same time, we have steadily given up the notion that we control our health.

If we eliminate some of the extreme approaches, we are able to see the value of both systems. Our modern technology and science have benefited us greatly and are essential to our development. Yet, responsibility for health must ultimately lie with each of us and our own behavior. By recognizing the value and the need for both systems, we must confront an age-old question: Is there a bridge that links the material and spiritual? Is there a way of linking the modern with the ancient?

The refusal of modern medicine to accept the value of the ancient systems is the reason our society is unable to define health. If we accepted the traditional approaches, we would be forced to embrace the invisible aspects of life, and of healing. Yet, we already know that our thoughts, emotions, and psychological outlook—the invisible influences—either enhance or detract from our health. The realms of the mind and spirit play vital roles in how the physical body functions. To exclude such realms is both arbitrary and wrong. Moreover, the traditional methods of health care have been shown to work. Diet, massage therapy, acupuncture, and herbs all have powerful enhancing effects on health.

How can we understand East and West to unify them? How can we define health so that it can embrace the physical, the mental, and the spiritual?

Physician and author Deepak Chopra says that the body is characterized by intelligence that is not limited to the intellect or the head, but permeates every cell. In his book *Creating Health,* he writes, "All disease results from the disruption of the flow of intelligence. Intelligence is not simply in the head, though. Its expression may be at the subcellular level, at the cellular or tissue level, or at the level of the central nervous system." The myriad enzymes, genes, hormones, immune constituents, and nerves are all "expressions of intelligence," says Chopra. "They regulate essential functions with perfect know-how and do it at the body's far outposts, so to speak, far from where intellect is seated. Although all these expressions of intelligence can be located, intelligence itself cannot . . . it is all-pervasive in us and universal in nature."

How this intelligence guides cells in their selective activities is still unknown, but there are interesting theories, which we will get to shortly.

Organs that are made up of healthy cells behave in the same orderly and efficient ways as the cells themselves. They do not routinely become hyperactive, or hypoactive, and when they become ill, they are capable of throwing off disease in a relatively short period of time.

Illness, on the other hand, is disorderly. At the atomic level, sick atoms break up and rapidly decay, a phenomenon called free radical formation. These degenerative atoms cause new chemical bonds to form within the cells, which can give rise to a wide array of illnesses, from arthritis and heart disease to cancer and Alzheimer's. What is remarkable is that disorderly cells do not act in harmony with the overall body, but behave according to their own specific patterns.

At the other end of the spectrum, we know that disorderly behavior also causes disease. Erratic or chaotic sleeping patterns, eating habits, thoughts, and lifestyle all may lead to illness of one kind or another. Sickness can be understood as disordered behavior at the macroscopic and microscopic levels.

We use order to treat sickness. More rest, more balanced eating, calmer thoughts, and less stress all contribute to better health. Of course, order can become dogmatic, rigid, and stagnant. Stagnation leads to the refusal to grow and to sickness. Indeed, all growth is made possible by the breakdown of old tissues and old behavior patterns, which are then replaced by stronger tissues or new ways of acting. Change and evolution depend upon old systems giving way to disorder and the construction of a new system. Life itself is not stagnant, but ever moving, ever flowing.

Therefore, we face the paradox of life at its most basic level once again. We cannot escape the adventure of change, made possible by the paradox of order and disorder, or regeneration and decay. We can easily become blinded to this reality, that opposites make up the fabric of life. Indeed, the more we build up one side of life, the more we deny the other. As physicist Fred Alan Wolf says in *Taking the Quantum Leap,* "For nature is dualistic; she behaves according to the Principle of Complementarity. . . . The more we determine or define a system in terms of one of these complements, the less we know about the other. . . . There was always a hidden, complementary side to everything we experienced."

Order must be challenged, systems must change, if health is to exist on any level, whether it be in the physical body or in institutions. In the same way, health is achieved by balancing paradoxical influences, so that both can exist to appropriate degrees. Here we come to another fact about health: Balance is essential for health to exist. Health cannot exist when extremes of behavior of any kind rule a person's life. Regeneration and degeneration must exist in balance. Excessive work, rest, worry, or criticism—all excess of any kind is the basis for illness.

In *The Stress of Life,* pioneering stress researcher Hans Selye took up the question of aging and pointed out that no one dies of old age, but of a breakdown of one or more vital organs upon which the entire body depends. "Among all my autopsies (and I have performed quite a few), I have never seen a man who died of old age. In fact, I do not think anyone has ever died of old age yet. To die of old age would mean that all the organs of the body would be worn out proportionately, merely by having been used too long. This is never the case. We invariably die because one vital part has worn out too early in proportion to the rest of the body. Life, the biological chain that holds our parts together, is only as strong as its weakest vital link."

Selye's advice is to spread the wear and tear around in a process he called deviation. "The human body—like the tires on a car, or the rug on a floor—wears longest when it wears evenly. We can do ourselves a great deal of good in this respect by just yielding to our natural cravings for variety in everyday life. We must not forget that the more we vary our actions the less any one part suffers from attrition." In short, live a balanced life.

Paradox and balance were the basis for all traditional medical systems. Whether it was the yin-yang system of the Chinese, or the four humors of the Greeks, the Hindu trinity of Brahma (creation), Vishnu (maintenance), and Shiva (destruction), health depends upon balancing opposing forces that exist in the body, and in all of life.

The ancients understood that health is not a static state, but a fluid one that is continually adapting to its environment. Why is health a flowing or moving condition? Because opposites or paradoxes are continually present in your life, to which you must continually adapt. Sometimes you need more rest, sometimes less; sometimes more of these foods, other times less; today you place greater emphasis upon work, tomorrow on play.

Opposites create movement and energy, the basis of life. This was the underlying realization that unified East and West in the traditional world. Nothing was more basic, nor more useful in physical and spiritual questions.

According to these systems, healing was accomplished through the abundant presence of this flowing life energy. Whether the problem was a cut or a cancer, life energy was the underlying force that caused the cells to close the wound or eliminate the illness. This life energy flowed best in a balanced physical, emotional, and spiritual life. Hence, the path toward

Never let a surgeon take out a "functionless" organ unless it is really diseased. Functionless organs have a way of turning into very useful ones as soon as researchers admit the possibility of function and try to document it.

ANDREW WEIL

greatest health, vitality, and spiritual development emanated from balanced behavior. The healing systems of the Chinese and Greeks were based upon balancing opposite forces. The Doctrine of the Middle Way is the Buddhist ideal for spiritual development. The Logos, truth, is followed by balancing opposites in daily life, said Greek philosopher Heraclitus. Balance allows life energy to flow and thus brings forth the healing process.

THE ERA OF ENERGY MEDICINE

As foreign as a life energy may sound to some, a new medical science is now emerging that supports this very concept. The science is being called energy medicine, or the understanding of how electromagnetic energy flows within the body.

As we have seen throughout this book, the body is more than a chemical and mechanical machine; it is also an electrical unit. For the most part, science has maintained that these electrical events are localized to specific organ functions, such as the heart or the nervous system. But new research is demonstrating that electromagnetic energy flows along pathways analogous to the meridians described in Chinese acupuncture. Moreover, scientific research is showing that electromagnetic energy may well be the underlying power that triggers the healing process.

In his book *Cross Currents: The Promise of Electromedicine; The Perils of Electropollution,* Dr. Robert O. Becker scientifically documents the presence of an underlying electromagnetic life force that animates the body, and causes it to grow and heal. Describing his work with technology that can measure minute electromagnetic energy, Becker demonstrates that the human body is a complex web of electrical currents. These currents trigger cells to restore health, repair wounds, and promote growth. The electromagnetic energy is itself the stimulus to the healing process, Becker found.

By combining biology, chemistry, and physics, Becker formulated an hypothesis and eventually proved how this repair process works. He showed that an injury causes the brain to send a low-level electrical signal to the wound that stimulates repair. As the repair process progresses, this original "stimulating signal" diminishes in intensity. The lower stimulating signal in turn

The scientific basis for energy medicine is often poorly understood, and body energies are still considered by many practitioners to be mysterious, unknowable entities. If energy medicine is to assume its rightful place as an effective form of medical therapy, it must be based on established scientific principles and careful scientific experimentation.

ROBERT BECKER

slows the repair activity. Eventually, when the wound is fully healed, the stimulating signal stops, at which point the repair process also stops.

This was just the beginning. Becker also has shown that the electrical web of the body corresponds to Chinese acupuncture meridians. The points along these acupuncture meridians enhance or reinforce the electromagnetic current flowing in the body. He says, "We found that about 25 percent of the acupuncture points on the human forearm did exist, in that they had specific, reproducible and significant electrical parameters and could be found in all subjects tested. Next, we looked at the meridians that seemed to connect these points. We found that these meridians had the electrical characteristics of transmission lines, while nonmeridian skin did not. We concluded that the acupuncture

The Body's Energy Field

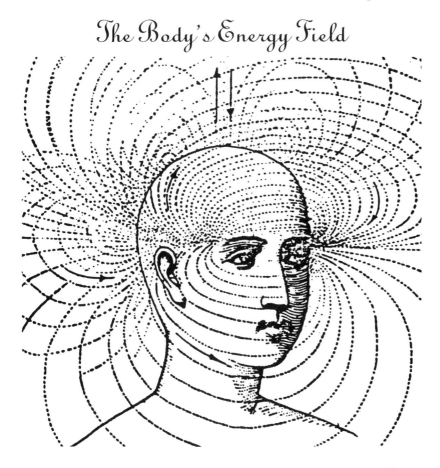

Scientists and alternative healers now envision the human body in not only chemical and mechanical terms, but as an electrical unit that both generates and is affected by electromagnetic fields. According to cell biologist Jim Oschman, "Parts of the whole may be interconnected by various types of energetic fields." Some scientists even speculate that electromagnetic energy may well be the underlying power that triggers the healing process.

system was really there, and that it most likely operated electrically. This system was quite likely the input route to the brain that transmitted the signal of injury."

Why doesn't a fingernail produce liver cells? What regulates DNA so that certain genes will be active while others remain dormant? Becker attempted to answer these questions by examining the ability of salamanders to regenerate. The salamander can regrow a leg in every detail. It can also regenerate an eye, ear, one-third of its brain, almost all of its digestive tract, and much of its heart. Remarkably, if you cut off a salamander's leg and remove the budding repair-cells of the leg and place them on a severed salamander tail, the salamander will grow a tail. If you cut off the tail and place it on a leg, the salamander will grow a new leg in every detail. Such experiments demonstrated to Becker that "there is some mechanism within the living salamander that contains an overall plan for the salamander's body and provides the information that instructs the blastema [newly formed cells] what tissue it should construct."

Essentially, Becker was asking how it is possible that the salamander's regenerative capacities act in so orderly a pattern, even when common sense might suggest that this would be the one place where disorder would reign.

Through rigorous scientific study, he demonstrates that these morphogenetic fields are actually electrical fields that permeate and surround the living organism. The fields contain complex information that directs the healing process and determines which cells will grow where. Such energetic fields are where intelligence may well lie.

Remarkably, the salamander is similar to humans in its skeletal and nervous systems. "The salamander's foreleg has the same bones, muscles, blood vessels, and nerves, in the same arrangement, as a person's arm," writes Becker. "The brain and the arrangement of nerves throughout its body are basically the same as ours, except that the thinking area of our brains is greatly expanded."

Becker, an orthopedic surgeon twice nominated for the Nobel Prize, has demonstrated that optimal amounts of electromagnetic energy flowing through the body determine the level of health. This discovery, he points out, is the basis for the birth of a new medicine—electromagnetic medicine.

A man laid on the operating table in one of our surgical hospitals is exposed to more chances of death than the English soldier on the field of Waterloo.

SIR JAMES YOUNG
SIMPSON

326

Electromagnetic medicine is essentially the enhancement or strengthening of the life energy within the body. Many ancient and modern healing techniques, including such diverse methods as shamanism and homeopathy, can enhance or strengthen the life energy within the body, Becker has shown. He has divided these many techniques into three groups.

The first is what he calls minimal energy techniques, which include visualization, placebo, shamanism, and hypnosis. The second is energy-reinforcement techniques, such as acupuncture, magnets, diet, homeopathy, herbs, and massage. The third is high-energy transfer techniques, which is the introduction of energy from outside the body. These include the use of machines that can transfer higher amounts of energy into the body and thus repair cells and restore health.

Proper use of these approaches works, says Becker, but much research remains to determine how they can be utilized best, especially the third category, high-energy transfer. Becker urges people to use caution in selecting practitioners of energetic medicine. The use of electrical acupuncture, for example, can be dangerous to cells, Becker points out, because only minute DC currents are active in the body. The introduction of excessive current can damage cells and create havoc. Though Becker is a pioneer in this field, many other scientists are now actively involved in developing electromagnetic medicine and its techniques, including scientists at the State University of New York Medical School, the University of California, and Syracuse University.

It may well be that electromagnetic medicine represents both the future of health care, and a bridge between East and West, ancient and modern, spirit and matter.

Healthy people look healthier and younger than unhealthy people. They're freer of disease and it shows. They're also happier, says Deepak Chopra. The reason: Health can exist only in an atmosphere of healthy thoughts. As the science of psychoneuroimmunology has demonstrated, thoughts profoundly affect the immune system and thus directly impact on health. Depression, chronic stress, anger, and loneliness weaken immunity and make the body more susceptible to a variety of illnesses, everything from the common cold to heart disease and cancer. Conversely, happy thoughts have health-enhancing effects on the body.

"It appears that happiness, which simply means having happy

The machine analogy has some plausibility in relation to adult organisms: machines, especially those containing feedback control systems, are indeed like artificial organisms or organs: airplanes are like birds, cameras like eyes, pumps like hearts, computers like brains. Machines, made by human beings to serve human purposes, reflect some of the organic, purposeful qualities of the people that make and use them. But the fact that machines are like artificial organisms does not mean that organisms are nothing but machines.

RUPERT SHELDRAKE

thoughts most of the time, causes biochemical changes in the brain that in turn have profoundly beneficial effects on the body's physiology," says Chopra. "For every state of consciousness, there is a corresponding state of physiology. If you are having hostile thoughts, for example, they will be reflected in your mood, your facial expression, your social behavior, and how you feel physically."

That true bible . . . the human body.

ANDREAS VESALIUS

In short, the condition we call health permeates every fiber of our being, every aspect of our lives. One of the best definitions of health, which also offers a glimpse of our potential, is offered by Michio Kushi. He defines health as having seven characteristics: experiencing abundant energy without fatigue, having an excellent appetite, enjoying deep and fully-restful sleep, having an excellent memory, never being angry, being ever joyous and alert, and having endless gratitude for life and other people.

Such a state describes someone fully equipped to enjoy life, and capable of realizing his or her full potential. That, said the great Swiss psychiatrist Carl Jung, is the purpose of life. For those willing to follow the path of life courageously and intelligently, life leads inevitably to one's own inner nature, the true center of being. Jung called such a path leading to self-knowledge the process of individuation.

"Individuation means becoming a single, homogeneous being, and, in so far as 'individuality' embraces our innermost, last, and incomparable uniqueness, it also implies becoming one's own self. We could therefore translate individuation as 'coming to selfhood' or 'self-realization.'"

That, said the ancients, is where health leads: to the knowledge of the inner you.

BIBLIOGRAPHY

Anatomy, Physiology, and Western Medicine:

The American Medical Association's Encyclopedia of Medicine. Random House, 1989.

Brody, Jane. *Jane Brody's New York Times Guide to Personal Health.* Times Books, 1982.

Gray, Henry. *Gray's Anatomy: Descriptive and Surgical.* Bounty Books, 1927.

Hooper, Judith and Dick Teresi. *The Three Pound Universe.* Jeremy P. Tarcher, 1986.

Juhan, Deane. *Job's Body: A Handbook for Bodywork.* Station Hill Press, 1987.

Steen, Edwin and Ashley Montagu. *Anatomy and Physiology,* vols. I and II. Barnes & Noble Books, 1985.

Early and Traditional Medical Systems:

Grossinger, Richard. *Planet Medicine: From Stone Age Shamanism to Post-Industrial Healing.* North Atlantic Books, 1987.

Preuss, Julius. *Biblical and Talmudic Medicine.* Trans. and edited by Fred Rosner, M.D. Sanhedrin Press, New York, 1978.

Thorwald, Jurgen. *Science and Secrets of Early Medicine.* Thames & Hudson, London, 1962.

Medical History:

Bettmann, Otto L., Ph.D. *A Pictorial History of Medicine.* Charles C. Thomas, Springfield, 1956.

Castiglioni, Arturo, M.D. *A History of Medicine.* Trans. from Italian and edited by E. A. Krumbhaar, M.D., Ph.D. Alfred A. Knopf, New York, 1947.

Clendening, Logan. *The Romance of Medicine: Behind the Doctor.* The Garden City Publishing Co., Inc., Garden City, New York, 1933.

Clendening, Logan, M.D. *Source Book of Medical History.* Dover Publications, Inc., New York, 1942.

Servetus, Michael. *A Translation of His Georgraphica, Medical and Astrological Writings.* Trans. by Charles Donald O'Malley. American Philosophical Society, Philadelphia, 1953.

Smith, Anthony. *The Body.* Viking Penguin, New York, 1986.

Chinese and Japanese Medicine:

Fierbrace, Peter, B.Ac. *Acupuncture: Restoring the Body's Natural Healing Energy.* Harmony Books, 1988.

Garvey, John W., N.D. *Introducing the Five Phases of Food: How to Begin.* Wellbeing Books, Brookline, Massachusetts, 1982.

Kaptchuk, Ted J., O.M.D., and Michael Croucher. *The Healing Arts.* Summit Books, New York. 1987.

Kaptchuk, Ted J. O.M.D. *The Web That Has No Weaver; Understanding Chinese Medicine.* Congdon and Weed, New York, 1983.

Kushi, Michio. *The Book of Macrobiotics.* Japan Publications, 1977.

Lu, Henry C., *Chinese System of Food Cures.* Sterling Publications Co., Inc., New York, 1986.

Matsumoto, Kiiko, and Stephen Birch. *The Five Elements and Ten Stems.* Paradigm Publications, Brookline, Massachusetts, 1983.

Muramoto, Naburo. *Healing Ourselves.* Avon Books, 1973.

Ohashi, Waturo, with Tom Monte. *Reading the Body.* Viking Penguin, 1991.

Von Durckheim, Karlfried Graf. *Hara: The Vital Centre of Man.* George Allen & Unwin, 1985.

Wing-Tsit Chan. *Chinese Philosophy, A Source Book.* Princeton University Press, 1963.

Wong, K. Chimin, and Wu Lien-Teh. *History of Chinese Medicine.* The Tientsin Press, Ltd., Tientsin, China, 1936.

The Yellow Emperor's Classic of Internal Medicine. Trans. with an introduction by Ilza Veith. University of California Press, Berkeley and Los Angeles, 1949.

Ayur-Veda:

Ballentine, Rudolph, M.D. *Diet and Nutrition.* The Himalayan International Institute, 1978.

Chopra, Deepak, M.D. *Creating Health: Beyond Prevention, Toward Perfection.* Houghton Mifflin, 1987.

Lad, Vasant, Dr. *Ayurveda: The Science of Self-Healing.* Lotus Press, Sante Fe, New Mexico, 1984.

Monro, Robin, Dr., et al. *Yoga for Common Ailments.* Fireside Books, 1990.

Svoboda, Robert E. *Prakruti: Your Ayurvedic Constitution.* Geocom, Albuquerque, New Mexico, 1989.

Naturopathy:

Trattler, Ross, Dr. *Better Health Through Natural Healing.* McGraw-Hill, 1988.

Homeopathy:

Panos, Maesimund B., M.D. and Jane Heimlich. *Homeopathic Medicine at Home.* Jeremy P. Tarcher, Inc., 1980.

Richardson, Sarah. *Homeopathy: Stimulating the Body's Natural Immune System.* Harmony Books, 1988.

Ullman, Dana. *Discovering Homeopathy: Medicine for the 21st Century.* North Atlantic Books, 1991.

Herbs and Supplements:

Hausman, Patricia, M.S. *The Calcium Bible.* Warner Books, 1985.

Hutchens, Alma R. *Indian Herbology of North America.* Shambhala, 1991.

Mairesse, Michelle. *Health Secrets of Medicinal Herbs.* Arco Publishing, 1981.

Mindell, Earl. *Vitamin Bible.* Warner Books, 1991.

Tierra, Michael. *Planetary Herbology.* Lotus Press, 1988.

Tierra, Michael, N.D. *The Way of Herbs.* Washington Square Press, Pocket Books, New York, 1983.

Greek Medicine:

Plato, Selections. Edited by Raphael Demos. Charles Scribner's Sons, 1927.

The Presocratics. Edited by Philip Wheelwright. The Odyssey Press, a division of Bobbs-Merrill Co., 1966.

The Republic of Plato. Translated by Frances MacDonald Cornford. Oxford University Press, 1975.

Alternative Approaches and Syntheses of East and West:

Becker, Robert O., M.D. *Cross Currents: The Perils of Electropollution; the Promise of Electromedicine.* Jeremy P. Tarcher, 1990.

Carlson, Richard, Ph.D., and Benjamin Shield, eds. *Healers on Healing.* Jeremy P. Tarcher, 1989.

Colbin, Annemarie. *Food and Healing.* Ballantine Books, 1986.

Diamond, John, M.D. *Your Body Doesn't Lie.* Warner Books, 1983.

Monte, Tom. *The Way of Hope.* Warner Books, 1989.

Samuels, Michael, M.D. *Healing with the Mind's Eye.* Summit Books, 1990.

Pearsall, Paul, Ph.D. *Super Immunity.* McGraw-Hill, 1987.

Price, Shirley. *Aromatherapy for Common Ailments.* Fireside, 1991.

Pritikin, Nathan, with Patrick McGrady. *The Pritikin Program for Diet and Exercise.* Grosset & Dunlap, 1979.

Pritikin, Nathan, et al. *Live Longer Now.* Grosset & Dunlap, 1974.

Sattilaro, Anthony J. and Tom Monte. *Living Well Naturally.* Houghton Mifflin, 1984.

———. *Recalled by Life: The Story of My Recovery from Cancer.* Houghton Mifflin, 1982.

Serinus, Jason, editor. *Psychoimmunity and the Healing Process.* Celestial Arts, 1986.

Weil, Andrew, M.D. *Health and Healing.* Houghton Mifflin, 1988.

INDEX

ABOUT THE AUTHOR

Tom Monte has written numerous books on health and environment. He coauthored *Recalled by Life: The Story of My Recovery From Cancer* and *Living Well Naturally,* both with Dr. Anthony Sattilaro (Houghton Mifflin, 1982 and 1984, respectively). He also wrote *Pritikin: The Man Who Healed America's Heart,* with Nathan Pritikin's widow, Ilene (Rodale Press, 1987); *The Way of Hope* (published by Warner Books, 1989); and *Reading the Body,* with Waturo Ohashi (Viking, 1991). Tom Monte's work has been published in many of the nation's leading magazines and newspapers, including *Life,* the *Saturday Evening Post, Runner's World, The Chicago Tribune, Natural Health, New Age Journal,* and many other well-known publications.

He is the former editor of *Nutrition Action,* a publication of Center for Science in the Public Interest and associate editor of *East West/Natural Health.*

He lives with his wife and three children in Amherst, Massachusetts.

ABOUT *NATURAL HEALTH* MAGAZINE

Natural Health: The Guide to Well-Being (formerly *East West Journal*) has been the leading national magazine on alternative health, herbalism, bodywork, personal growth, and natural foods for over two decades. *Natural Health* provides more than half a million readers in the U.S. and around the world with practical information on health and longevity. As a recent magazine review by *USA Today* noted, *Natural Health* "is far too splendid to be confined to a health-food store shelf."

The magazine's awards include the 1989 Alternative Press Award for Service Journalism. *Natural Health* is one of only three magazines listed under the Health and Nutrition Magazines category in *The New York Public Library's Desk Reference* of "The Ultimate One-Volume Collection of the Most Frequently Sought Information."

The editors of *Natural Health* have written numerous books on natural healing and whole foods cooking, including *Quick and Natural Rice Dishes; Meetings with Remarkable Men and Women: Interviews with Leading Thinkers on Health, Medicine, Ecology, Culture, Society, and Spirit; Sweet and Natural Desserts; Shopper's Guide to Natural Foods;* and *Natural Childcare.*

Natural Health is produced bimonthly in Brookline, Massachusetts. For subscription information write or call Natural Health, 17 Station St., P.O. Box 1200, Brookline Village, MA 02147; (617) 232-1000.